The Autistic Spectrum

The Autistic Spectrum

Characteristics, Causes and Practical Issues

Jill Boucher

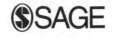

Los Angeles | London | New Delhi
Singapore | Washington DC

First published 2009
Reprinted 2011, 2012

SAGE Publications Ltd
1 Oliver's Yard
55 City Road
London EC1Y 1SP

SAGE Publications Inc.
2455 Teller Road
Thousand Oaks, California 91320

SAGE Publications India Pvt Ltd
B 1/I 1 Mohan Cooperative Industrial Area
Mathura Road, New Delhi 110 044

SAGE Publications Asia-Pacific Pte Ltd
3 Church Street
#10-04 Samsung Hub
Singapore 049483

Library of Congress Control Number: 2008922349

British Library Cataloguing in Publication data

A catalogue record for this book is available from the British Library

ISBN 978-0-7619-6211-3
ISBN 978-0-7619-6212-0 (pbk)

Typeset by C&M Digitals (P) Ltd, Chennai, India
Printed in Great Britain by the MPG Books Group
Printed on paper from sustainable resources

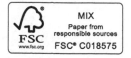

CONTENTS

Preface   vii
Publisher's Acknowledgements   ix

PART I   WHAT IS AUTISM?   1

1   The Subtypes Model of Autism: Concept and Definitions   3
2   The Spectrum Model of Autism: Concept and Definitions   22
3   Filling in the Picture: From Conformity to Diversity   42
4   Facts and Figures: Epidemiology and Lifespan Development   70
5   What is Autism? Personal View   87

PART II   WHAT CAUSES AUTISM?   95

6   A Framework for Explaining Autism   97
7   First Causes and Brain Bases   114
8   Explaining the Social, Emotional, and Communication
    Impairments   142
9   Explaining the Repetitive Behaviours and Lack of Imaginative
    Creativity   166
10 Explaining Other Universal or Common Behavioural
    Characteristics   188
11 Explaining Autism as a Whole: Attempts at a Synthesis   209
12 What Causes Autism: Personal View   232

PART III   PRACTICAL ISSUES   255

13 Assessment, Diagnosis and Screening   257
14 Intervention   279
15 Care   307

Glossary   331
References   364
Index   401

PREFACE

My aim in writing this book is to provide an account of autism that people with little or no specialist knowledge will find comprehensible and digestible, but which at the same time offers more advanced readers a clear summary of existing knowledge with pointers to more detailed reading. In brief, the book is intended as both an introduction and a source. I have tried to keep in mind parents whose child has just received a diagnosis of autism and who are seeking a full but not too technical account of the 'what', the 'why' and the 'how' of autism; also undergraduate and graduate students who need a crib before embarking on more detailed and specialised reading relevant to their essay, project, or dissertation; and trainee professionals, whether careworkers or classroom assistants, teachers, therapists, or doctors, who need the overall picture as a context for more detailed study related to their specialist practice. For non-specialist readers a Glossary of possibly unfamiliar terms or usages is included. Glossary items are in bold font on their first mention in the text.

I also wanted to write an account that was as impartial as I could make it. There are many books that present an author's particular 'take' on autism, and these can contribute greatly to advanced discussion of the nature, causes, treatment etc. of autism. However, they do not make good starting points, and – unless several such books are read – they can leave the reader with an incomplete or biased understanding. It is of course impossible to be completely objective and impartial, and my own biases inevitably leach through the main text. However, I have tried to control them by including sections entitled 'Personal View' at the close of each main part of the book, in which I express my own views concerning issues covered in preceding chapters.

There are some other underlying principles or themes that may make the book a little different from some others. In particular, I try to put current views into the perspective of a continuing search for answers, in which much can be learned from past research and much remains to be learned in the future. I try to take a non-adversarial approach in which research and practice are seen as working together to make life as good as possible for people with autism, their families and other carers, whilst accepting some differences in priorities and terminological preferences across research and practice. Similarly, where there is a controversy with supporting evidence on both sides of a theoretical argument I try to find ways of reconciling the opposing evidence and argument, rather than taking sides one way or the other. Finally, much of the illustrative material is provided by people with autistic spectrum disorders themselves, either within disguised descriptions or with their own or their families' agreement: I have specifically not included illustrations of several well-known psychological tests, illustrations of which can be found in many other books on autism (for example, Frith, 2003; Bowler, 2007).

The book covers more material than most beginning students will need, and lecturers using it as a basic text, whether to back up a single lecture or as the basis for a term's course on autism, should use the text selectively according to their student group. For example, for students on a non-vocational psychology course, Part III could be made optional reading. For students on vocational courses, on the other hand, some of the more theory-laden chapters in Part II might be omitted.

I am enormously grateful to Rita Jordan, Dermot Bowler and Jon Brock who reviewed the book between them, providing invaluable comments based on expert knowledge; and to Sophie Lind who drew the pictures. I am also grateful to Cathy Grant, Don and Ann Locke, Patty Cowell, and Sally Bigham who read and commented on parts of the book at various stages of drafting; and to Steve Metcalf of the Newlyn Rythmes Gallery in Winchester and Anthony Frost who between them helped us to identify and use the Terry Frost picture on the cover. Finally I am grateful to Michael Carmichael and Kate Wood at Sage for their exceptional patience.

PUBLISHER'S ACKNOWLEDGEMENTS

The author and publishers wish to thank the following for the permission to use copyright material:

We thank the American Psychological Association for granting us permission to use material from Waterhouse, L., Fein, D., & Modahl, C. (1996). Neurofunctional mechanisms in autism. *Psychological Review, 103,* 457–489 (Figure 1). Adapted with permission from the APA.

We thank Blackwell Publishing for granting us permission to use material from Plaisted, K., O'Riordan, M., & Baron-Cohen, S. (1998). Enhanced visual search for a conjunctive target in autism: A research note. *Journal of Child Psychology and Psychiatry, 39,* 777–783 (Figure 1). Adapted with permission from Blackwell Publishing.

We thank Cambridge University Press for granting us permission to use material from the following: Boucher, J., Mayes, A., & Bigham, S. (in press). Memory, language and intellectual ability in low-functioning autism. In J. Boucher & D. M. Bowler (Eds.), *Memory in Autism.* © Cambridge University Press, reprinted with permission; Dawson, G., Webb, S., Schellenberg, G., Dager, S., Friedman, S., et al. (2002). Defining the broader phenotype of autism: Genetic, brain, and behavioural perspectives. *Development and Psychopathology, 14,* 581–611 (Figure 2). Reprinted with permission from Cambridge University Press.

We thank Elsevier for granting us permission to use material from Mottron, L. & Belleville, S. (1993). A study of perceptual analysis in a high-level autistic subject with exceptional graphic abilities. *Brain and Cognition, 23,* 279–309 (Figure 2). Reprinted with permission from Elsevier.

We thank IOS Press and Joe and Marilynn Henn for granting us permission to use material from Henn, J., & Henn, M. (2005). Defying the odds: You can't put a square peg in a round hole no matter how hard you try. *Journal of Vocational Rehabilitation, 22*(2), 129–130. Reprinted with permission from IOS Press.

We thank MIT Press for granting us permission to use material from Baron-Cohen, S. (1995). *Mindblindness: An Essay on Autism and Theory of Mind,* (Figure 4.1). © 1995 Massachusetts Institute of Technology, by permission of The MIT Press.

We thank Sage Publications for granting us permission to use material from Preissler, Melissa (in press), *Autism.* Reprinted with permission from Sage.

We thank Springer for granting us permission to use material from Hughes, C. (1996). Brief Report: Planning problems in autism at the level of motor control. *Journal of Autism and Developmental Disorders*, 26, 101–109 (Figure 1). Reprinted with permission from Springer.

PART I

WHAT IS AUTISM?

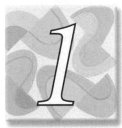

THE SUBTYPES MODEL OF AUTISM: CONCEPT AND DEFINITIONS

AIMS

••••

HISTORICAL BACKGROUND
Early Case Histories
The First Attempts to Identify Autism as a Distinct Condition
Two Blind Alleys
Back to Kanner
The First Official Definitions

••••

CURRENT DEFINITIONS BASED ON A SUBTYPES MODEL
DSM-IV and ICD-10
The Group of Pervasive Developmental Disorders
DSM-IV Criteria for Autism-related Pervasive
Developmental Disorders

••••

MANIFEST BEHAVIOUR
Generalised vs. Particular Behaviours
Manifest Behaviours: Some Examples
Manifest Behaviours in Relation to Diagnostic Criteria
Manifest Behaviours as Clues to Diagnosis

••••

SUMMARY

AIMS

The aims of this chapter are to provide some historical background to the concept of a set of autism-related conditions that we are familiar with today; to provide a concise account of current definitions of autism-related disorders based on a subtypes model of autism as in the internationally recognised diagnostic manuals; and to emphasise and illustrate the complexity and variety of behaviours that may be seen in different individuals, all of whom have some form of autism. An underlying aim is to counteract the view that the past has nothing to tell us about autism, by demonstrating that early definitions and descriptions of autism prefigure those in use today.

HISTORICAL BACKGROUND

Early Case Histories

Autism has almost certainly always existed in human populations. However, it was not recognised as a distinct condition until the mid-twentieth century. Prior to that, less able people with autism were included within an undifferentiated group of those who were described as simpletons, or imbeciles, or feeble-minded (people were not sensitive to stigmatising language in those days). More able people with autism – those who might now be described as having **Asperger syndrome** – were merely seen as withdrawn or eccentric.

A few reports of individuals whom we might now recognise as autistic survive from as early as the eighteenth century. Notable amongst these are reports of feral children, that is to say children who had been abandoned by their parents but who had managed to survive in the wild. The earliest well-documented case of a feral child is that of the 'Wild Boy of Aveyron', found in the late 1780s at about the age of 12, living like an animal alone in a forest. Victor, as the boy was named by those who rescued him, had no language, nor was he responsive to human beings. Significantly, Victor never became responsive to other people despite the fact that from the time of his rescue until the time that he died in middle age he was kindly cared for, and energetic attempts were made to educate him (Frith, 1989). Other detailed accounts of children who might nowadays be diagnosed with autism survive from the nineteenth century (Waltz & Shattock, 2004).

The First Attempts to Identify Autism as a Distinct Condition

Kanner's and Asperger's seminal accounts

Autism was first identified by an American psychiatrist named Leo Kanner in a paper published in 1943 entitled 'Autistic disturbances of affective contact'.

One year later an Austrian medical student called Hans Asperger published a paper entitled 'Die Autistischen Psychopathen im Kindesalter' ('Autistic psychopathy in children') (Asperger, 1944/91). The individuals described by Kanner and by Asperger in their separate papers differed from each other in some respects. However, there was also considerable overlap between the descriptions, as is clear from Box 1.1.

BOX 1.1   Kanner's and Asperger's early descriptions

KANNER	ASPERGER
'Early infantile autism'	'Childhood autistic psychopathy'
Profound lack of affective [i.e., emotional] contact with others.	Severe impairment of social interaction, shown in odd, inappropriate behaviour rather than aloofness and indifference.
Intense resistance to change in routines. Fascination with manipulating particular objects, but not using them for correct function.	All-absorbing, narrow interests, often to the exclusion of other activities. Imposition of repetitive routines on self and others.
Muteness or abnormalities of language.	Good grammar and vocabulary but inappropriate use of speech. A tendency to engage in monologues on special interests. Limited or inappropriate non-verbal communication.
Superior rote memory and visual-spatial skills	Motor clumsiness. 'Mischievous' behaviour.

Kanner's paper was immediately influential in English-speaking countries. However, Asperger's paper was not brought to the attention of English-speaking researchers for nearly 40 years (Wing, 1981) and was not readily available in English until 1991. For 40 years, therefore, answers to the question 'What is autism?' were largely shaped in English-speaking countries by Kanner's original descriptions, although Asperger's paper was influential in psychiatric circles in parts of Europe.

Origins of the subtypes model of autism

Kanner and Asperger were both medical practitioners. It came naturally to them, therefore, to think of autism in terms of a physical illness, and to apply a **medical model** in their descriptions and discussions of autism. The term **model**, as used here, means a way of envisaging the nature of the condition under discussion – the kind of thing, or collection of things, that it is, with some implications concerning causes and kinds of treatment that might be effective. As noted later in this chapter, some other clinicians envisaged autism in terms of a **psychoanalytic model**. Others for a brief period attempted to fit autism into a **behaviourist model**, claiming that autism results from learning inappropriate behaviour patterns. Models, in this special sense, tend to be associated with particular sets of terms. Some terms associated with the medical model are listed and defined in Box 1.2.

BOX 1.2   Medical model terms and concepts

Symptoms	Physical or behavioural signs of illness
Diagnosis	The identification of an illness by its symptoms
Syndrome	A disease or disorder characterised by a particular cluster of symptoms
Etiology	The original cause, or causes, of an illness
Prognosis	The predicted course and outcome of an illness
Treatment	Intervention designed to alleviate the symptoms or causes of illness
Patient	Someone with an illness
Nosology	The classification of diseases

The medical model classifies physical diseases and mental disorders according to categories and subcategories, rather as biology classifies living things into a hierarchy of categories and subcategories with definable boundaries, such as 'animals' (main category), 'lions, mice, people...' (subcategories). This was the way in which autism was first conceptualised. For this reason, the medical model, as applied to autism, is sometimes referred to as a **categorical** or **subtypes model** (for a discussion of the appropriateness or otherwise of applying this type of model to autism, see Sonuga-Barke, 1998).

Two Blind Alleys

In the years following the publication of Kanner's and Asperger's initial papers, two groups of professionals concerned with childhood mental health problems each tried to describe and understand autism in their own particular and rather different terms – and both got it wrong.

Autism as a neurotic condition

On the one hand the psychoanalysts and psychotherapists who were frequently asked by desperate parents to help their problem child, concluded that autism was a **neurotic** condition caused by disturbed mother–child relationships (Mahler, 1952; Bettelheim, 1967). The unfortunate term 'refrigerator mothers' indicates the supposed origins of the impaired relationship.

Psychoanalysis or other forms of psychotherapy were at that time the only available treatment on offer for children with social and emotional problems. Psychoanalysis is an expensive form of treatment, and this probably explains why the children who were brought to psychoanalysts for **diagnosis** and treatment tended to come from well-off families. These families also tended to be well educated and in a position to find out about those few clinical centres where autism was recognised as a distinct condition, and where at least some form of treatment was offered. It is perhaps not surprising, therefore, that at this period autism was widely (and incorrectly) supposed to occur mainly in affluent and well-educated families.

Autism as a form of psychosis

On the other hand, child psychiatrists and psychologists with a medical background conceived of autism as a **psychotic** condition with an organic (biological) cause (e.g., Bender, 1956). These medically minded practitioners were very concerned with issues of definition and diagnosis, and in the UK a committee was set up to establish a set of diagnostic criteria for what was interchangeably referred to as 'childhood schizophrenia', 'childhood psychosis', or 'early infantile autism'. The result was what became known as Creak's 'Nine Points' (Creak, 1961; see Box 1.3).

BOX 1.3   Creak's 'Nine Points'

Diagnostic criteria for 'childhood schizophrenia'

1   Gross and sustained impairment of emotional relationships
2   Serious retardation, with islets of normal or exceptional intellectual function
3   Apparent unawareness of personal identity
4   Pathological preoccupation with particular objects
5   Sustained resistance to change
6   Abnormal response to perceptual stimuli
7   Acute and illogical anxiety
8   Speech absent or underdeveloped
9   Distorted motility [movement] patterns

It is instructive to note that there is not one of Creak's nine points that would not be accepted today as descriptive of the problems of individuals with complex forms of autism. Moreover, all of the issues raised in the Nine Points continue to be discussed by diagnosticians and researchers and will come up as topics at various points in this book. This demonstrates the continuity between early theorists' attempts to define and describe autism, and those of the present day.

Retreat from the two blind alleys

Early suggestions that autism is either a neurotic condition or a form of childhood psychosis had been disproved by the early 1970s, on the following grounds.

Evidence that autism is not a form of neurosis   The notion of autism as a neurosis was disconfirmed by evidence that autism is associated with brain abnormalities, as demonstrated by **electroencephalography (EEG)** (Hutt, Hutt, Ounsted, & Lee, 1965), and by the high incidence of epilepsy in autistic teenagers and young adults with autism (Rutter, Greenfield, & Lockyer, 1967). It was also observed that autism could result from **maternal rubella** (German measles during pregnancy) (Chess, 1971), which was clear evidence that at least some cases of autism have an organic cause.

Evidence that autism is not synonymous with childhood schizophrenia, or with other forms of childhood psychosis   The suggestion that autism constitutes early onset schizophrenia was disproved by a study of children with 'childhood psychosis' (Kolvin, 1971). This study showed clearly that those children whose abnormal behaviours were apparent before the age of three years conformed to Kanner's (1943) description of children with 'early infantile autism' whereas those children whose development was essentially normal until the school years showed the hallucinations, delusions, and other behavioural abnormalities associated with schizophrenia. The parents of this latter group also showed an unusually high incidence of schizophrenia or **schizoid personality**, whereas this was not the case for parents of children in the early onset group. The relationship between autism and schizophrenia/schizoid personality has remained a topic of interest (C. Frith, 1992; see also Chapter 2). However, from the early 1970s onwards the conflation of autism with childhood schizophrenia ceased.

Two other subtypes of childhood psychosis, **childhood disintegrative disorder** and **Rett syndrome**, both of which are characterised by some autistic-like behaviours, were also studied and described during the 1950s and 1960s. It was clear from these studies that the manifestations and especially the course of both of these disorders differ from the typical manifestations and course of autism.

In sum, the more carefully the different subtypes of childhood psychosis were studied the less tenable it became to call children with autism 'psychotic', and reference to children with autism as 'psychotic' declined rapidly during the 1970s.

Further evidence of what autism is not The early attempts to define autism did not take place in a vacuum. On the contrary they were part of a burgeoning concern with children's mental health and educational needs which occurred during the third quarter of the last century. Over this period, for example, the first in-depth psychological investigations of **Down syndrome** were undertaken, and numerous other syndromes involving **intellectual disability (mental retardation)** began to be investigated and described by psychologists as well as by medical practitioners. The existence of **specific language impairments (SLI)** in children of normal intelligence became generally recognised during this period, as did **developmental dyslexia**. Similarly, 'hyperkinetic syndrome', now known as **attention deficit and hyperactivity disorder (ADHD)** was first identified and researched during the 1950s.

Thus, the group of what we now know as **neurodevelopmental disorders** emerged and became increasingly well defined at just the time when autism was first identified and described. This helped to differentiate autism from other childhood conditions some of which sometimes occur with autism but are not themselves core aspects of autism. As is the case with autism and childhood schizophrenia, the relationship of autism to other neurodevelopmental conditions remains a topic of interest, although less confusion between autism and other childhood disorders now exists (see Chapter 2 for further discussion).

Back to Kanner

The accumulation of evidence concerning what autism is *not*, cleared the way for a substantial return to Kanner's original view that autism is a condition in its own right, characterised by a distinctive set of behavioural abnormalities. Moreover, Kanner had suggested as early as 1943 that autism is a brain-based condition with a biological origin: in other words he anticipated the view, now universally accepted, that autism is a biologically based neurodevelopmental condition.

Once it became generally accepted that autism is a distinct neurodevelopmental condition, rather than a neurotic or psychotic disorder, attention turned back to Kanner's original description, and modified versions of Kanner's diagnostic criteria began to appear in the English-language literature. The most influential of these were those of Rutter (1968) in the UK and of Ritvo and Freeman (1977) for the National Society for Autistic Children in the USA, which were based on extensive research and discussion. These attempts to formulate an authoritative definition of what autism is, based on a set of diagnostic criteria, paved the way for the first official recognition of autism as a distinct condition, nearly 40 years after Kanner had first described it.

The First Official Definitions

DSM-III

Autism was first formally recognised as a distinct condition in 1980, in the third edition of the American Psychiatric Association's influential *Diagnostic and Statistical Manual of Mental Disorders* (DSM-III). What was called 'infantile autism' was defined in terms of the following diagnostic criteria.

- Lack of responsiveness to others.
- Impaired language and communication skills.
- Bizarre responses to aspects of the environment.
- Early onset (prior to 30 months).

It is worth noting that language abnormalities were considered central to autism at the time that DSM-III was published, remembering that this definition was produced before Asperger's work became known in the English-speaking world.

DSM-III(R)

In 1981, just one year after the first official definition of autism was published in DSM-III, Wing published a paper on 'Asperger's syndrome', which made Asperger's description of children with 'autistic psychopathy' accessible to English-language readers for the first time. Wing's paper was influential, not just because Wing herself was a highly respected clinician and academic in the field, but also because what she wrote in that paper was instantly recognised by many clinicians and others as matching their own intuitions and experience. In her paper, Wing summarised Asperger's (1944/1991) descriptions of people with **autistic psychopathy** and described individuals known to her who had the problems of social relating, communication, and behavioural flexibility described by Kanner, but who did not have significant language impairments, nor were they less intelligent than average. Indeed some had precociously large vocabularies and were highly intelligent. Wing suggested that these able people should be described as having 'Asperger's syndrome'.

As autism-related conditions became increasingly well-recognised through the 1980s, with child psychologists and psychiatrists in developed countries seeing more and more children with previously undiagnosed autism, and with the special educational needs of children with various forms of autism being increasingly recognised and catered for in schools, it was universally accepted that autism affects people who have no language or learning difficulties, as well as those who do have such difficulties. This was reflected in the diagnostic criteria for autism in a revised edition of DSM-III, known as DSM-III(R) (APA, 1987). However, the committee of experts whose responsibility it was to redefine autism in the DSM-III(R) did not go so far as to recognise Asperger syndrome as a form of autism. Instead, they reduced the emphasis on language impairment as a diagnostic criterion and increased the emphasis on impaired communication. Absent or delayed language was mentioned in the list of the kinds of impairments of communication that *might be* associated with autism. However, impaired language development was no longer seen as an *essential* characteristic without which a diagnosis of autism should not be made.

Thus, nearly 50 years after Asperger published his paper, people with the kinds of behaviours he had originally described could be diagnosed as autistic, as well as people with the fuller set of problems as originally described by Kanner. However, the diagnosis of 'Asperger syndrome' was not officially recognised until 1994, when the next edition of the *Diagnostic and Statistical Manual* was published. This edition has not yet been superseded, and its definitions, and those published by the World Health Organisation in the tenth edition of the *International Classification of Disorders* (ICD-10) (WHO, 1992, 1993), therefore count as current. These current definitions, framed in terms of sets of diagnostic criteria, are described next.

CURRENT DEFINITIONS BASED ON A SUBTYPES MODEL

DSM-IV and ICD-10

Succcessive editions of the American Psychiatric Association's *Diagnostic and Statistical Manual* and of the World Health Organisation's *International Classification of Diseases* are internationally recognised as offering the most authoritative classification schemes and diagnostic criteria for all recognised mental health disorders.

At the time of writing, the most recent version of the *Diagnostic and Statistical Manual*, first published in 1994 as DSM-IV, is the Text Revised version known as DSM-IV-TR, published in 2000. DSM-IV-TR provides a more detailed description of Asperger syndrome, in particular, than is given in the original version of DSM-IV. However, the subtypes of autism-related conditions and their criterial definitions remain the same in the two versions. A fifth edition of the manual is due to be published in 2011, and readers need to be aware that some changes to definitions of autism-related conditions are certain to be made.

The *International Classification of Diseases* (ICD-10) published in 1992 provides diagnostic criteria for use by mental health professionals, and the edition published in 1993 provides diagnostic criteria for use by researchers. ICD-10 is updated annually, the most recent version (at the time of writing) being referred to as ICD-10-2007. However, no major revisions have been made to the ICD-10 diagnostic criteria for autism-related disorders since1992/1993. The ICD-10 (1993) research criteria are more detailed and precise than the clinical definitions in ICD-10 (1992). However, the subtypes of autism-related conditions and their definitions are essentially the same.

Although there are some differences of detail and of terminology in the classification schemes in DSM-IV and in ICD-10, there are more similarities than differences. In what follows, therefore, only the DSM-IV classification scheme and diagnostic criteria are presented and discussed.

The Group of Pervasive Developmental Disorders

DSM-IV classifies autism-related conditions as members of a group of **pervasive developmental disorders (PDDs)**. Three subtypes of autism are identified within this group:

- autistic disorder;
- Asperger disorder;
- pervasive developmental disorders not otherwise specified (PDD-NOS).

The group of PDDs also includes:

- Rett syndrome;
- childhood disintegrative disorder.

Rett syndrome and childhood disintegrative disorder (which were mentioned above) are characterised by some autistic-like behaviours. However, both these disorders are degenerative conditions, with a later onset and different course and outcome when compared with the three autism-related PDDs, and are not therefore considered to be forms of autism. For this reason, neither Rett syndrome nor childhood disintegrative disorder will be further considered here.

DSM-IV Criteria for Autism-related Pervasive Developmental Disorders

Diagnostic criteria for autistic disorder

DSM-IV diagnostic criteria for autistic disorder are shown in Box 1.4.

BOX 1.4   DSM-IV diagnostic criteria for autistic disorder

A.   A total of six (or more) items from (1), (2), and (3), with at least two from (1), and one each from (2) and (3):
   (1)   Qualitative impairment in social interaction, as manifested by at least two of the following:
      (a)   marked impairments in the use of multiple non-verbal behaviours such as eye-to-eye gaze, facial expression, body postures, and gestures to regulate social interaction;
      (b)   failure to develop peer relationships appropriate to developmental level;

Autistic disorder as defined in DSM-IV closely resembles Kanner's original descriptions of children with autism. For this reason, the terms **Kanner's syndrome** or **classic autism** are sometimes used to refer to this constellation of behavioural impairments.

Diagnostic criteria for Asperger disorder

For **Asperger disorder** to be diagnosed, an individual must have at least two of the social interaction impairments listed under A (1) in Box 1.4. In addition, the individual must have at least one of the four types of restricted and repetitive behaviour listed under A (3), and they must not qualify for a diagnosis of autistic disorder.

There is no requirement that any of the communication impairments listed under A (2) should be present, and it is in fact specified that for a diagnosis of Asperger disorder to be made there should be no clinically significant general delay in language. It is also stated that there should be no clinically significant delay in **cognitive** (intellectual) development, or in the development of age-appropriate daily living skills, **adaptive behaviour** (other than in social interaction) and curiosity about the environment in childhood.

The term 'Asperger disorder', used in DSM-IV, never entered popular usage, and in what follows, 'Asperger syndrome', with lower-case 's' (or the acronym AS) is used in place of Asperger disorder. (Note that it is usual to talk about 'Asperger syndrome' without the additional / 's' /, and pronounced with a hard 'g' as in the original German.)

Diagnostic criteria for pervasive developmental disorder not otherwise specified

DSM-IV states that the diagnosis of **pervasive developmental disorder not otherwise specified (PDD-NOS)** is appropriate when there is severe and pervasive impairment in the development of reciprocal social interaction, *or* of verbal and **non-verbal communication** skills, *or* when stereotyped behaviour, interests, and activities are present. In other words, the diagnosis can be used when some but not all of the core features of autistic disorder are present. The diagnosis is also appropriate when a child presents with all the behaviours associated with autism, but these behaviours are atypical in some way, or very mild, or of late onset (after the age of three years). **Late-onset** autism is currently quite widely discussed, and is sometimes referred to as **regressive autism**.

In ICD-10 the term PDD-NOS is not used, **atypical autism** being used instead. A subtype of atypical autism, **pathological demand avoidance syndrome (PDA)** (Newson, Le Maréchal, & David, 2003) is recognised by some practitioners.

MANIFEST BEHAVIOUR

Generalised vs. Particular Behaviours

The descriptions of the criterial features of behaviour presented in diagnostic manuals such as DSM-IV are highly *generalised*. So, for example, 'lack of social and emotional reciprocity' is listed as one of the impairments of social interaction likely to be present in individuals with an autism-related condition, but there is limited indication of the range of behaviours that might come under this generalised description. This is necessarily the case because the descriptions in the diagnostic manuals are designed to apply equally to children and adults; to those with high intelligence and good language as well as to those with profound language and learning impairments; and to individuals with their own personalities and past experiences in all the different environments in which they might be observed – at home, at school, at work, on holiday, when well, when ill, etc.

In the following sections, thumbnail sketches of some individuals with autism-related conditions are given to illustrate the great diversity of *particular* behaviours that might be seen and would qualify as examples of the generalised behavioural impairments diagnostic of autism. These particular behaviours will be referred to as **manifest behaviours**, to differentiate them from the generalised descriptions given in DSM-IV. In the tables following the brief sketches, the manifest behaviours described for each individual will be listed under the headings of impaired social interaction, impaired communication, and repetitive and restricted behaviours, respectively. The examples given in the thumbnail sketches are, of course, only a minute sample of the innumerable actual behaviours that can be indicative of autism. Readers who know someone with an autism-related condition, or who have watched a TV programme featuring people with autism, will easily think of their own quite different examples.

Manifest Behaviours: Some Examples

Mandy, age eight years observed in the school playground at break time   Mandy is sitting on a swing, passively. When another child approaches, she doesn't look at the child, but gets off the swing and moves to a corner of the playground with her back to the other children. She rocks from foot to foot. At one point she utters an odd squeal and flaps her hands excitedly, for no apparent reason. Then she begins to hit her own head with her hand. The adult on playground duty approaches, takes Mandy's hand to stop her hitting herself, and says: 'Did you want to have a swing, Mandy? Look, there's a swing free now.' Mandy removes her hand from the adult's and turns away saying 'free now'. But she doesn't go towards the vacant swing. Instead she runs off, with a clumsy gait, bumping into a smaller child who falls over and begins to cry. Mandy stops running, puts her hands over her ears and stands looking at the weeping child, with an uncomprehending, distressed expression on her face.

Damien, age 16 years, observed at home   Damien is sitting at the dining room table, tracing a map of New Zealand. He tells the observing adult that he is interested in geology, and asks, rhetorically: 'Do you know the difference between a fjord and a sound?' The adult smiles and says: 'That's a funny question! They're quite different sorts of things, aren't they?' Damien ignores the observer's response and continues with what he was going to say anyway, providing the textbook definitions of a fjord as opposed to a sound (as in Queen Charlotte Sound, in New Zealand). Damien's mother comes in to lay the table for tea, and asks Damien to move his things and feed the dog before tea. Damien complies without objecting, putting away his pencils, ruler, tracing pad, etc. carefully in different compartments of a drawer. He opens a tin of dog food, fills the dog's bowl, and puts it in the usual place, but does not call the dog in from the garden. He tells the observer that he is taking four subjects in his next set of school exams and expects to get straight 'A's and go to university to study geology. The observer volunteers the information that her own son is, by chance, already studying geology at university, but Damien doesn't follow this up. Instead he asks: 'Did you know that New Zealand is 268,000 square kilometres in size, and two thirds the size of California?' When it is time for the observer to leave, Damien's mother says: 'See the lady to the door, Damien'. Damien rises reluctantly to his feet and walks behind the observer as far as the front door, immediately turning back without returning her wave.

John, age three, observed during free play in his nursery school John is sitting on the cushions in the play area, with a toy car in his hands. He is making the wheels spin over and over again, sometimes holding the car to the side of, but close to, one eye. When another child sets up a toy garage on the floor in front of John, John scrambles off the cushions and sits by the garage with the car in his hand. 'Make your car get petrol', says the other child. John puts the car on the floor, moving it along and saying 'brroom brroom', without letting the car out of his hand. 'No', exclaims the other child. 'Put it by the petrol pump'. John gets the car wheels to spin hard by running it over the floor, then puts the spinning wheels close to his ear, listening and smiling. The other child grabs the car from John, who sits crying, but without retaliating or seeking comfort from an adult. One of the nursery helpers comes to the rescue and picks John up to sit on her knee. He changes his position so he has his back to the adult, but remains on her knee. The helper picks up a book and says: 'Shall we look at some pictures? Where's the monkey?' John points to the correct picture, but doesn't turn to check the helper's face for approval. 'Get your coat' he says. John says this often, because he has learned that the instruction 'Get your coat' sometimes signals that it is time to go home. The helper ignores John's remark, and continues to get him to point to animals in the picture book, which he does successfully but without enthusiasm.

Malcolm, a physicist, observed with his wife Sheila in a counselling session Malcolm says of himself: 'I hated school. I couldn't get on with the other boys – I didn't understand their slang and their jokes, and I was hopeless at sport. I got bullied a lot, and teased for being a "swot". At secondary school I got permission to sit in the library during breaks, and that was a great relief. I used the time to study. I was never interested in fiction – I still don't read novels. Once I was in the sixth form I got friendly with another boy, who had a stammer, and was interested in science, like me. This made life a lot easier because I had a friend to do things with, in and out of school. We took up hiking. I still enjoy walking, and I met Sheila through a local hiking group.' Sheila butts in here to say: 'There are certain things we do together, like walking, and listening to music. Otherwise we live very separate lives. I sometimes think it's a good thing we never had children, because Malcolm wouldn't have known how to cope. If I'm feeling poorly or upset about something, he really hates it, because he sees it as me putting demands on him. He does buy me flowers on my birthday and our wedding anniversary – but a hug when I'm feeling low would be much more welcome. I never get a hug unless I ask for one!'

Usman, aged 11, observed in class in his special school Usman is in a class of eight, with a teacher and one assistant. Seven of the children are working at tables set in a square. Usman is seated apart, with his back to the room and facing a blank wall partly because he is easily distractable, and also because he has a compulsion to pull other children's hair. Each child is working through a maths exercise, and the adults are moving from one child to another to check progress. Suddenly Usman gets up, pushing his chair back noisily and crashing his book down on to the table shouting 'Can't do it! Got it WRONG!' Before either adult can stop him he has walked rapidly to the window with his arm raised and his hand clenched, as if to put his fist through the glass. But he doesn't actually do it, and as the teacher and the assistant reach him, Usman smacks the wall between the windows with the palm of his hand. He is red in the face and close to tears. The teacher signals to the assistant that she can cope, and, without touching Usman (who might lash out at her if she did), she says quietly: 'Well done Usman: you hit the wall instead of the window. And that doesn't hurt anyone, does it? Do you want to walk up and down the corridor with me for a bit, until you feel better?' When the teacher and Usman have left the room, the assistant explains to the observer that Usman is a perfectionist and on a very short fuse. If he makes a mistake in his work he used at one time to tear it up. When prevented from doing this, he would bite his own arm, sometimes drawing blood, and on one occasion he did actually put his fist through a window, without seeming to feel any pain. To release his emotions harmlessly, he has been taught to slap the table, or to slap against a wall when he feels unbearably frustrated and angry, as on this occasion. He is quite a clever boy, the assistant adds, but difficult to get through to, even for an adult; and the other children are scared of him.

Manifest Behaviours in Relation to Diagnostic Criteria

The tables below suggest how particular examples of behaviour described in the above sketches might fit under the three main headings of autism-related behaviours listed in DSM-IV. Table 1.1 picks out instances of impaired social interaction; Table 1.2 shows instances of restricted and repetitive behaviours, including impaired play; and Table 1.3 identifies instances of impaired communication.

Table 1.1 *Manifest behaviours exemplifying impaired social interaction*

Mandy	Sits on swing alone, not interacting with peers.
	Does not make eye contact with the child who approaches her on the swing, and avoids possible social approach by, or confrontation with, this child by moving away.
	Turns her back towards others in the playground, as if to shut them out.
	Does not respond to friendly approach by a familiar adult; removes hand from adult's, and moves away.
	Bumps into, rather than running round, another – and smaller – child.
	Does not understand that the other child is hurt, simply dislikes the noise the child is making; neither offers comfort nor looks apologetic or guilty.
Damien	Asks a rhetorical question: doesn't need a reply.
	Doesn't respond to the observer's smile, or her remark 'That's a funny question!'
	Does not infer – or care? – that the dog is unaware that food has been put down for it, and that it would be appropriate to call the dog in.
	Does not appreciate that boasting is socially inappropriate.
	Does not show socially appropriate interest in the observer's remark about her son.
	Egocentric obsession with own topic of conversation.
	Does not follow the social convention in seeing someone off at the door.
John	Joins other child, but does not (cannot?) participate in the other child's pretend play. Does not retaliate when other child takes car from him.
	Does not seek redress or comfort from an adult.
	Moves to avoid face-to-face positioning on adult's knee.
	Doesn't check adult's face for approval of correct pointing.
	Doesn't appear to get pleasure from interaction with the familiar adult.
Malcolm	Lifelong difficulty in making peer relationships – a conspicuous loner at school.
	Single schooldays friendship made with another (probable) loner.
	Friendship motivated at least in part by the desire to appear less conspicuously alone – to be more like other people.
	Hobbies relatively non-social – walking, listening to music.
	He and wife live 'very separate lives'.
	Dislikes having to respond to someone else's emotional needs.
	Gives stereotypical gifts, but fails to offer spontaneous affection or comfort.
Usman	'Difficult to get through to', as reported by classroom assistant.

Table 1.2 *Manifest behaviours exemplifying restricted, repetitive behaviours*

Mandy	Inactive on swing – no spontaneous play.
	Rocks; flaps hands.
	Repetitive self-injuring behaviour – hitting her own head.
Damien	Obsessive interest in one particular topic – accumulation of facts.
	Inflexible conversationalist: no topic shift; no reciprocity. Unusually tidy with objects he values – has compartments for each item.
John	Obsessive interest in parts, only, of the toy car.
	Manipulates toy, rather than using it for pretend play.
	Such pretend play as he produces (running the car along the ground making car engine noise) is limited and repetitive – a taught routine?
	No evidence that he can engage in the kind of pretend play the other child suggests.
	Repetitive utterance 'Get your coat' used non-communicatively.
Malcolm	Limited and unchanging interests: academic study, walking, listening to music.
	Date-triggered, conventional giving (flowers for birthdays, wedding anniversaries).
Usman	Compulsion to pull other children's hair.
	Tendency to self-harm – and apparent unawareness of pain.
	'Perfectionist' – extreme intolerance of imperfection or failure.

Table 1.3 *Manifest behaviours exemplifying impaired communication*

Mandy	Avoids interaction/communication with the child, then the adult, who approach her. Bizarre vocalisation (squealing), unconnected with any obvious stimulus. Does not respond to the adult's question, either verbally or by moving towards the now-vacant swing – does not understand what the adult said? Echoes the adult's final words – further indication of lack of comprehension? Does not understand the smaller child's emotion-expressive crying or bodylanguage.
Damien	Failure to appreciate double meaning of the word 'sound', and the observer's puzzlement. No response to observer's smile as she hints at a possible misinterpretation. Lack of response to the observer's question; says what he was going to say anyway. Highly factual conversational content – impersonal. Literal interpretation of mother's request to feed the dog: failure to infer 'and call the dog in to eat its food'. Conversational egocentricity: no response to observer's remark about her son. Literal interpretation of mother's instruction to 'See the lady to the door' – does not infer 'and say good-bye to her' or 'Stand at the door and wave'. Failure to engage in non-verbal looking and waving as someone leaves.
John	Does not respond appropriately to other child's suggestions for play – may not understand; or may not know how to engage in the suggested play. Does not complain verbally or gesturally when car taken from him, either to the other child or to an adult: instead expresses feelings by crying. Delayed language: understands single words, and can point to pictures – but no evidence of phrasal understanding. Repetitive utterance 'Get your coat' used out of context. Echoed pronoun 'your' suggests personal pronoun usage not understood.
Malcolm	Problem in understanding non-literal language (slang and jokes). No interest in fiction – (problem with narrative structure? and/or imagination?). Avoidance of situations involving communication – preference for solitary pursuits. Lack of spontaneous communicative behaviours expressing sympathy or affection; preference for the conventional, impersonal gesture of giving flowers.
Usman	Social interaction/communication with others, whether peers or adults, limited and abnormal. Habitually expresses emotions inappropriately.

Manifest Behaviours as Clues to Diagnosis

It would of course be absolutely wrong to base a diagnosis on the scraps of information given in the thumbnail sketches above. Proper clinical diagnosis involves in-depth information-gathering and actual observation of, and interaction with, the individual who is being assessed (see Chapter 13). However, there is enough information in the thumbnail sketches to suggest that it might not be surprising if subsequent full investigation were to show the following.

- Mandy fits the DSM-IV diagnostic criteria for autistic disorder: she has very poor social and communication skills, various kinds of repetitive behaviours, little language, and low learning ability.
- Damien fits the criteria for Asperger syndrome: he has good academic ability and normal language in the sense of vocabulary and sentence structure, but poor communication and social skills, restricted interests and a tendency towards obsessive behaviours.

- Malcolm probably has relatively mild and well-compensated Asperger syndrome that could have gone undiagnosed had his marriage not highlighted his social inadequacies.
- John probably has autistic disorder, though his desire to interact with another child (even though he lacks the requisite skills), his tolerance of physical contact by an adult, and the fact that he has some comprehension of language, suggest that he is less severely affected than Mandy.
- Usman possibly has PDD-NOS: there are hints of intractable social interaction difficulty; and his compulsive hair-pulling, his perfectionism, and his self-injuring tendencies are consistent with a certain kind of obsessiveness and behavioural rigidity not uncommon in association with autism. However, his inappropriate communication could be explained in terms of emotional problems rather than autism, and further investigation might well indicate that Usman has emotional and behavioural difficulties, and perhaps attentional difficulties, not associated with any form of autism.

The fact that individuals such as Mandy at one extreme, and Malcolm at another, can be seen as fitting into one or other of the subtypes of autism listed within the DSM-IV and ICD-10 classification schemes, suggests that these schemes have considerable theoretical **validity** as well as practical usefulness for the diagnosis of autism. Nevertheless, as an answer to the question 'What is autism?', the DSM-IV and ICD-10 descriptions are very limited. They are also open to certain theoretical criticisms, and these criticisms are reflected in some of the difficulties in applying a subtypes model in practice. Some of the limitations, theoretical problems, and practical difficulties are described in the next chapter.

SUMMARY

Cases of autism-related conditions were first described by Kanner in 1943 and by Asperger in 1944. However, Asperger's work did not become well known in the English-speaking world until the early 1980s, and for 40 years Kanner's view that autism was always associated with language and learning impairments was universally accepted. Initially, autism was conceptualised as either a form of neurosis associated with inadequate mothering, or as a form of psychosis synonymous with childhood schizophrenia. Both these views were abandoned during the 1960s in the face of contrary evidence. There was then a return to Kanner's original view that autism is a brain-based, neurodevelopmental condition characterised by a distinctive set of behavioural abnormalities.

This view was officially recognised when 'infantile autism' was included in the third edition of the *Diagnostic and Statistical Manual* (DSM-III), published in 1980. Shortly afterwards, Asperger's work became known, and it was realised that autism-related conditions included people with normal language and intelligence. However, Asperger syndrome as a subtype of autism was not recognised in the diagnostic manuals until the 1990s.

There are currently two internationally recognised, authoritative diagnostic manuals, DSM-IV (APA, 1994) and ICD-10 (WHO, 1992, 1993). Definitions of autism in these two manuals are quite similar and DSM-IV definitions are referred to unless otherwise stated. DSM-IV conceives of autism as consisting of three subtypes of pervasive developmental disorder (PDD): autistic disorder, Asperger syndrome, and pervasive developmental disorder not otherwise specified (widely referred to as PDD-NOS). The diagnostic criteria for autistic disorder centre round three types of abnormal behaviour: impaired social interaction, impaired communication, and restricted and repetitive behaviour. Some abnormalities of language are included under the heading of impaired communication. The diagnostic criteria for Asperger syndrome also focus on the three core impairments. However, Asperger syndrome can be diagnosed only if early language development was normal, and if language and intellectual abilities are currently normal, and if the individual does not qualify for a diagnosis of autistic disorder. The criteria for PDD-NOS allow for partial, atypical or late-onset forms of autism.

It is important to make a distinction between the generalised descriptions of behaviour given in the diagnostic criteria for autism-related conditions, and the particular manifest behaviours that fall within the generalised descriptions. The range of actual manifest behaviours that may qualify as forms of impaired social interaction, communication, and restricted and repetitive behaviours is enormous, varying widely across individuals and within individuals at different stages of development and in different situations.

THE SPECTRUM MODEL OF AUTISM: CONCEPT AND DEFINITIONS

AIMS

••••

PROBLEMS ASSOCIATED WITH THE SUBTYPES MODEL
Limited Description
Theoretical Problems
Practical Problems
A Defence of the Subtypes Model
Conclusion

••••

THE SPECTRUM CONCEPT OF AUTISM
Origins of the Spectrum Concept
Wing's Description of the Triad of Impairments
Wing's Descriptions of Additional Problems Associated
with Autism
Critique of the Spectrum Concept and its Usefulness
Relative to a Subtypes Model

••••

TERMINOLOGY
Terminological Instability and its Causes
Terminology in this Book

••••

SUMMARY

AIMS

This chapter has two main aims. The first is to indicate certain problems associated with the subtypes model of autism as used in DSM-IV and ICD-10. The second is to describe the alternative, spectrum model, and to compare and contrast the two models. An underlying aim is to stress that both models have advantages and disadvantages, and that both are useful but for different purposes.

PROBLEMS ASSOCIATED WITH THE SUBTYPES MODEL

Limited Description

The DSM-IV and ICD-10 diagnostic criteria provide a limited answer to the question 'What is autism?' This is intentional, as the aim of the experts who drew up the definitions and supplementary descriptions was to identify a minimal set of behavioural characteristics necessary and sufficient for diagnosis of an autism-related condition. It was not their intention to provide a comprehensive description of autism. Such a description would have to cover the kinds of additional problems that sometimes occur, even if quite rarely, but which can radically alter the way in which an individual's autism-related characteristics are manifested. A comprehensive description would have to cover areas of strength as well as areas of weakness; also the changes in behaviour that occur with development. All of these aspects of autism will be considered in subsequent chapters, mainly in Chapter 3, entitled 'Filling in the Picture', but also in Chapter 4, in which **developmental** changes are discussed. Meanwhile, some more serious problems associated with the subtypes model underlying DSM-IV and ICD-10 are considered.

Theoretical Problems

Autism as a pervasive developmental disorder

It is widely questioned as to whether autism is appropriately placed within a group of pervasive developmental disorders. People with autism are not, in general, pervasively impaired: the most able differ from members of the general population in only a small number of ways; and many of those who have additional language and learning impairments are nevertheless more healthy and 'normal' than they are 'disordered' or 'abnormal'. Nor does autism sit comfortably alongside two degenerative disorders, Rett syndrome and childhood disintegrative disorder, which have predictably poor outcomes. Most individuals with an autism-related condition respond positively to appropriate intervention, education and care to the extent that their autism-related behaviours become less debilitating over time, and good quality of life can be achieved. It may be that when a fifth edition of the *Diagnostic and Statistical Manual* is published, autism-related conditions will no longer be placed within the group of pervasive developmental disorders.

Autism, and autism subtypes, as clear-cut categories of disorder

The subtypes model used in DSM-IV and ICD-10, which is derived from the kinds of classification schemes that work well in physical medicine, implies:

- autism-related disorders are distinct from normality;
- subtypes of autism are distinct from each other;
- subtypes of autism are distinct from other disorders.

However, none of these implications holds true in terms of behaviour, as argued below.

Autism and normality Evidence that there is no sharp cut-off point between 'normality' and autism comes from studies of families in which there is someone with a diagnosis of an autism-related condition (Pickles et al., 2000; Wilcox, Tsuang, Schurr, & Baida-Fragoso, 2003; Dawson, G. et al., 2007). These studies show that it is quite common for other family members to show mild signs of one or other kind of autism-related behaviour, although there has never been any question of that individual being diagnosed as autistic. An aunt, for example, may have had speech and language therapy as a child, and was slow to learn to read; a brother or sister may have had difficulty in making friends at school and have chosen a career with minimal contact with other people; the father may be an avid collector of something, with unusual factual knowledge relating to his hobby. The discovery that very mild signs of autism can be found in some of the relatives of a person with autism, led to the concept of a **broader autism phenotype (BAP)**, sometimes referred to as **lesser variant autism**.

Distinctness of subtypes There is currently no evidence of clear cut-off points between Asperger syndrome (AS) and autistic disorder in terms of language ability or overall intellectual ability, these being the two behavioural areas that differentiate these subtypes according to DSM-IV. Rather, there is a steady decline in language ability and overall intellectual abilities from superior in the most highly able people (likely to be diagnosed with AS) through average, to low average or mild impairment, all the way down to moderately, severely, and finally profoundly impaired. It is not the case, of course, that there are no clear-cut differences between language and learning abilities in the most able as compared with the least able individuals with autism-related conditions; rather that there are many borderline cases.

One attempt to establish clear-cut behavioural differences between AS and autistic disorder has focused on possible differences in **motor** skills. Asperger himself included impaired motor skills as one of the universal characteristics of the individuals on whom he based his original paper. More recently, others have followed Asperger in arguing that impaired motor skills should be included as a defining feature of AS, and one that distinguishes AS from autistic disorder (Ehlers & Gillberg, 1993; Klin, Volkmar, Sparrow, Cicchetti, & Rourke, 1995). Some careful reviews of the research evidence have, however, failed to find unambiguous support for this claim (see for example Ozonoff & Griffith, 2000) although the majority of individuals with AS are markedly clumsy (Green, Baird, Barnett, Henderson, Huber, & Henderson, 2002; Jansiewicz et al., 2006). In fact authoritative reviews of all the evidence relating to possible qualitative, as opposed to quantitative, differences between AS and autistic disorder have found no such differences (Frith, 2004; Macintosh & Dissanayake, 2004; see also the books on Asperger syndrome edited by Klin, Volkmar, and Sparrow (2000) and by Prior (2003)). It is not surprising, therefore, that ICD-10 describes the subtype of Asperger syndrome as being of 'doubtful **nosological** validity'.

Distinctness from other neurodevelopmental disorders   The question here concerns whether or not the social and communicative impairments and the restricted and repetitive behaviours that define autism are unique to autism or can be found in qualitatively similar form in other childhood disorders. Several conditions appear to overlap with autism in significant respects. Three such disorders are described in Box 2.1.

BOX 2.1   Three disorders that share some behavioural characteristics with autism

Non-verbal learning disability (NVLD or NLD) is a neurodevelopmental disorder characterised by normal language ability including good verbal memory and a tendency to verbosity, in combination with a range of visual–spatial–tactile perceptual and constructional impairments, poor motor skills, social interaction deficits, and resistance to change (Rourke, 1989). The resemblance to Asperger syndrome is obvious, and some investigators have concluded that non-verbal learning disability and AS are virtually the same disorder (see, for example, Rourke & Tsatsanis, 2000). It seems more likely, however, that they are

(Cont'd)

overlapping conditions, with sensory– perceptual and motor abnormalities being a more prominent and pervasive feature of non-verbal learning disability, whereas lack of empathy and restricted interests are more marked features of AS.

Pragmatic language impairment (PLI) is characterised by problems of language use rather than problems of language acquisition. Again, the overlap with Asperger syndrome is obvious. Nevertheless, pragmatic language impairment and AS can be differentiated (Bishop & Norbury, 2002; Botting & Conti-Ramsden, 2003).

Schizoid personality disorder is characterised by emotional coldness and impaired reciprocal social interaction, abnormalities of verbal and non-verbal communication, and obsessive interests. Once again, there is clear descriptive overlap with autism, although the two conditions are not identical when the problems of social interaction etc. are examined in detail (Tantam, 1988; Wolff, 2000).

In sum, it does not appear to be the case that there are clear-cut differences between the autism subtypes and other childhood neurodevelopmental or mental health conditions. Rather, to quote Klin and Volkmar:

> It is currently unclear whether these concepts describe different entities or, more probably, provide different perspectives on a heterogeneous, yet overlapping, group of individuals sharing at least some common aspects. (Klin & Volkmar, 1995: 3)

Practical Problems

The theoretical problems associated with DSM-IV, outlined above, may seem academic and unimportant. However, the theoretical problems are reflected in practical problems of diagnosis.

For example, the lack of a clear boundary between autism and normality means that the decision to diagnose someone with Asperger syndrome may depend on circumstances such as whether or not the diagnosing clinician is alert to the fact that AS can occur in mild and well-compensated forms. The lack of clear boundaries between the named subtypes means that a decision to diagnose a child with AS or autistic disorder may depend on a clinician's judgement as to how the parents may react to the one or the other diagnostic label. Similarly, the lack of clear boundaries between autism and other neurodevelopmental disorders can lead to one clinician diagnosing a child with, for example, non-verbal learning disability, whereas another clinician diagnoses the same child with PDD-NOS.

Practical difficulties associated with diagnosing autism, and ways in which clinicians may respond to these difficulties, are discussed in greater detail in Chapter 13.

A Defence of the Subtypes Model

Do the problems associated with the subtypes classification system imply that this type of model is inherently inappropriate to apply to autism, and that the attempt to define and diagnose autism in such terms should be abandoned? The answer to these questions is 'No', for the following reasons.

In the first place, behavioural criteria such as are used in DSM-IV are never likely to yield the clear-cut distinctions implied by this model. The case of Down syndrome illustrates this point. Down syndrome is a (relatively) clear-cut diagnostic category because the patterns of chromosomal abnormality associated with the syndrome are well known and easy to ascertain. Moreover, there are clear physical appearance and health-related markers associated with the syndrome. If Down syndrome were to be identified by behavioural characteristics alone, it might be difficult to distinguish the most able people with Down syndrome from 'normal' people with low average ability; and it could be difficult to distinguish Down syndrome from other intellectual disability syndromes. Autism-related conditions may become much more sharply distinguishable if and when physical markers such as genetic abnormalities become available, as they are in Down syndrome.

In the second place, behavioural differences or physical markers are not the only criteria that can be used to differentiate one disorder from another. Other criteria include causal agents, age of onset, the course and outcome of the condition, and response to treatment. Age of onset is already used to differentiate autism-related conditions from schizoid personality disorder and childhood schizophrenia. Both age of onset, course and **prognosis** are used to differentiate autism-related conditions from Rett syndrome and childhood disintegrative disorder. A few cases of autistic-like behaviour resulting from encephalitis in late childhood or adulthood have been reported in the literature suggesting that a subtype of **acquired autism** might eventually prove valid and useful. Regressive autism (mentioned in the previous chapter) is another example of a subtype that might prove to be distinctive in terms of causal factors and age of onset.

Thirdly, if autism-related conditions do at some future time prove to be clear-cut categories similar to measles or mumps, then this will only be discovered by assuming that AS, autistic disorder, regressive autism, etc. exist as clear-cut entities, selecting research participants on the basis of current subtype criteria, and investigating possible differences between the hypothetical subtypes. Diagnostic systems such as those in DSM-IV and ICD-10 are essential for this type of research, whilst posing many practical problems for practitioners. The different needs of researchers as opposed to practitioners are explicitly recognised in the two different versions of ICD-10 (WHO, 1992 and 1993) (see Jordan, 2005a for further discussion).

Conclusion

The tremendous advances in the recognition of autism-related conditions made possible by the definitions and diagnostic criteria formulated in the official diagnostic manuals must not be underrated. It is easy, a decade and more later, to identify the limitations of these schemes. However, at the time of publication (in 1994 for the original DSM-IV; 1990 for ICD-10) they represented a significant advance over what had gone before. Moreover, it is certain that the next editions of the manuals will be modified to take account of the most widely accepted criticisms of the current formulations relating to autistic conditions. DSM-IV and ICD-10 have proved immensely fruitful as a step towards answering the question 'What is autism?', DSM-V and ICD-11 (when they appear) are likely to continue to be central to our understanding of these complex conditions.

Meanwhile, a rather different way of answering the question 'What is autism?', one that circumvents the limitations and the theoretical and practical difficulties associated with the DSM-IV and ICD-10 classification schemes, has gained widespread acceptance in the autism field, especially amongst practitioners. This is the **dimensional**, or **profiling, model** that conceives of autism as a **spectrum** of related disorders. The spectrum concept of autism is described next.

THE SPECTRUM CONCEPT OF AUTISM

Origins of the Spectrum Concept

In 1979, Wing and Gould published a report of a large-scale study of special needs children living in the London district of Camberwell. In the Camberwell study, Wing and Gould identified some children who had all the behavioural impairments originally described by Kanner (1943), including impaired language and low learning ability (see Box 1.1). However, the researchers also found another group of children who had impaired social interaction, communication, and **behavioural flexibility** but whose language and learning abilities were normal. Moreover, they identified a large group of children who had some but not all of the behavioural impairments described by Kanner. It might be said that Wing and Gould identified one group of children who would now be seen as conforming to DSM-IV criteria for autistic disorder, one group conforming to the criteria for Asperger syndrome, and another conforming to the criteria for PDD-NOS. However, in describing the children in their study, Wing and Gould went beyond the DSM-IV criteria and descriptions in several important ways.

First, they explicitly noted that the severity of each of the three core impairments varied along a continuum from mild to severe in individual children. For example, one child might be severely socially withdrawn, but have only mild problems of behavioural flexibility; whereas another child might be only mildly socially impaired, but be markedly obsessive and resistant to change.

Secondly, Wing and Gould explicitly noted that intellectual ability and language ability across the whole group of children whom they were assessing also varied along continua, covering the full range from entirely normal to profoundly impaired.

Thirdly, they explicitly noted that some but not all of the children had additional physical disabilities, medical problems, or developmental difficulties. These, too, might be more or less severe.

In making these additional observations Wing and Gould did not discover anything that the experts who formulated the DSM-IV or ICD-10 criteria did not know. But whereas the diagnostic criteria identified in the subtypes definitions were designed to isolate and identify only those features of behaviour that uniquely define autism, Wing and Gould were interested in encompassing the diversity that characterises people who have one or more of the typical autism-related impairments. Stated succinctly, whereas the DSM-IV and ICD-10 definitions emphasise the **homogeneity** that can be found in whole groups of individuals with autism-related conditions, Wing and Gould emphasised the **heterogeneity** of the individuals themselves.

Wing and Gould (1979) thus conceived of autism as a multi-dimensional condition, each dimension corresponding to a different facet of behaviour including social interaction, communication skills, and capacities for creative social imagination; also language ability, learning ability, and many other dimensions of behaviour, health, and development. They saw each individual as having a different dimensional profile depending on the degree to which the individual differed from the average for the general population on each dimension. Some contrasting profiles of individuals, all of whom have an autism-related condition, are shown in Figure 2.1. The horizontal axis in the figure shows examples of dimensions that might be included in a profile for an individual with an ASD, and the vertical axis shows notional values from low to high where 100 = average.

Wing and Gould initially coined the phrase the **autistic continuum** to refer to the varied forms this multi-dimensional, multi-profile condition might take. However, in later publications Wing preferred the term **autistic spectrum disorders (ASDs)**. Whereas 'continuum' captures the continuous variation in severity that occurs along individual dimensions of behaviour associated with autism, 'spectrum' captures the lack of clear boundaries between different forms of autism. Just as red merges into orange merges into yellow in the spectrum of light, so the different forms of autism are not clearly separable from one another. Thus, although Wing sometimes identifies certain behavioural profiles with labels such as 'Kanner's syndrome' or 'Asperger syndrome' (which roughly correspond to the profiles representing 'LFA' and 'AS/HFA' in Figure 2.1), she does not consider that these profiles correspond to distinct clinical entities.

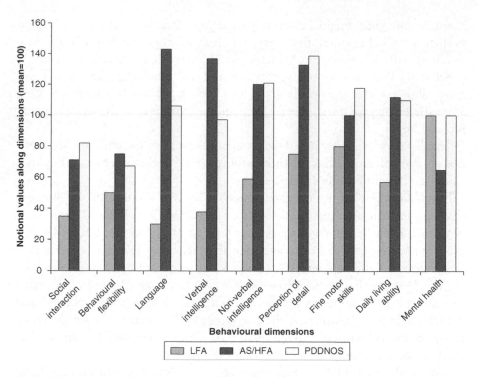

Figure 2.1 Examples of contrasting dimensional profiles of individuals all of whom qualify for a diagnosis of an autistic spectrum disorder

Wing and Gould (1979), and later publications by Wing (1988, 1996) went beyond the 'bare bones' approach of DSM-IV in other ways, some of which are described next.

Wing's Description of the Triad of Impairments

In their report of the Camberwell study, Wing and Gould referred to a **triad** of social impairments affecting:

- social interaction;
- social communication;
- social imagination and creativity.

In her later publications, Wing refers simply to impairments of social interaction, communication, and imagination, and has spelt out the kinds of behaviour that typically go to make up each of the three elements of the triad, as outlined below.

The social interaction impairment

Wing emphasises that the abnormalities of social behaviour which occur in people with autistic spectrum disorders are quite varied, and she identifies four subgroups of individuals with qualitatively different types of social abnormalities: the aloof group, the passive group, the 'active but odd' group, and the overly formal, stilted group. Key characteristics of each subgroup as described by Wing are shown in Box 2.2.

BOX 2.2   Wing's four types of autism-related social behaviour

The *aloof group* 'behave as though other people did not exist.'
The *passive group* are 'not completely cut off from others. They accept social
    approaches and do not move away from others but they do not initiate social
    interaction.'
The *active but odd group* 'make active approaches to other people...
    but do so in a peculiar one-sided fashion to make demands or to go on and on
    about their own concerns.'
The *overly formal, stilted group* are highly able older adolescents or adults who are
    'excessively polite and formal....They try very hard to behave well and cope by
    sticking rigidly to the rules of social interaction.'

(From Wing, 1996: 35 – 38)

The additional detail given by Wing in her description of social interaction impairments is important, because it counteracts the myth that all individuals with ASDs are completely asocial. This is not the case, as anyone who has spent time with a variety of people with ASDs will know. For any reader who has not spent time with people with ASDs, the first table in Chapter 1 illustrates the range of manifest behaviours, all of which fall under the broad general description of impaired social interaction.

It is important to note that Wing does not see the aloof, passive, active-but-odd, and stilted groupings as constituting discrete, clear-cut subtypes of ASD, if only because an individual's social interaction often changes over time. For example, the child who tolerates being pushed on a trike may grow into an adolescent who seeks to make social contact, even if clumsily; and the child who buries her head in her arms to escape other people may grow into an adult who can tolerate being with others, even though rarely initiating social contact. Thus, Wing's terms are descriptive rather than categorical, in keeping with her overall approach to diagnosis and definition.

The communication impairment

Wing's (1996) description of the communication impairment does not differ in broad outline from that of DSM-IV. However, she is particularly clear about the distinction between the acquisition of a language system, and the use of language for communication (for details of this distinction, see Box 3.5). Wing emphasises that not everyone with an ASD has an impaired language system in the sense of impaired vocabulary and grammar; but that everyone with an ASD *uses* such language as they have in limited and unusual ways. For example, the content is often repetitive, and even able adults tend to monologue about their own preferred interests. Less able individuals do not truly converse with others. They may answer or ask questions, state facts, or make their views known, but they cannot sustain the normal to and fro of social chat or everyday discussion. An example of a conversation with a young man with low average ability, including relatively normal language, is shown in Box 2.3.

BOX 2.3   A sample of conversation between Tom, a young man with an ASD and low average ability, and a visitor

Visitor:	What did you do with your dad this weekend? Did you go anywhere special?
Tom:	I don't think we did – apart from the pub for a meal.
Visitor:	Did you have something nice to eat?
Tom:	Can't remember.
Visitor:	You can't remember?
Tom:	Sirloin steak, I think.
Visitor:	That sounds nice.
Tom:	S'pose it is.
	[*Pause*]
Visitor:	What's your dad like, Tom?
Tom:	He has the same thing…steak….maybe something else.
Visitor:	Is he nice, your dad?
Tom:	S'pose he is.
Visitor:	And do you see him every weekend?
Tom:	Every weekend.
	[*Pause*]
Visitor:	Have you got any brothers and sisters, Tom?
Tom:	One called Michael and one called Susan, but they live far away now.
Visitor:	Oh, right. How old are they then?
Tom:	Michael's about 28 and I'm 26.
Visitor:	And what about Susan?
Tom:	…older than that – born in 1967.

(From Dobbinson, 2000, with kind permission)

In the sample of conversation reproduced in Box 2.3 it is conspicuous how little Tom contributes to the conversation (he would have said much more if asked about space travel or military equipment, two of his particular interests).

As it is, the visitor has to work hard to keep the conversation going. Even then, there are glitches: for example when Tom misinterprets the question 'What's your dad like?' and when he provides unasked for information about his own age in place of the expected information about his sister's age.

In addition to emphasising impaired use of language, Wing observes that the speech of people on the autistic spectrum is frequently monotonous in tone, or marked by inappropriate inflexion: the 'vocal tunes' and speech rhythms are odd. To use the technical term, **prosody** is almost always abnormal. Moreover, there are sometimes peculiarities of voice such as being overloud, or too soft, or using a 'special' voice to say certain things. 'Abnormalities in the pitch, stress, rate, rhythm and intonation of speech' are, in fact, included in ICD-10 (1993) criteria for childhood autism, although this characteristic has been relatively little researched (McCann & Peppé, 2003; Paul, Augustyn, Klin, & Volkmar, 2005).

Finally, Wing comments on the fact that communication problems are much broader than impaired use of spoken language. She points out that conventional gestures rarely develop beyond the simplest, such as shaking or nodding the head, and that manual signs are not generally acquired more readily than spoken words. She also comments on the marked problems of understanding and using non-verbal communication signals such as facial expressions or body movements. Research studies suggest that facial expressions are not intuitively understood by people with ASDs (e.g., Gross, 2004), although more able individuals learn to compensate to some extent (Grossman, Klin, Carter, & Volkmar, 2000). The difficulty with comprehending facial expressions is consistent with the fact that people with ASDs are generally bad at recognising faces (Boucher & Lewis, 1992; Boucher et al., 2005). However, it is at odds with relatively good ability to tell one face from another (face discrimination), and with anomalously good ability to recognise photographs of faces presented upside down (Hobson, Ouston, & Lee, 1988). For research findings on the perception, discrimination, and recognition of faces, and on the ability to comprehend the emotions conveyed by facial expressions see reviews by Dawson, Webb, and McPartland (2005) or Jemel, Mottron, and Dawson (2006).

The impairment of imagination

Wing identifies a lack of imaginative activities such as pretend play with miniature objects, inventive role-play, and the ability to enter imaginatively into a story, as central to the third impairment in the triad. She also identifies the inability to enter imaginatively into other people's experiences and feelings as part of this impairment, which is no doubt why she sometimes writes of 'an impairment of social imagination'. Wing mentions, also, impaired ability to imagine the future, a characteristic feature of autistic behaviour not mentioned in DSM-IV. (This characteristic is discussed at some length in Chapter 12.) Repetitive and restricted behaviours are recognised as occurring, but are seen as just 'the other side of the coin of impairment of imagination' (Wing, 1996: 45). This direction of cause and effect is the exact opposite to that assumed in DSM-IV or ICD-10, where lack of creative and imaginative behaviour is seen as resulting from the preoccupation with a restricted set of repetitive behaviours.

It is worth noting another difference between Wing's description and the DSM-IV criteria. This is a difference of opinion as to whether lack of pretend play should belong under the heading 'impaired imagination' (Wing), or under the heading 'communication impairment' as in DSM-IV (see Box 1.4). This difference of opinion reflects a lack of understanding of the cause or causes of impaired pretence in children with ASDs: it could result from difficulties to do with imagination (as Wing implies) or from impaired ability to use **symbols**, an ability that is necessary for both language and pretend play (as assumed in DSM-IV). This issue is discussed more fully in Chapter 5.

One might ask if differences such as the above between Wing's and DSM-IV's descriptions matter. For practical purposes, such as making a diagnosis, differences in the allocation of particular abnormalities of behaviour to particular members of the triad of impairments are unimportant: repetitive behaviours are indicative of an autism-related condition whether they are the *result* of a lack of social imagination and creativity, as suggested by Wing, or the *cause* of a lack of novel, imaginative behaviour, as is implicit in DSM-IV. Similarly, impoverished pretend play is indicative of autism regardless of whether theoreticians assume that it is related to impaired imagination or to inability to symbolise.

For theoretical purposes, however, differences in the allocation of particular abnormalities of behaviour to particular members of the triad are important for two reasons. First because they demonstrate the gaps in our knowledge of the causes of much of autistic behaviour (about which much more is said in Part II). Secondly, differences in the way particular abnormalities are allocated shows that characterising ASDs in terms of a triad of impairments, whether within a subtypes or a spectrum model, does not fully succeed in assigning the most typical behaviours to three distinct groups. One may conclude that the convention of diagnosing autism in terms of a triad of impairments is open to revision, a possibility that is discussed in Chapter 5.

Wing's Descriptions of Additional Problems Associated with Autism

Wing's description of the triad of impairments, summarised in the previous section, was taken from her book *The Autistic Spectrum* (Wing, 1996). Later in her book Wing describes other features of behaviour, additional to the triad of impairments, which are commonly though more variably present in people with ASDs. The other features of behaviour she describes include motor abnormalities affecting gait and posture, problems in imitating body movements, unusual responses to sensory stimulation, and uneven cognitive (intellectual) abilities with **rote memory** and encyclopaedic memory for facts being strikingly good in some people with an ASD, with rarer instances of special skills in drawing, music, or mathematical ability.

Wing also comments on certain physiological anomalies, including the unusual prevalence of food fads and excessive thirst, and the frequent occurrence of sleep disturbance, especially in younger or less able individuals. She notes the vulnerability to certain mental health problems, especially anxiety and fears, and has a whole chapter on medical conditions that may co-occur with autism.

Wing's model of autism allows for these additional impairments, special skills, and **co-morbid** physiological, mental, or physical health problems, in that all of them are seen as potentially contributing to the dimensional profile of an individual with an ASD. In Chapter 3 more detail is provided about the additional problems and anomalies that either universally or commonly occur in association with the triad of impairments.

Critique of the Spectrum Concept and its Usefulness Relative to a Subtypes Model

The term autistic spectrum disorders, and the dimensional concept of autism that it embodies, has proved popular and is now widely used. For practitioners making a diagnosis it has the advantage that it is more flexible and less committing than the DSM-IV classification scheme. For those caring for and working with people with ASDs the profiling approach is attractive because it emphasises individuality and provides detailed information about current strengths and needs. The spectrum concept also avoids some of the theoretical problems that were identified in a previous section.

For theoreticians, on the other hand, a diagnosis of autistic spectrum disorder, however well profiled, may have disadvantages. In particular, it is not designed to probe the possibility that autism may, in the long term, prove to be divisible into distinct subtypes. The search for subgroups has potential importance for medical treatments, and eventually for prevention of autism, and the loose and inclusive nature of the spectrum concept is not useful for guiding this kind of research. Similarly, the intentionally loose and inclusive concept of autistic spectrum disorders lacks the potential to convey information about differences in **etiology, neurobiology**, prognosis, and likely response to various forms of intervention that may in the longer term be found to apply to different subgroups of individuals with different dimensional profiles.

In sum, the spectrum model and the subtypes model both have their advantages and disadvantages. Roughly speaking, where the spectrum model is strong the subtypes model is weak, and vice versa. There is currently no way of knowing which model, each with its slightly different set of diagnostic criteria and slightly different diagnostic labels, will in the long term prove more consistent with what will eventually be understood as a full description and understanding of 'autism'. Meanwhile, both approaches are useful, and the lesson to take away is not that one model is right and the other wrong. If both are useful to people with ASDs, their families, and those who work with or for people with ASDs, then both should be valued for what they can do, and they should be seen as mutually complementary concepts.

TERMINOLOGY

Terminological Instability and its Causes

Before moving on to look at characteristics of autism in more detail in Chapter 3, and to consider facts and figures concerning autism and how people with ASDs change over the lifespan in Chapter 4, it is necessary to consider terminology in the field; not least to say how terms will be used in the main body of this book.

Terminology centring on autism is something of a minefield. In the first place, as is clear from the content of this book so far, different models or concepts of autism use slightly different sets of terms. Moreover, the historical background presented in Chapter 1 demonstrates that terminology changes as more becomes known and concepts of autism develop and change. For example, describing children as 'psychotic' or 'schizophrenic' turned out to be quite simply wrong. Similarly, terms such as 'early infantile autism' and 'early childhood autism' were rejected not because autism is not an early-onset condition that affects children, but because it was increasingly realised that autism is not confined to infancy or childhood. Terms relating to people who are different from the majority also change because these terms tend to become stigmatised over time, and there is repeated need to refresh the vocabulary and free it (temporarily) from stigma.

These processes of change are continuing, and possible future changes in concepts of autism and in related terminology are considered below and again, briefly, in Chapter 5.

There are also some macro- and some micro-cultural differences in preferred terminologies. At the macro-cultural level, different countries use slightly different terminologies. This is the case even amongst English-speaking developed countries that share literatures, as is the case in the field of autism. For example, the UK and US differ in the terms most widely used when discussing individuals who are slow to learn: whereas 'mental retardation' is widely used in the US it is infrequently used in the UK, except by some members of the medical professions. The UK equivalents of mental retardation include intellectual disability, **learning disability** and **general learning difficulty**. However, 'learning disability' is used in the US to refer to what in the UK would be termed **specific learning difficulty/disability** (for example, developmental dyslexia, or specific language impairment), and this can lead to misunderstandings unless one is aware of the different interpretations. Similarly, the overarching term **special educational needs** that is widely used in the UK translates as **exceptional children** in the US.

Different usages at the micro-cultural level are hinted at in the remark that 'mental retardation' is only used by members of the medical profession in the UK. This is a very ancient profession with historically entrenched attitudes and vocabularies as exemplified in some of the terms listed in Box 1.2. For reasons that will be touched on below, many medical model terms are judged to be inappropriate and objectionable by members of some other professions, and also by some people with ASDs themselves.

Finally, terminology is influenced by changes in social attitudes that may cut across professional and national cultures. In recent decades, social attitudes to disability have been changing largely as a result of the refusal of able and articulate people with disabilities to be defined in terms of their disabilities and accordingly objectified, undervalued, discounted, and patronised. Some practitioners anticipated the need for attitude change. The Warnock Report (1978) into special education in the UK introduced the term special educational needs precisely to move the emphasis away from children's disabilities to their strengths and needs and a memorable book *People not Patients*, by Peter Mittler, an educationalist, was published in 1979.

In the autism field there were corresponding changes during the last decades of the twentieth century, away from using terms such as 'autistics' or 'autists' to using less objectifying terms such as 'children with autism', 'teenagers with ASDs', placing emphasis on the person rather than on the condition. More recently, some of the most able and articulate people with Asperger syndrome have argued against this, pointing out that their autism is precisely what makes them the person they are. These articulate people have also argued vehemently against the application of medically derived terms such as 'disorder', 'disability', 'deficit' and 'impairment' to people with ASDs. They argue that autism is more comparable to a different way of life than a disorder, and that a value-free vocabulary of difference should be preferred to the inherently devaluing language of disease (Mottron, Dawson, & Soulières, 2008). More is said about changing social attitudes to autism in Chapter 15.

Terminology in this Book

Given the changing nature and cultural variations of terminology in the field, decisions concerning terminology have to be made and justified when writing an introductory book such as the present one, which may be read by people with a range of different experiences of autism.

Autism-related terminology

In the chapters so far, I have tended to use old-fashioned terminology when discussing historical background; medical model language when discussing the subtypes concept of autism; and spectrum model language when discussing the spectrum concept, on the principle 'when in Rome do as the Romans do'. To some extent I will continue to do this. If, for example, I am discussing some research that investigated cognitive abilities in people diagnosed with Asperger syndrome according to DSM-IV criteria, I must obviously refer to 'people with Asperger syndrome'. If, on the other hand, I am describing a study investigating differences in outcomes in children who were initially described as 'aloof', 'passive' or 'active but odd', then use of these terms is essential.

When, however, as in much of the remainder of the book, I am discussing autism/autistic spectrum disorders regardless of any particular concept or model, spectrum terminology will be preferred to DSM-IV terminology. This is because the former is less theoretically committing than the latter: it leaves important unanswered questions open. Thus, the phrase 'autistic spectrum disorders' (ASDs) will be used to refer to the set of autism-related conditions, however conceptualised, with the plural form being used when describing groups of people with autism to avoid the implication that autism is a single, or **unitary**, condition. The singular form 'autistic spectrum disorder' (ASD) will be used when referring to any one individual or any one particular subtype.

In place of the DSM-IV terms 'Asperger syndrome' and 'autistic disorder', I will tend to use the loosely descriptive terms high-functioning autism (HFA) and low-functioning autism (LFA), and sometimes 'very high-functioning', 'moderately high-functioning', 'lower functioning', 'very low-functioning' and so on, consistent with the continuous variation of language ability and intelligence from the highest-functioning to the lowest-functioning people with ASDs. However, I will generally use the combined abbreviations AS/HFA to refer to individuals at the most able end of the spectrum, because the diagnostic category of Asperger syndrome is theoretically important, widely used in clinical practice, and unlikely to be abandoned, despite current difficulties of definition.

I have decided not to anticipate what may be a major change in terminology over the next decade. This major change, if it comes about, will involve using the word 'autism' to apply only to what has been variously termed Kanner's syndrome, classic autism, autistic disorder, or low-functioning autism, whilst using 'Asperger syndrome' synonymously with high-functioning autism, and retaining the category of PDD-NOS. A demotion of the term 'autism' from its historic role as the generic term covering all ASDs to refer only to one subtype of ASD, is likely to be slow to percolate into popular usage, if indeed it ever does. It is partly for this reason that I have decided against using the term in this narrowed sense in this book. An additional reason for not using autism to refer to a subgroup is that I prefer not to use terms that imply a set of as yet unproven subtypes.

Other terms

Some other terms I have opted to use reflect UK usage, rather than US usage. In particular, I will use the term 'intellectual disability', and sometimes 'learning disability/difficulty' rather than 'mental retardation'. And I will use the phrase 'special educational needs' rather than 'exceptional children'.

The phrase 'restricted and repetitive behaviours and lack of creativity' is cumbersome. It is also subtly inaccurate as a description of a set of behaviours characteristic of people with ASDs, because some individuals with an ASD (notably **savants**, as discussed in Chapter 3) are undeniably creative in certain specific spheres and ways. To minimise these difficulties I will sometimes use the expression 'behavioural inflexibility' in place of the longer phrase. I will also use the word 'imagination' rather than 'creativity' when discussing what it is that *all* people with ASDs lack in terms of producing novel and varied forms of behaviour.

Regarding the use of 'difference' terminology as opposed to 'disorder/ deficit' vocabulary, I take as made the case for Asperger syndrome as constituting a different constellation of cognitive strengths and weaknesses from that most commonly found in the general population (see Baron-Cohen, 2000, for discussion). Terms such as 'disorder', 'disability', 'abnormality', 'deficit', 'impairment' will therefore be avoided when discussing able people with ASDs, except in certain circumstances. These include circumstances in which such terms might equally well be applied to people in the general population who do not have Asperger syndrome. So, for example, I have a bad memory for faces, as does my friend JS, who is an exceptionally high-functioning person with an ASD: we might both be described as having impaired face recognition. JS himself uses the 'impairment/disability' terms to describe some of his own problems, but does not see this as bearing on his value as a person. Another situation in which the more medicalised 'disorder/deficit' terminology might be used when referring to people with high-functioning autism or AS is when I am reporting the work of others who use this terminology.

I do not, however, consider as made the case for 'difference' terminology to be extended to individuals with those forms of ASD that include language and learning impairments, and possibly multiple additional problem behaviours and physical conditions; nor in my experience do many parents, siblings, and others close to such people believe that the individuals they care for and love are merely different (see the anecdote reported in Box 2.4). The terminology of disorder, deficit, and abnormality will therefore be used more freely when discussing more complex and severe forms of autism. More is said in Part III about the balance to be achieved between fully valuing every individual whilst not underplaying – essentially denying – the seriousness of the difficulties they may face.

BOX 2.4 Parents' preferences

A few years ago I was invited to give a talk to a group of parents, all of whom had adult children with severe intellectual disabilities, with or without autism. In preparing my talk I was careful to avoid using terms such as mental retardation, mental handicap, disorder and so on, planning to use instead the set of terms that give a less medical and less negative view of people with learning problems.

However, when I came to give my talk I had not been speaking for more than a few minutes, referring as planned to 'people with learning difficulties', when one parent interrupted to say that in her view, 'learning difficulties' was not an appropriate description of her son's problems. Other parents instantly joined in, in support. They told me that talk of 'difficulties' underestimated the severe and intractable problems their sons and daughters faced, and that in their view this actually reduced their ability to make a strong case for the support needed to help them to care and provide for their children. There was unanimous agreement that the stronger, albeit negative, terminology of disability, disorder, and mental handicap was both descriptively more appropriate and also more useful to them than what they termed the 'politically correct' terminology of difficulty and difference.

I took away three lessons from this little incident. First, as an outsider to the real world of living with ASD (or similar condition), whether as a person with an ASD or as a parent, sibling, or other closely involved person, one should always be sensitive to, and adopt, the individual's or family member's preferred terminology. Second, terminology relating to diagnosis and description is a tool, and as such should be selected to have maximum usefulness for individuals and families (see also Chapter 13). Third, although terminology reflects and reinforces attitudes, and 'politically correct' terminology has the laudable aim of changing attitudes for the better, respecting the views of insiders and giving them the strongest possible tools for obtaining the help they need is more immediately important than changing social attitudes.

SUMMARY

Despite the respect accorded to the DSM-IV and ICD-10 classification schemes, and despite their worldwide influence and usefulness, there are certain problems associated with these schemes. These include the incomplete accounts of autistic behaviour provided by the diagnostic criteria and descriptions; the fact that autism does not fit comfortably within the group of pervasive developmental disorders; nor does it, at least in the current state of knowledge, fit comfortably with the assumptions of the medical, subtypes model concerning distinctness from normality and from other neurodevelopmental disorders, and distinctness between the suggested subtypes of autism. These theoretical problems lead to difficulties in using the DSM-IV/ICD-10 criteria in practice. It should not be concluded, however, that autism will never be amenable to description in terms of a set of distinct subtypes, because greater understanding may clarify some of the boundaries.

The dimensional model of autism as a spectrum of related disorders can be traced back to a study carried out by Wing and Gould in the 1970s. This study showed that, although groups of children could be identified whose behaviour fitted with either Kanner's or Asperger's descriptions of autism, some children did not clearly fit either description. Moreover, the severity of each individual child's impairments varied along continua, from mild to severe, and many of the children had additional medical, mental health or developmental problems. These observations led Wing to propose the concept of a spectrum of autism-related disorders based on a dimensional model. According to the dimensional model, the spectrum of autism-related disorders consists of a heterogeneous set of behavioural profiles with one or more of the triad of impairments as an essential feature. Wing's descriptions of the triad of impairments differ in minor ways from those of DSM-IV, notably in her identification of four types of social interaction impairment; also in her emphasis on lack of imagination as a cause of the restricted and repetitive behaviour that is described in the subtypes model.

The spectrum concept has various advantages over the subtypes concept of autism embodied in DSM-IV. These include the ability to capture the diversity amongst individuals all of whom have one or more features of autistic behaviour of varying severity, plus or minus a range of additional problems. The spectrum concept also avoids the theoretical problems associated with the subtypes model of autism embodied in DSM-IV. It is also easier to apply in diagnostic practice and more informative concerning each individual's strengths and needs. For these reasons, the spectrum concept and terminology may be preferred by practitioners. However, the spectrum model is not useful to researchers investigating possible distinctions between subtypes of autism, for which DSM-IV criteria are needed. Until such time as more is known about autism it is not therefore possible to make a judgement concerning the spectrum concept as opposed to the subtypes concept in terms of capturing the true nature of autism. For the time being, the two models are best viewed as having complementary uses.

Terminology in the autism field changes, as concepts of autism change and understanding increases. There are also cultural differences in terminology: for example, between terms used in the American literature as opposed to the UK literature; and between terms used by members of the medical professions as opposed to members of the teaching professions. Terminology is also influenced by changes in social attitudes, most recently by the arguments of able and articulate people with ASDs for the use of language that recognises them as different rather than as defective. The ways in which terms are used in the remainder of the book are identified, with reasons given for the sometimes difficult choices made.

FILLING IN THE PICTURE: FROM CONFORMITY TO DIVERSITY

AIMS

••••

INTRODUCTION

••••

ADDITIONAL CHARACTERISTICS THAT MAY BE UNIVERSAL
Emotion Processing: Strengths and Weaknesses
Sensory-perceptual Processing: Strengths and Weaknesses
Motor Skills: Strengths and Weaknesses
Other Spared Abilities

••••

CHARACTERISTICS THAT DISTINGUISH LFA FROM AS/HFA
Language Ability
Intellectual Ability

••••

CO-MORBID CONDITIONS
Physical and Medical Conditions
Mental Health Problems
Neurodevelopmental and Behavioural Problems
Multiple Difficulties

••••

INDIVIDUAL DIFFERENCES

••••

SUMMARY

AIMS

The main aim of this chapter is to provide a fuller picture of autism, both in terms of characteristics that all or most people with ASDs share but that are not covered, or minimally covered, in the DSM-IV/ICD-10 diagnostic criteria; and in terms of the many characteristics that are shared by some but not all individuals across the spectrum, and which progressively introduce diversity and uniqueness amongst individuals. The fuller picture of autism is important for establishing 'What has to be explained' in Part II; also for identifying intervention needs to be discussed in Part III. Subsidiary aims of the chapter are to stress the unevenness that exists within all domains of behaviour in people with autism, with conspicuous areas of strength as well as specific impairments and anomalies; and to emphasise the fact that people with ASDs are more different from each other than they are alike.

INTRODUCTION

In Chapter 2 it was suggested that as an answer to the question 'What is autism?' the DSM-IV description of autism is limited in that it gives a 'bare bones' definition, focusing on the most striking and consistent behavioural characteristics that people with ASDs have in common with each other, whilst intentionally ignoring much of the detail. It was also pointed out that one of the strengths of the spectrum concept of autism is that it takes into account a range of additional characteristics that contribute to answering the question 'What is autism?' In the present chapter, some of these additional characteristics are described.

In the opening section, characteristics that probably occur universally in people with ASDs are described, contrasting the peaks and troughs of ability within three domains of behaviour:

- emotion processing;
- sensory-perceptual processing;
- motor skills.

In the second section of the chapter, language and intellectual abilities in people with ASDs are described, focusing mainly on the linguistic and intellectual impairments that distinguish low-functioning from high-functioning autism. In the third section medical, mental health, and **developmental disorders** that may co-occur with the triad of impairments are outlined. Some of these are relatively common, but others affect only a small percentage of people with ASDs. The final section of the chapter is headed 'Individual Differences', and marks the end-point in moving from characteristics that confer some degree of conformity on groups of people with ASDs, to characteristics that increasingly introduce diversity and uniqueness.

ADDITIONAL CHARACTERISTICS THAT MAY BE UNIVERSAL

Emotion Processing: Strengths and Weaknesses

To understand the pattern of emotion processing abilities and disabilities in people with ASDs it is necessary to establish some key terms and concepts. These are presented in Box 3.1.

BOX 3.1 Terms used in the psychological study of emotion

Affect is a term used by psychologists to mean emotion.

Basic emotions are those that are universal in humans: happiness, sadness, anger, fear, and disgust (surprise is sometimes included).

Complex emotions are those that are dependent on understanding how others see us, for example, pride, guilt, embarrassment.

Emotion contagion refers to the most primitive form of emotion processing, or affect processing, and consists of the involuntary sharing of others' basic emotions. Emotion contagion produces physiological changes such as increased heart rate, or sweating, which may be accompanied by involuntary behaviours such as laughing or crying along with the laughter or tears of another person. This 'infectious behaviour' can occur in the absence of knowing what the other person is laughing or crying about.

Sympathy – literally 'feeling with' – is sometimes used with the same meaning as emotion contagion. However, because 'sympathy' is used in general conversation with a much wider meaning, it will be avoided here.*

Empathy is the term used to describe intuitive knowledge of the cause or 'content' of an experienced emotion: knowing what the emotion is about. The fact that experiencing an emotion can be differentiated from knowing what the emotion is about is evident from the common experience of waking in the morning with a sinking feeling but momentarily not knowing the cause of the feeling (e.g., the exam to be taken, the bad news received the previous day).

* Narrow and quite specific usages of 'sympathy' and 'empathy' are used in this book. However, these terms are used more broadly and variously both in everyday speech and also in the specialist literature (for example see the discussion of 'empathy' in Singer, 2006).

Empathy is almost certainly impaired: people with autism do not appear to understand the causes, or content, of other people's emotions (Sigman, Kasari, Kwon, & Yirmiya, 1992; Ben Shalom, 2000a). Mandy, for example, one of the children described in the thumbnail sketches in Chapter 1, does not appear to understand that the child she knocks over is crying because she is hurt: she has failed to acquire the usual unconscious association between being hurt and crying.

The problem of knowing what another person's emotion is about may extend to knowing what one's own emotion is about (Hill, Berthoz, & Frith, 2004; Faran & Ben Shalom, 2008). This may explain why children with ASDs ask questions such as 'Did I like it when I went on the bouncy castle?' or 'Was I frightened when I went on the aeroplane?' They may remember going on the bouncy castle or the trip on the aeroplane, but have no memory of whether it was frightening or fun.

The ability to understand **complex emotions** is also impaired (Baron-Cohen, 1991; Capps, Yirmiya, & Sigman, 1992). So, for example, many adolescents and adults with autism have to be taught that completing a task successfully may win praise, or that appearing in public in states of undress will embarrass others.

The ability to experience **basic emotions** is, by contrast, undoubtedly spared. People with ASDs smile when they are happy, cry when they are sad, scowl and shout when they are angry – even if the actual sounds they make, the facial expressions and bodily gestures they produce, are not always quite like those of other people (Yirmiya, Kasari, Sigman, & Mundy, 1989). **Emotion contagion** is also probably spared in people with ASDs (Blair, 1999; Ben Shalom et al., 2006). Children with autism are not oblivious to the emotion of others, and one screaming child in a room full of children with autism will produce signs of **arousal** and even distress in the other children. Similarly, experienced teachers will often say that children with autism whom they teach, even those who are quite severely learning disabled, are quick to pick up nervousness or apprehension in a novice teacher and, completely unconsciously, behave in an anxious or disorganised way as a 'contagious' response.

Sensory-perceptual Processing: Strengths and Weaknesses

Sensory information may be understood as raw, or unelaborated, data from the senses, in contrast to **perception**, which involves the elaboration and interpretation of sensory data – making sense of it. **Sensation** and perception are, however, so closely linked and interactive, including **top-down** influences from perception to sensation, as well as **bottom-up** input from sensation to perception, that for present purposes the two will not be differentiated.

(In Chapter 10, however, where possible causes of sensory-perceptual anomalies in autism are considered, the distinction will sometimes be made.)

Sensory-perceptual experience in people with ASDs

First-hand accounts of what it is like to be autistic invariably emphasise problems to do with the processing of sensory-perceptual information. Some excerpts from first-hand accounts are shown in Box 3.2.

BOX 3.2   First-hand accounts of sensory-perceptual experiences in very high-functioning individuals with autism-related characteristics

Darren White (quoted in White & White, 1987: 224) 'I was rarely able to hear sentences because my hearing distorted them. I was sometimes able to hear a word or two at the start and understand it and then the next lot of words sort of merged into one another and I could not make head or tail of it.... Sometimes when other kids spoke to me I could scarcely hear them, and sometimes they sounded like bullets. I thought I was going to go deaf. I was also frightened of the vacuum cleaner, the food mixer and the liquidiser because they sounded about five times as loud as they actually were. Life was terrifying... '

John van Dalen (quoted in Boucher, 1996a: 84, 85) 'My way of perceiving things differs from that of other people. For instance, when I am confronted with a hammer, I am initially not confronted with a hammer at all but solely with a number of unrelated parts: I observe a cubical piece of iron near to a coincidental bar-like piece of wood. After that, I am struck by the coincidental nature of the iron and the wooden thing resulting in the unifying perception of a hammerlike configuration. The name "hammer" is not immediately within reach but appears when the configuration has been sufficiently stabilised over time. Finally, the use of a tool becomes clear when I realise that this perceptual configuration known as a "hammer" can be used to do carpenter's work.'

Temple Grandin (Grandin & Scariano, 1986: 32) 'Wool clothing is intolerable for me to wear. ... I dislike nightgowns because the feeling of my legs touching each other is unpleasant.'

Jim (reported in Cesaroni & Garber, 1991) 'Sometimes the channels get confused, as when sounds come through as colour. Sometimes I know that something is coming in somewhere, but I can't tell right away what sense it's coming through.'

Donna Williams (Williams, 1994: 22) 'In my dark cupboard ... the bombardment of bright light and harsh colours, of movement and blah-blah-blah, of unpredictable noise and the uncontrollable touch of others were all gone. Here there was no final straw to send me from overload into the endless void of shutdown.'

Hearing Under-responsiveness to sound can occur even in individuals with ASDs whose hearing is normal. At the same time, over-sensitivity to sound, or **hyperacusia** is not uncommon (Rosenhall, Nordin, Sandstroem, Ahlsen, & Gillberg, 1999), and particular sounds may become the focus of a phobic resistance to certain places or situations such as travelling on the underground, or going to an event where there are balloons that may burst.

Certain aspects of the perception of sound may be better than those of ordinary people of similar age. For example, people with ASDs have a better sense of musical pitch than people in the general population (Heaton, Hermelin, & Pring, 1998).

Vision **Peripheral vision** may be utilised to an unusual extent (Lord, Cook, Blumenthal, & Amarel, 2000; Mottron, Dawson, Soulières, Hubert, & Burack, 2006). Over-sensitivity to visual stimuli also occurs. For example, some people with ASDs prefer to watch television with the brightness turned down. Impaired processing of visual motion (seen movement) has been reported in several studies (Gepner & Mestre, 2002; Milne, Swettenham, & Campbell, 2005).

Visual detail may be perceived in place of whole objects or scenes, making the perception of whole objects effortful and slow, as described by John Van Dalen in Box 3.2. However, good perception of detail has some advantages: for example, it enables people with ASDs to notice small changes in familiar surroundings, and to outperform people without autism in certain **visual search tests**. Further evidence of the processing of detail as opposed to wholes will be presented and discussed in Chapter 10. A comprehensive review of research on visual processing in ASDs can be found in Dakin and Frith (2005).

Taste, smell and touch These are hypersensitive according to parental reports and first-hand accounts. One girl with autism commented that nearly everyone has bad breath (Stehli, 1992). A child I worked with had a habit of approaching strangers and putting her face close to theirs in order to sniff them.

Pain Sensitivity to pain, on the other hand, is low, making people with ASDs vulnerable to injury, and it has been suggested that **self-injurious behaviours (SIBS)** such as in hand-biting or head banging are experienced as pleasurable self-stimulation, rather than as painful.

Synaesthesia and overload Information from the various senses may be confused, as in the condition known as **synaesthesia**, where, for example, sound may be perceived in terms of colour, or colours may be perceived in terms of taste and smell. Information arriving from the different sensory channels can also be experienced as confusing to the point of being overwhelming, as vividly described in the last quote in Box 3.2.

Wendy Lawson, a very able person with an ASD, has suggested that people with ASDs have **monotropic attention**, in the sense of only being able to attend to a limited range of sensory inputs at any one time (Murray, Lesser, & Lawson, 2005). This suggestion is consistent with early studies reporting **over-selective attention** in people with ASDs (Rincover & Ducharme, 1987) and is also consistent with some of the superior perceptual abilities noted above, such as unusual sensitivity to musical pitch and to visual detail. It might also help to explain why complex or multi-sensory inputs are experienced as confusing and overwhelming, leading to the defensive reaction of **shutdown** referred to by Donna Williams (Box 3.2) and endorsed in many other first-hand accounts. However, an understanding of the precise nature of processes associated with **attention** in ASDs has proved elusive, as discussed in Chapter 9.

A comprehensive review of evidence on sensory-perceptual processing in people with ASDs can be found in Iarocci and McDonald (2006).

Motor Skills: Strengths and Weaknesses

The term motor skills covers a wide range of abilities involving not only nerves and muscles, but also an internalised self-image, **or body schema**, derived from **proprioceptive** and **kinaesthetic** awareness, and complex psychological processes of planning, temporal organisation, and control. **Fine motor skills**, such as are involved in, for example, doing up buttons or typing, involve a different set of underlying abilities from **gross motor skills** such as walking or climbing stairs. Balance is important for some kinds of motor skills; hand-eye co-ordination for others. Well-learned, unconsciously executed movement patterns such as doing up buttons or climbing stairs utilise a partly different set of abilities from those required for novel willed actions such as fashioning a clay figure or negotiating an obstacle course.

Motor abnormalities are very common and possibly universal in people with autism-related disorders (Jansiewicz et al., 2006). Common areas of difficulty include the following.

- Motor stereotypies such as finger flicking, hand flapping, toe-walking, head banging, or rocking are named in DSM-IV and ICD-10 as diagnostic features of autistic disorder.
- Clumsiness, or poorly co-ordinated gross movement, is cited in the diagnostic manuals as an associated (but not necessary) feature of Asperger syndrome, and was included in Asperger's original criteria (see Chapter 1). However, the majority of individuals with autistic disorder (lower-functioning autism) are also clumsy, with awkward gait and posture (Ghaziuddin & Butler, 1998; Rinehart, Tonge et al., 2006). Other studies point to there being impairments of motor planning and control such as would cause clumsy and ill-directed movements (Hughes, 1996; Rinehart, Bradshaw, Brereton, & Tonge, 2001a; Schmitz, Martineau, Barthelemy, & Assaiante, 2003; Rinehart, Bellgrove et al., 2006).

These studies are described and discussed in the section on explanations of uneven motor abilities in Chapter 10.

- Movement imitation in people with ASDs is impaired, but not in all respects. A **meta-analysis** of studies of imitation in people with ASDs suggested that whilst object-oriented actions (such as pointing to a picture or picking up a spoon) are relatively spared, the imitation of bodily actions not involving an object (such as touching one's nose with a finger or pulling a face) is severely impaired (Williams, Whiten, & Singh, 2004). Acting on objects in ways that involve relationship with the body (for example, holding a music box close to one ear) is also impaired (Meyer & Hobson, 2004). Imitation involves multiple abilities many of which are social or cognitive. It is not certain, therefore, that imitation impairments in people with ASDs stem from motor deficits, strictly defined.

Despite the common occurrence of motor abnormalities of one kind or another in people with ASDs, some aspects of motor functioning are relatively unaffected in most individuals, and peaks of motor skill are occasionally observed. Wing (1996) reports, for example, that some young children with ASDs, including some who are not particularly able, are strikingly well co-ordinated, and may be agile climbers with excellent balance and no apparent fear of heights. Individuals with good piano-playing ability or those who are skilful in speed-dependent video games may also be inferred to have good fine manual control and hand–eye co-ordination.

Other Spared Abilities

Uneven abilities are, in fact, very characteristic of people with ASDs, with peaks and troughs occurring within quite limited domains of behaviour, as evident in the foregoing sections. Even people with very low-functioning autism tend to have one or more things that they do better than would be expected on the basis of their overall level of functioning, even if not completely normally. In such instances it can be said that some of their abilities are *relatively* spared, or *relatively* intact. In people with AS/HFA, spared and often superior abilities greatly outnumber behavioural impairments and underlie the high achievements of many individuals in one or more fields. For individuals across the spectrum, spared abilities provide possibilities for compensatory mechanisms, and may be maximised in ways that enhance identity and self-esteem.

Pairs of closely related spared and impaired abilities are referred to in the autism literature as **fine cuts** (see Frith & Happé, 1994a, for examples). Fine cuts are theoretically important because they are informative about the root causes of autism: if skill A is impaired but closely related skill B is unimpaired, this narrows down possibilities concerning the cause of the impairment of skill A.

Some spared abilities commonly or universally occur even within the areas of social interaction, communication, and imagination, where impairments are most indicative of autism. There are also some well-known peaks of intellectual ability. Examples of a spared ability in each of these domains are described next.

Spared social interaction ability: Attachment

An important area of predominantly spared social ability is **attachment**. A definition of attachment and a description of attachment-related behaviours are given in Box 3.3.

BOX 3.3   Attachment and attachment behaviours

Attachment is the word used in psychology to refer to the emotional bond between two people, especially between young children and primary carers. In adults, attachment generally implies a mutual dependency for the satisfaction of emotional needs. However, between young children and their carers the bond is asymmetrical and based in the first instance on the satisfaction of basic needs and desires for food, warmth, and freedom from discomfort or pain. Familiarity provides predictability, and with it the sense of security that is central to attachment. Later, appropriate stimulation also helps to create and sustain attachments between young children and their close carers (Bowlby, 1973).

Attachment behaviours. Young children reveal their attachments in their behaviour: they will go to an attachment figure if in distress; they are relaxed in their company and are anxious if separated from them, especially if left with a stranger; on reunion with their attachment figure after a separation, they greet and approach them, seeking proximity or contact to soothe their anxiety or distress (Ainsworth, Blehar, Waters, & Wall, 1978). Children who show these normal attachment behaviours may be described as being securely attached. Children who do not show the usual behaviours are described as being insecurely attached, and this can show up in behaviour that is avoidant (the child moves away or hides when the parent returns); ambivalent (the child might hide but peep out; or move towards the parent then stand at a little distance); or disorganised (the child might approach, veer away, pick up toys and fiddle with them before moving back to the parent).

Several studies have shown that young children with ASDs do form attachments to their primary carers, although there are some differences in the ways in which attachment is expressed, and less able children with autism are less securely attached than more able children (Rutgers, Bakermans-Kranenburg, Ijzendoom & Berckelaer-Onnes, 2004).

Spared communicative ability: Protoimperatives

Most individuals with ASDs, again excluding those who are most profoundly intellectually impaired, will communicate wants and needs intentionally, whether by using language, or by gesture (pointing to something they want), or by manipulating another person's hand towards a desired object or to carry

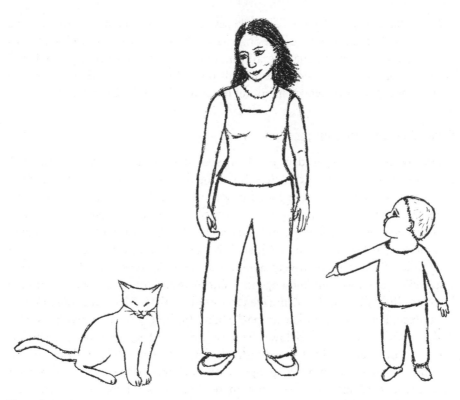

Figure 3.1 Protodeclarative pointing

out a desired action, such as opening a door. Pointing, or otherwise indicating, a desired object or action is called **protoimperative** pointing, because it constitutes a demand. Protoimperative or 'demand' communication contrasts with **protodeclarative** communication in which the intention is to *share* something of interest. Protodeclarative pointing is illustrated in Figure 3.1. Lack of protodeclarative communication is one of the earliest and most reliable signs of autism, contrasting sharply with spared or relatively spared use of protoimperatives.

Spared imagination: Prompted or instructed pretend play; savant creativity

Children with ASDs *can* produce novel ideas for pretence, such as making a box into a boat, or using a piece of wood as if it were a spoon, if strongly prompted or actually instructed to do so (Lewis & Boucher, 1988). The fact that they *do not* spontaneously do so is part of the pervasive pattern of underuse of available abilities, sometimes referred to as 'underutilisation'. Underutilisation of intact, or relatively intact, abilities is discussed further in Chapter 9, in connection with possible problems of action initiation.

Remarkable capacities for certain kinds of creativity occur in some autistic savants, as described below. Although rare, these isolated examples of outstanding creative ability may be informative about the nature and origins of autism or of some aspects of autism. This possibility is discussed in the section on the theory of **enhanced perceptual function (EPF)**, in Chapter 10.

Spared cognitive abilities

There are numerous spared, or relatively spared, cognitive abilities common to all or most individuals with ASDs. Some of these were noted in the earliest descriptions of autism and included in some early definitions (see Chapter 1). In particular, rote memory is generally spared, as is evident from children with autism's good echoing ability, and their ability to memorise advertising jingles or tunes or (if able to acquire language) lists of factual information such as bus timetables. Spared, or relatively spared, visual-spatial reasoning and constructional skills are also well known, and occur even in individuals with profound learning difficulties and autism (DeMyer et al., 1974). **Mechanical reading**, or **hyperlexia**, is another well-known peak ability (although some individuals with ASDs are dyslexic – see below). In people with LFA, hyperlexia takes the classic form of an ability to read individual words accurately with no understanding of their meaning; in people with AS/HFA, hyperlexia manifests as mechanical reading that is superior to reading comprehension (Grigorenko, Klin, Pauls, Senft, Hooper, & Volkmar, 2004; Nation, Clarke, Wright, & Williams, 2006).

Many other, less well-known, areas of spared or relatively spared ability have emerged from detailed research designed to investigate the psychological causes of autism, and some of these spared abilities will be described in Part II.

Savant abilities

A small minority of individuals on the autistic spectrum have abilities that are very significantly superior to their overall level of function, which is often low, and also significantly superior to abilities found in the general population. These special talents are referred to as savant abilities, and the people in whom they occur are referred to as savants. Most frequently, savant abilities involve feats of perception, memory or calculation. Very occasionally, however, a savant with autism, or features of autism, shows genuinely creative ability in, for example, musical improvisation, art and design or poetry composition. As noted in the previous chapter, savant creativity calls into question use of the phrase 'lack of creativity' as a diagnostic feature of autism, raising important questions concerning the kinds of creativity that can and cannot occur in association with ASDs. An account of savant abilities can be found in Hermelin (2001). Greater detail is not given here, because savants are in fact rare, and not always autistic. However, an example of an unusual peak of ability (even if not truly 'savant') is described in Box 3.4.

BOX 3.4   Grace: A young woman with a special talent for humour

Grace is a woman whose autism and mild intellectual disability are combined with a striking capacity for humour. Humour is not generally considered to be characteristic of people with ASDs, which makes Grace all the more unusual. Examples of her jokes are shown below.

Puns
(On approaching the weaving centre when showing a visitor around her residential village): 'Here's the weavery looming up'.
(When asked to write in a local church visitor's book): 'Smashing windows'.

Riddles
Question: 'What does the ant aerial get called?' Answer: '*Antenna*'.
Question: 'What happens if a boa constrictor argues with another boa constrictor?' Answer: 'A boa war'.

Nonsense talk
(Describing two train passengers who were sitting when Grace had to stand, which she resented): 'There was a man chatting to a colly-girl with miniscule lips and sloping bum, while womping through a burger. God! I thought he was going to burst his trouser-buttons!'

(From Werth, Perkins, & Boucher, 2001)

CHARACTERISTICS THAT DISTINGUISH LOWER- FROM HIGHER-FUNCTIONING PEOPLE WITH AUTISM

Language Ability

Terminology

For a clear understanding of what is and what is not impaired across the spectrum, it is essential to be clear about what is meant by communication as opposed to language; and about the distinction between language and the input–output systems used to receive and convey language. These distinctions are explained in Box 3.5.

BOX 3.5 Distinctions between communication, language, and speech

Communication is something that humans – and animals – *do*. They do it to convey, receive, and share feelings, thoughts, information, etc., or simply to oil social wheels or pass the time. It can be involuntary (for example, yawning during a boring conversation; laughter), or voluntary (escaping from a boring conversation by making a verbal excuse; telling a joke). Communication is closely related to social interaction: all communication involves social interaction, whether directly or indirectly; and all social interaction involves communication of some kind or another.

Language is something that humans *have*. Languages consist of a set of symbols (the words or signs), plus rules for combining symbols meaningfully (the grammar). Linguistic knowledge can be stored in the brain, or described in dictionaries and grammar books. Language is the uniquely human means or method of communicating. However, it is not the only means of communicating. Non-linguistic, or non-verbal, signals are more primitive but particularly informative about the speaker's real feelings and intentions. Language may be used to mislead or deceive, but non-verbal signals rarely lie.

Speech is the output channel for spoken language, just as writing is the output channel for written language, and hand postures and movements are the main output channel for signing. Speech is the product of vocalisation (sounds made by the vocal cords), which are modified by changes in the positioning of the jaw, lips, tongue, teeth, and hard and soft palates to articulate the sound patterns of a spoken language. Speech is therefore a motor activity subserving language: it is not part of the language system itself, any more than hearing, the input system that subserves spoken language, is part of the language system.

Communication across the spectrum

Communication is always, by definition, impaired in people on the autistic spectrum, including the most able. It could not be otherwise, given that impaired social interaction is at the heart of autism, and communication is involved in every form of social interaction. The rules and conventions for using non-verbal communication signals and language to communicate come under the heading of **pragmatics** (Leinonen, Letts, & Smith, 2000; Perkins, 2007). Because of its intimate relation to social and communication skills, pragmatics is invariably impaired across the spectrum (for a short review, see the section on 'Language Use' in Tager-Flusberg, Paul, & Lord, 2005). The kinds of communication skills that come under the heading of pragmatics are assessed within Bishop's (1998) 'Children's Communication Checklist', relevant sections and items of which are reproduced in Box 3.6.

In addition to the communication impairments that are unique to people with ASDs, a communication impairment called **selective, or elective, mutism** occasionally co-occurs with autism. In this condition, which is not confined to people with ASDs, the individual understands at least some spoken language, and speaks in some environments and situations, but not in others. So, for example, a child may speak at home but not at school; or with adults but not with other children. Selective mutism is generally an anxiety-related or phobic condition (Cline & Baldwin, 2004).

Speech across the spectrum

High-functioning individuals with autism generally have correctly articulated speech. In lower-functioning people with LFA, **articulation** may be impaired, but usually only to the same extent as in other individuals with a comparable degree of intellectual disability (Bartolucci, Pierce, Streiner, & Tolkin-Eppel, 1976; Boucher, 1976). However, neuromuscular impairment is a little more common in people with ASDs than in the general population (see the section on 'Co-morbid Conditions', later in the chapter), and can cause speech output problems in a minority of high-functioning as well as lower-functioning individuals.

A small minority of individuals with ASDs have a form of mutism that appears to result from a physical difficulty in initiating actions required for language output, regardless of whether speech, writing, signing or typing is used. People with this kind of **pervasive mutism** can understand at least some spoken or written language, but can only express themselves non-verbally.

Language in people with high-functioning autism

Language, including language onset, is normal in people with Asperger syndrome, according to DSM-IV diagnostic criteria. Sometimes, however, a child with an ASD who has average or above-average intelligence is slow to acquire language (Rapin & Dunn, 2003), or, more rarely, has persistent language impairment (Kjelgaard & Tager-Flusberg, 2001). Such individuals cannot be described as having Asperger syndrome, strictly speaking, but are more appropriately described as having high-functioning autism with language impairment. Persistent language problems in HFA are referred to briefly in Chapter 10, where possible causes of language impairment in ASDs are considered.

Language in people with low-functioning autism

A proportion of low-functioning individuals with ASDs never develop meaningful language, displaying little or no understanding of speech, written language or signs, and using few or no meaningful sounds, words or signs. Some of these individuals are profoundly intellectually impaired, often with multiple physical as well as intellectual disabilities. However, other individuals in this group are not profoundly intellectually disabled, as shown by their relatively good self-care and daily living skills (Carter et al., 1998; Kraijer, 2000).

People with middle to low-functioning autism generally acquire some useful language. Language profiles in this group are very varied. This is because co-morbid conditions such as hearing loss are commonly present, and cause particular patterns of language impairment. Syndromes such as **Fragile-X syndrome** or Down syndrome may also occasionally co-occur with autism, causing their own distinctive sets of language acquisition impairments and anomalies.

Underlying the diversity of language profiles in LFA, however, some common characteristics can be perceived. These emerge only from large-scale group studies in which the diversity amongst individuals is outweighed by the shared characteristics of all the individuals in the group (see, for example,

Rapin, 1996; also Rapin & Dunn, 2003; see also the extensive review of communication and language by Tager-Flusberg et al. (2005) or the short review by Boucher (2003)). Shared characteristics of language in lower-functioning autism include the following.

- The language impairment is **amodal**: in other words, it affects language in all modalities, whether spoken, signed, written or otherwise conveyed.
- The impairment is characterised first and foremost by problems of comprehension and meaning, or **semantics**. In a review of early studies of language in young children with LFA, Fay and Schuler (1980) wrote 'the vocal product, whether echoic or otherwise noncommunicative, continues unimpinged by the meaning system' (p. 49). Linguistic meaning for older or more able individuals tends to remain abnormally narrow and literal, revealing 'limited ability to integrate linguistic input with real-world knowledge' (Lord & Paul, 1997: 212).
- Expressive language (language output) may appear to be superior to comprehension as a result of the tendency to reproduce echoed or rote-learned chunks of language verbatim. For example, the phrase 'Time to go home' may be uttered when the bell rings at the end of afternoon school, or 'Do you want some juice' may be used to ask for a drink, echoing sentences frequently addressed to the individual. Truly productive language output is, however, not superior to comprehension. Thus, a child using the echoed sentences in the examples above would be unlikely to produce spontaneous utterances recombining parts of those sentences, for example: 'Time / for some juice' or 'Do you want' [meaning 'I want'] / 'to go home'.
- Expressive language is also characterised by some distinctive features including **echolalia** in younger or less able people, the use of idiosyncratic words or phrases and also **neologisms** (made-up words), and problems with **deictic** terms, the meaning of which is dependent on the speaker and the speaker's location in space and time, for example, 'you'/'me', 'here'/'there', 'now'/'then' (Bates, 1990).
- Impairments of grammar may be present (Eigsti, Bennetto, & Dadlani, 2007), but are less pervasive and severe than the impairments of comprehension and meaning.
- Knowledge of the sound system of spoken language (**phonology)** is largely unimpaired. This is evident from the fact that speech articulation is usually appropriate for **mental age**, which would not be the case in the absence of age-appropriate phonological knowledge.

Intellectual Ability

Intellectual ability may be analysed and described in two ways: first in terms of cognitive abilities such as attention, perception, memory, and reasoning (Sparrow & Davis, 2000), and second in terms of intelligence as assessed by **standardised** intelligence tests. Most research into cognitive abilities in people with ASDs has been carried out with high-functioning individuals and has little to say about intellectual abilities across the whole spectrum. For present purposes, therefore, intellectual ability across the spectrum will be described in terms of intelligence and the results of intelligence tests. Cognitive abilities in people with AS/HFA will be considered at some length in various chapters in Part II, where the causes of ASDs are discussed.

Intelligence and intelligence tests

We all know what we mean when we say that someone is 'intelligent' and another person 'not so intelligent' or 'not so bright'. However, actually pinpointing what it is that makes people more or less intelligent is very difficult, and psychologists have argued about this for over a century (see Mackintosh, 1998, for a full account of the psychology of intelligence).

However, many intelligence tests are based on a broad distinction between genetically determined general reasoning ability, or possibly speed of thinking, referred to as **general intelligence** ('**g**'), or, **fluid intelligence**; as opposed to acquired knowledge, referred to as **crystallised intelligence**. Broadly speaking, fluid intelligence is reflected in tasks that assess **non-verbal abilities** such as pattern perception and visual-spatial reasoning, whereas crystallised intelligence is reflected in tasks that assess **verbal abilities** and the kinds of knowledge acquired via language.

The most widely used tests of intelligence are the Wechsler scales (the Wechsler Adult Intelligence Scale (WAIS) and the Wechsler Intelligence Scale for Children (WISC)). These scales were first published in the US in the mid twentieth century, but have been updated on a regular basis with different editions that take account of differences in language and culture. The Wechsler scales are based on the verbal–non-verbal distinction, and a summary of subtests comprising the Verbal and Performance (non-verbal) scales from the WISC is given in Box 3.7, plus an explanation of how **intelligence quotients (IQs)** and mental ages (MAs) are calculated.

BOX 3.7   The Wechsler scales: Subtests and interpretation

Verbal Subtests
   Information assesses general knowledge.
   Vocabulary assesses the ability to define words.
   Comprehension assesses knowledge of social and cultural conventions.
   Arithmetic assesses mental arithmetic skills.
   Similarities assesses the ability to say in what way two things are alike.
   Digit Span tests the ability to repeat back a string of numbers in the correct order, and in the reverse order.

Performance Subtests
   Picture Completion involves spotting the missing detail in a picture.
   Picture Arrangement involves placing a set of small pictures in order, to tell a story.

Object Assembly is a timed jigsaw puzzle test.

Block Design involves using nine cubes, each with two red, two white, and two diagonally red and white faces, to copy a given red and white pattern; the test is timed.

Digit Symbol (adult scale) and *Coding* (children's scale) provides a symbol (e.g., square, oblique line) for each of the digits 1–9, to be written against a randomised string of digits within a given time.

Measures

Raw scores are calculated for each subtest.

Standard Scores (SS) and *Full Scale IQ (FSIQ)* can be identified from the raw scores, using a table representing how the participant's raw score rates in terms of the average for the general population in a given age range. Note: Intelligence Quotient (IQ) is calculated in some other tests by dividing an individual's MA by their Chronological Age (CA) and multiplying by 100. Thus, if an individual's MA and CA are identical, their IQ = 100 which is, by convention, the exact average for the population on which the test has been standardised.

Verbal IQ (VQ/VIQ) can be identified as for FSIQ (above) using scores from Verbal subtests only.

Performance IQ (PQ/PIQ) can be identified as for FSIQ (above) using scores from Performance subtests only.

Mental Age (MA) or Age-Equivalent (AE) is calculated by taking the individual's combined subtest scores (to ascertain overall MA) and using a table to identify the chronological age for which the score is the exact average. To ascertain Verbal MA (VMA), or Performance/Non-verbal MA (NVMA), scores on the relevant set of subtests are used.

Intelligence test profiles in people with ASDs

The Wechsler scales have been used more frequently than other intelligence tests to assess intellectual abilities in individuals with ASDs. A summary of past findings on these tests can be found in Siegel, Minshew, and Goldstein (1996). Later studies using the Wechsler scales to assess intelligence in groups that include individuals from across the spectrum can be found in Dickerson-Mayes and Calhoun (2003) and in Minshew, Turner, and Goldstein (2005). Certain broad generalisations can be drawn from these studies, as listed below. It should be borne in mind, however, that individuals with severe or profound language impairments and intellectual disability cannot be assessed using formal tests, and the generalisations listed are therefore drawn from findings that exclude the least able individuals. Moreover, there is – as always when considering people with ASDs – considerable individual variation. The following broad generalisations will not, therefore, apply to every individual – just to the majority.

- Intelligence test scores in people with ASDs tend to be uneven. However, the unevenness has a different pattern in people with AS/HFA as compared to people with LFA. Specifically, as follows.
- People with AS/HFA quite often have higher **verbal quotients (VQs)** than **performance quotients (PQs)** (Lincoln, Courchesne, Allen, Hanson, & Ene, 1998).
- People with LFA, by contrast, almost invariably have higher PQs than VQs (Siegel et al., 1996; Lord & Paul, 1997).

Typical profiles of Wechsler subtest scores for individuals with AS/HFA compared to those with LFA are shown in Figure 3.2.

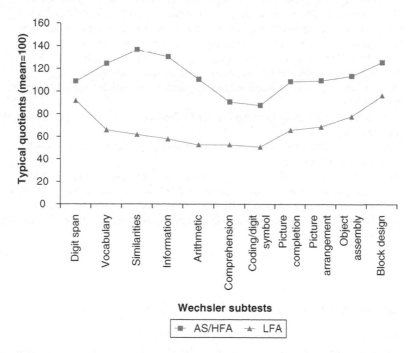

Figure 3.2   Typical profiles of Wechsler subtest scores in lower- and high-functioning individuals

The fact that scores on most non-verbal ('performance') subtests are consistently better than performance on verbal subtests in lower-functioning individuals, suggests that 'g', or fluid intelligence, is less affected than crystallised intelligence in people with LFA. This is consistent with a finding from a study by Scheuffgen, Happé, Anderson, and Frith (2000) that showed speed of processing (an ability sometimes identified with 'g') was completely unimpaired in children with middle-functioning ASDs and significantly better than in a group of children of comparable ability without autism. A study by Dawson, Soulières, Gernsbacher, and Mottron (2007) also provides evidence that fluid intelligence is relatively unimpaired in lower-functioning individuals, at least compared to crystallised intelligence. Possible implications of this observation are considered in Chapter 10, where possible causes of intellectual disability in lower-functioning individuals are considered.

CO-MORBID CONDITIONS

Co-morbidity is a medical term that refers to the co-occurrence of two or more identifiable conditions or disorders, where one is not an integral component of the other. Several co-morbid conditions appear to be related to autism in the sense that they co-occur with the triad of impairments more often than they occur in the general population, and therefore more often than can be explained in terms of chance. This need not imply that the rate of co-occurrence with autism is high. **Tuberous sclerosis**, for example, which is described below, occurs in 0.01 per cent of the general population, but in approximately 2 per cent of all people with ASDs. Thus, none of the conditions described in this section are universally associated with autism; few are as commonly associated with autism as are language impairment or intellectual impairment; and some are rare.

Some related co-morbid conditions are outlined under the following subheadings:

- physical and medical conditions;
- mental health problems;
- neurodevelopmental and behavioural problems.

Physical and Medical Conditions

Sensory impairments Hearing impairment occurs in approximately 13 per cent of people with ASDs (Rosenhall et al., 1999). Visual impairment in the sense of decreased visual acuity is also relatively common (Dakin & Frith, 2005; see also chapters in Pring, 2005).

Neuromuscular problems Both exaggerated muscle tone (**hypertonia**) (Damasio & Maurer, 1978) and abnormally low muscle tone (**hypotonia**) (Rapin, 1996) have been reported.

Apraxia, or **dyspraxia**, as it is sometimes called, is an impairment of voluntary movement in the absence of hyper- or hypotonia. It can differentially affect the limbs, hands or mouth areas. Someone with limb apraxia may without thinking scratch the back of their neck if it itches, but have great difficulty in voluntarily bringing a brush or comb into contact with the back of their head to tidy their hair. Similarly, someone with oral apraxia may blow out a match or lick an ice-cream without thinking, but if asked to copy someone rounding their lips to make the sound 'oo', or if instructed to stick their tongue out, they struggle to achieve these movements voluntarily. Rates of between

25 per cent and 75 per cent of various forms of dyspraxia have been reported in various studies, with higher rates in lower- than in higher-functioning individuals (Rapin, 1996; Dzuik et al., 2007). Limb dyspraxia may contribute to the clumsiness commented on earlier in the chapter; and oral and manual dyspraxia contribute to language output problems (speech or manual signing) in some individuals (Seal & Bonvillian, 1997; Page & Boucher, 1998).

Epilepsy This occurs in an estimated 20–35 per cent of individuals with ASDs, more commonly in those with low-functioning rather than high-functioning forms of autism; with onset often, though not exclusively, occurring in adolescence or adulthood (Tuchman & Rapin, 2002).

Immune system disorders **Autoimmune disorders** occur when the immune system attacks normal body components as if they were foreign invaders. Some autoimmune disorders are well-known and easy to identify, such as asthma, eczema, rheumatoid arthritis, and Type-1 diabetes. Other, less immediately detectable, immune disorders operate by producing antibodies that can cause biochemical and tissue abnormalities, as in the case of inflammatory bowel disease (see below). When brain chemistry and tissue are affected, there are consequences for behaviour. There are many anecodotal and some research reports of raised prevalence of autoimmune disorders in people with ASDs. However, these reports have yet to be confirmed in methodologically rigorous studies (see Krause, He, Gershwin, & Shoenfield, 2002, and Ashwood & Van de Water, 2004, for reviews).

Gastrointestinal disorders Gut and bowel disorders became a much-debated topic in the autism literature when it was suggested that inflammatory bowel disease and autism might result from administration of the measles, mumps, and rubella (MMR) vaccines (Wakefield et al., 1998). As with other suggested immune system disorders, the evidence for a raised prevalence of gastrointestinal disorders is mixed. However, parents and other carers commonly report symptoms such as abnormal stools (see Box 3.8); also constipation, diarrhoea, food faddiness, and excessive thirst (**polydipsia** in medical terminology), all of which could be related to digestive problems. A review of reported gastrointenstinal disturbances can be found in Erickson, Stigler, Corkins, Posey, Fitzgerald, and McDougle (2005).

BOX 3.8   Home truths

Working in the field of autism provides some treasured moments, often provided by parents' humorous anecdotes. One such moment occurred at a conference many years ago, when researchers began – belatedly – to share conferences with parents and practitioners for mutual benefit. After several scholarly presentations

---

by academics, a parent stood up and stated that their child's stools were abnormally large and that they floated: could the academics comment, please. There was instant endorsement of this observation by other parents in the hall, with bemused silence from the academics. It was the most memorable observation emerging from that conference.

Observations made by parents that remain at the level of anecdote, but are intriguing and possibly important for an understanding of autism as a whole, include the observations that, when a child with an ASD has a fever, they become less 'autistic' until the fever subsides; that challenging behaviours can be seasonal, e.g., mild in good weather, severe in the winter; and that people with ASDs are not well in tune with the 24-hour day-night cycle, one parent commenting that his son got in phase with everyone else about once in three weeks, then slipped out of phase again. Other reports are of individuals who have never before spoken in their lives uttering a fully formed sentence when coming out of an anaesthetic before relapsing into mutism again; or of individuals with very low ability escaping from school and walking several miles to their home without getting lost.

This latter group of observations concern rare incidents. The evidence of digestive abnormalities, on the other hand, is endorsed by many parents.

Metabolic disorders A number of **metabolic** disorders have been reported as co-occurring with autism, the best authenticated link being between autism and **phenylketonuria (PKU)** (Baieli, Pavone, Meli, Fiumara, & Coleman, 2003).

Tuberous sclerosis Tuberous sclerosis is a rare genetic disorder in which benign growths occur in various organs of the body, including the brain. It is frequently associated with seizures, intellectual disability, and autistic features (Gutierrez, Smalley, & Tanguay, 1998).

Cerebral palsy, Fragile-X syndrome, Down syndrome, Williams syndrome, Prader-Willi syndrome, Turner syndrome These and various other syndromes of genetic origin also co-occur with autism more often than can be explained by chance, although infrequently.

The above-chance levels of association between ASDs and various co-morbid medical disorders have implications for understanding the causes of autism, and several of the disorders named above will be referred to again in Chapter 7.

Mental Health Problems

Certain mental health problems are relatively common in people with ASDs, as is evident from data shown in Table 3.1.

Table 3.1 *Mental health problems in people with ASDs (Medical Research Council, 2001) compared with the general population*

	Depression	Anxiety disorders	Bi-polar disorders	Schizophrenia
Prevalence in autism (percent)	39	17	10	7
Prevalence in the general population (percent)*	17	15	0.5	0.5

*UK estimates

Depression   This is more common in people with AS/HFA than in less able individuals, suggesting that depression is partly or mainly a reaction to an appreciation that being different from others entails many difficulties and frustrations. It seems the capacity for self-awareness and self-knowledge that is of such benefit in some ways can at the same time bring great unhappiness, which less able people with ASDs are largely spared.

Anxiety disorders   These may also be at least in part a reaction to the experience of autism. In particular, the experience of sensory-perceptual 'overload' (see Box 3.2) is described as highly stressful, and fear of experiencing overload as well as the experience itself may be related to anxiety in some individuals.

Sources of anxiety more likely to affect lower-functioning individuals are the fears and phobias that get attached to certain stimuli, such as fear of loud sounds or of getting wet or even of a certain colour or a certain number. These fears are usually acquired as a result of some single past experience, and may be difficult to eradicate, in which case they can become a dominant factor in that individual's daily existence. However, although anxiety in people with ASDs is often reactive and situation-specific, some individuals appear to be anxious most of the time, for physiological reasons.

Obsessive-compulsive disorder   Table 3.1 does not include figures on **obsessive-compulsive disorder (OCD)**. However, in an overview of diagnostic issues, Volkmar, Klin, and Cohen (1997) note the frequency with which compulsive behaviours have been reported in studies of people with ASDs (e.g., Zandt, Prior, & Kyrios, 2007). Some of these compulsions are self-destructive or bizarre, such as pulling out hair (**trichotillomania**) or eating non-edible substances (**pica**); others are harmless in themselves, but disruptive to normal life, such as constant handwashing.

Neurodevelopmental and Behavioural Problems

Abnormal activity levels and attentional abnormalities   Hyperactivity, impulsivity and distractibility sometimes co-occur with ASDs, and high levels of co-morbidity are reported in some studies (Sturm, Fernell, & Gillberg, 2004; Gadone,

DeVincent, & Pomeroy, 2006). However, the precise rates of co-morbidity of autism with **attention deficit and hyperactivity disorder (ADHD)** or **attention deficit disorder (ADD)** are not well established.

Moreover, some individuals with ASDs are hypoactive (underactive), and **catatonic states** (in which activity either effectively ceases or is alternatively ceaseless and chaotic) have been occasionally reported (Hare & Malone, 2004). It may also be the case that distractibility is part of a wider set of attentional abnormalities in people with autism, rather than occurring only as a component of co-morbid attention deficit disorder or attention deficit with hyperactivity disorder. Indeed, contemporary research increasingly suggests that impairments of attention are an integral component of autism, a possibility that is discussed in Chapters 9 and 10.

Self-injurious and other maladaptive behaviours Self-injurious behaviours such as head banging, eye poking or hand-biting quite commonly occur in severely learning disabled people with and without ASDs (Collacott, Cooper, Branford, & McGrother, 1998). Self-injurious behaviours may be responses to a lack of external stimulation and/or high pain threshold or, conversely, to an excess of stimulation that the individual cannot process (see the section above relating to anxiety disorders). Some self-injurious behaviours may result from internally generated compulsions such as occur in obsessive-compulsive disorder and in other rare syndromes. However caused, these behaviours are always an issue of serious concern for those caring for the affected individual. Moreover, the behaviours can cause secondary health problems of bruising, bleeding, and infection that may cause additional distress.

Other **maladaptive** or 'unwanted' behaviours can also occur as a reaction to overstimulation, anger or frustration. For example, instead of injuring themselves, some people with ASDs may vent their anger or frustration on others (but this is rare). More common maladaptive behaviours are antisocial, such as spitting or having a temper tantrum. Behaviours such as these may be judged by us to be 'maladaptive', 'unwanted' or 'antisocial'. However, when such **challenging behaviours** occur in severely intellectually disabled people who have little or no effective control over their own lives, and who have little or no means of communicating their own desires and preferences, such behaviours are more appropriately understood as expressive and communicative. So for example hitting may express 'Go away: leave me alone'; spitting may express 'I'm frightened: get me out of here'. Such communicative acts are not, of course, intentional or under voluntary control, let alone 'naughty' or 'malicious'. (It takes some degree of insight to be naughty or malicious, and although more able children with ASDs may on occasion do things that they know will hurt or annoy, this is uncommon.) Many of the bizarre or undesirable behaviours that can occur in people with ASDs should rather be seen as responses to being autistic, vulnerable to stress, powerless, and – in very young children or less able adults – with limited ability to communicate (Jordan & Powell, 1995).

Sleep disturbance   Sleep disorders are common in people with ASDs, especially in those who are lower functioning, in common with other groups of children with intellectual disabilities (Richdale, 1999; Stores, 1999). There may be problems in getting to sleep at an appropriate time or problems of night-time waking. Abnormalities of rapid eye movement (REM) sleep in people with ASDs have been demonstrated in several studies (see for example Elia et al., 2000). Sleep disturbances are extremely wearing for parents and other close carers to cope with, and may create more problems for families than any other aspect of their child's autism.

Specific learning impairments   Specific language impairment (SLI) co-occurs with autism significantly more often than could occur by chance, although prevalence estimates vary (Bartak, Rutter, & Cox, 1975; Kjelgaard & Tager-Flusberg, 2001). The relationship between autism and SLI is controversial, as is discussed in Chapter 10. Developmental dyslexia is also more common in people with ASDs than in the general population (Nation et al., 2006).

Multiple Difficulties

The occurrence of one or more co-morbid conditions is common in people with autism, especially in the less able. Indeed, many less able individuals can appropriately be described as having multiple disorders/difficulties, and the behaviours associated with autism may not even constitute those of most concern to those caring for an individual. For example, if someone has both cerebral palsy and autism, their cerebral palsy may dictate their needs to a greater extent than their autism. Box 3.9 describes a child with multiple problems, including autism, whom I came to know a few years ago.

BOX 3.9   Craig: A child with multiple difficulties

Craig was initially diagnosed as having Williams syndrome, a rare genetic disorder usually characterised by overall intellectual disability in combination with hyper-sociability and relatively good language. Williams syndrome, like Down syndrome, is easy to detect in early infancy because it is associated with distinctive facial features and also some health problems that may need early medical attention. It can also, like Down syndrome, be diagnosed using a physical test.

   When I first met him at age eight years, Craig was very clearly a Williams syndrome child: in appearance, in some of the health problems he had, and also in the fact that he had marked intellectual disability. However, he had no language, either spoken or signed: in fact he could not even communicate using pictures – for example pointing to a picture of a biscuit to ask for a biscuit; or to a picture of

---

his coat if he wanted to go outside. Failure to acquire language is very unusual in a child with Williams syndrome, and in his junior school years Craig was found to meet DSM-IV criteria for autistic disorder (Boucher, Leekam et al., unpublished data). This did not mean that he had been wrongly diagnosed as having Williams syndrome. Rather, it showed that he suffered from Williams syndrome and autism simultaneously. In addition to his autism and Williams syndrome, Craig suffers from various problems, including a heart abnormality, dyspraxia and psoriasis, a truly unfair load.

Now aged 15, however, Craig has finally learned to communicate using pictures, and is as demonstrateively affectionate towards his parents as he always was, which was probably what masked his autism for so long.

(With thanks to Craig's parents, Karen and Michael Winterbourne, for permission to publish this description.)

INDIVIDUAL DIFFERENCES

A common stereotypic view of someone with autism is of a person who never looks you in the eye, who rocks or bangs their head on the wall, and who is generally 'out of it' to the extent that they are unmanageable and an embarrassment in public places. An alternative stereotypic view, largely derived from the kind of fictional presentations of autism exemplified in the film *Rain Man* and the novel *The Curious Incident of the Dog in the Night*, is of a slightly quaint, quirky character with some amazing (savant) abilities. Individuals fitting both these stereotypes can be found in reality. However, this alone emphasises the very great range of people who fit under the large umbrella word 'autism'. It also illustrates just how wrong any one stereotypic view of people with autism can be.

There is no reason, in fact, why people with autism should conform to any stereotype. Imagine a room full of people with hearing impairment, or who are of short stature. They would have certain things in common by virtue of the fact that they all have hearing impairment or a growth deficiency. However in all other respects they would be different from each other: in detailed physical characteristics; in temperament and personality; in abilities, education, and interests, likes and dislikes; all with different histories and formed by different experiences. Exactly the same is true of people with ASDs: they have a few things in common by virtue of the fact that they all have to a greater or lesser extent some specific impairments and some strikingly spared abilities, but in other respects they differ from each other. They differ from each other partly because of differences in the severity of their autism, in their language and intellectual abilities, and in the presence or absence of co-morbid disorders; but pre-eminently because they differ from each other in all the usual ways that make individuals unique.

SUMMARY

Individuals with ASDs generally have some specific difficulties in emotion processing, sensory-perceptual abilities, and motor skills, additional to the triad of core impairments. At the same time, most have certain spared abilities or abilities that are simply different to those of most people. Spared, or relatively spared, abilities include some facets of social interaction, communication, and creativity; some facets of emotion processing, sensory-perceptual abilities, and motor skills; and also many cognitive abilities, some of which may be superior to those of people without autism. Where a spared ability is closely related to an impaired ability this can be referred to as a 'fine cut'. Fine cuts are common in autism, typifying the uneven ability profiles that are so characteristic. Commonly spared abilities should not, however, be confused with savant abilities, which are rare.

Language impairment and intellectual impairment frequently occur in association with the triad of impairments, but are not universal as is evident from the excellent language ability and high intelligence of people with AS/HFA. Both language impairment and intellectual impairment in people with LFA have a characteristic pattern of strengths and weaknesses, although the typical profiles change with age and development, and are often masked by additional problems associated with co-morbid conditions. Most typically, however, language impairments in LFA are amodal, with comprehension and meaning (semantics) most severely and persistently affected. Pragmatics is always impaired, because it is primarily associated with *use* of language, that is to say with communication, rather than with the language system itself. IQ profiles across the spectrum are conspicuously uneven. However, the typical profile in higher-functioning individuals differs from the typical profile in lower-functioning individuals. In people with AS/HFA verbal intelligence is often equal or superior to non-verbal intelligence, with the reverse being true for people with LFA.

Various medical, mental health, and developmental conditions occur in association with ASDs more often than can be explained by chance. Some of these co-morbid conditions are relatively common and may occur in high-functioning as well as in lower-functioning individuals: for example hearing impairment, dyspraxia, and anxiety. Others are fairly common but more likely to occur in lower-functioning individuals: for example epilepsy, behaviour problems, and sleep disturbance. Some other co-morbid conditions are rare, though still occurring more often than in the general population. Most of these rarer conditions are more likely to occur in, and to contribute to, low-functioning autism, and include various genetic syndromes such as Fragile-X syndrome and Prader-Willi syndrome. Some lower-functioning individuals with ASDs have multiple difficulties, of which autism may not be the most important for dictating the individual's needs.

Additional and co-morbid conditions, as outlined above, contribute to the great diversity amongst individuals with ASDs. However, the largest contribution to diversity comes from individual differences of temperament, experience and so on, as in the general population.

FACTS AND FIGURES: EPIDEMIOLOGY AND LIFESPAN DEVELOPMENT

AIMS
••••
EPIDEMIOLOGY
Frequency of Occurrence of ASDs
Distribution of ASDs
••••
LIFESPAN DEVELOPMENT
Age of Onset
The Developmental Trajectory: Continuities and Change
Adult Outcomes
Judging Long-term Outcomes
••••
SUMMARY

EPIDEMIOLOGY

Epidemiology translates literally as 'the study of epidemics', and refers to the frequency of occurrence and the distribution of diseases or disorders in particular populations. The frequency of occurrence of ASDs will be considered first, followed by a section on the distribution of ASDs across gender, race and social class.

Frequency of Occurrence of ASDs

Frequency of occurrence can be calculated either in terms of **incidence** or in terms of **prevalence**, words with slightly different meanings when used by epidemiologists.

- Incidence refers to the number of new cases of a disease or disorder reported in a given period of time.
- Prevalence refers to the total number of cases of a disease or disorder in a specified population at a particular point in time.

An easy way to remember this distinction is to think of incidence as referring to 'incidents', or 'happenings', that is to say new cases; whereas prevalence refers to a prevailing, or ongoing, situation.

There are some problems in calculating either the incidence or the prevalence of ASDs. The problem for calculating incidence is that ASDs rarely have a clear date of onset, and the process of identification and diagnosis may occur late or be long and drawn out. For this reason, the incidence of new cases in any one year, or even over a five-year period, is difficult to calculate with certainty.

The problem for calculating prevalence is that it risks giving an underestimate of the actual numbers of people with an ASD. This is because some people who are autistic will not be diagnosed: perhaps because they are too young to have received a diagnosis; or because their autism is mild and they are coping well; or because they are severely physically and intellectually disabled and their needs are dictated mainly by these handicaps rather than by their autism.

The problem in calculating the incidence of ASDs is usually considered harder to overcome than the problem of calculating prevalence, which can be mitigated by calculating prevalence for an age group that specifically excludes very young children, and by **screening** all individuals in that age group within the general population. To answer the question 'How common are ASDs?', therefore, measures of prevalence are generally preferred, and will be used in the figures quoted below.

Rising prevalence estimates

Prior to the 1980s, Kanner's syndrome or classic autism was consistently estimated as affecting between 0.4 and 0.5 children in every 1,000. From the 1980s, when Asperger syndrome became recognised and the concept of a spectrum of autism-related disorders was increasingly accepted, estimates of the prevalence of ASDs began to rise. This is not surprising, because people who had not been included previously because they had normal language and intellectual ability, now began to be diagnosed and counted in to the prevalence estimates (see Fombonne, 1999 for a review).

More surprising is the continuing rise in the estimated prevalence of ASDs. Three studies published shortly after Fombonne's review (Baird, Charman, Baron-Cohen, Swettenham, Wheelwright, & Drew, 2000; Chakrabati & Fombonne, 2000; Betrand, Mars, Boyle, Bove, Yeargin-Allsop, & Decoufle, 2001) suggested that approximately 6 out of every 1,000 individuals have an autistic spectrum disorder. The most recent authoritative study at the time of writing produced a prevalence figure nearer to 10 per 1,000, or 1 per cent, using a broad definition of ASDs (Baird et al., 2006). Significantly, however, the prevalence rate was more than halved when narrower definitions based on more demanding diagnostic criteria were used.

The reported rise in the frequency of occurrence of ASDs is important for two highly practical reasons. First, a real increase in the proportion of the general population who have an autism-related condition would have implications for the financing and provision of additional diagnostic, educational, family support and care resources. Secondly, if there has been a real and significant rise in the prevalence of autism, there must be a reason. Moreover, because the gene pool of a stable population does not change over decades, any explanation of increased prevalence must invoke environmental factors that, once identified, might be counteracted. Thus it might be possible to halt and subsequently to reverse any real rise in numbers of people with ASDs. If, for example, it were reliably shown that a rise in prevalence resulted from the combined measles, mumps and rubella (MMR) vaccination, then abolishing use of the MMR vaccination should cause the prevalence of autism to decline.

No such evidence exists, however, as will be discussed in Chapter 7. Nevertheless, it is easy to see how the large rises in prevalence estimates over recent years have fuelled the debate concerning the possible role of the MMR vaccination programme and indeed other possible causal factors, which might be remediable, some of which will also be discussed in Chapter 7.

Possible reasons for the rise in prevalence estimates

Given the practical importance of any real rise in the frequency with which ASDs occur, it is essential to consider whether the rise in prevalence estimates reflects a genuine increase in frequency or only an apparent increase. If the latter, then one could conclude that there have always been around 1 per cent of the population with an ASD, broadly defined, but that in the past many of these people have gone undiagnosed.

Possible causes of an apparent rather than real rise in prevalence are discussed in papers by Charman (2002), Wing and Potter (2002), and Rutter (2005a). Possible causes include the following.

- Changed diagnostic practices that could allow a much broader group of individuals than previously to be described as having an ASD.
- Greater public awareness of autism through films, TV programmes, and newspaper articles, reducing the likelihood that cases of ASD go undetected.
- Improved availability of health-related services such as encourage families to bring their child to the attention of clinicians, or adults to self-refer.
- Greater willingness amongst clinicians to diagnose autism in individuals who have some other significant condition, for example intellectual disability or **Tourette's syndrome**.
- Improved methods in prevalence studies, including more careful screening and ascertainment procedures.

All authoritative commentators including those cited above agree that it is not possible to conclude that there has been a real rise in prevalence until the above explanations have been ruled out. At the same time, all commentators agree that it is important to keep an open mind, and that there is an urgent need to clarify this issue.

Distribution of ASDs

Gender distribution

Autistic spectrum disorders are more common in males than in females by a ratio of approximately 4:1, a ratio that has not changed significantly from the time of Kanner (Fombonne, 1999). However, this is a whole-spectrum average, which masks the fact that males outnumber females by about 6:1 at the high ability end of the spectrum, but by less than 4:1 at the low ability end of the spectrum.

Autism is not the only neurodevelopmental condition in which males are considerably more likely to be affected than females: language and literacy disorders, for example, are also more common in boys than in girls. Reasons for the excess of males in autism and other neurodevelopmental disorders, and for the changes in gender distribution from high-functioning to low-functioning autism, are not understood. However, some possible causes are considered in Chapter 7.

Geographical and racial differences

There is insufficient evidence to determine whether there are any geographical or racial differences in the distribution of ASDs. With regard to geographical differences, some differences in prevalence rates in various developed countries have been reported (Wing & Potter, 2002). However, these differences may stem from the methods used to assess prevalence. There have been no large-scale studies undertaken in developing countries. With regard to racial differences, such evidence as there is comes from studies of populations that include a significant proportion of immigrant families, and the evidence is ambiguous and clouded by other issues (Medical Research Council, 2001).

Social class differences

A once common belief about autism was that it occurred more frequently in families with middle or high socio-economic status than in families with lower socio-economic status. However, this has now been disproved in numerous studies (Fombonne, 1999). The myth arose because wealthier families were more likely than less well-off families to obtain a diagnosis for their child in the 1950s and 1960s when autism was not universally recognised, and diagnostic and educational services for children with autism were both rare and expensive (see Chapter 1).

It remains possible, however, that high-functioning autism or Asperger syndrome is more common in families with relatively high socio-economic status than in families with lower socio-economic status. There have been no studies of the social class distribution of ASDs according to intelligence level, so this possibility is currently speculative.

LIFESPAN DEVELOPMENT

Age of Onset

Early-onset autism

The majority of individuals with an ASD have **early-onset autism**. By this is meant that they show signs of abnormality within the first year of life even if these signs are not noticed at the time, but only remembered retrospectively (Wing, 1996). Babies who are subsequently diagnosed with an ASD may turn their head to the side when having a nappy changed, and fail to respond to the parent's voice by, for example, wriggling and gurgling in a display of welcome and pleasure. Some may feed poorly, cry a lot, and fail to establish a sleep–wake pattern. Others, however, are unusually easy, demanding little attention.

Home videos of children subsequently diagnosed with an ASD reveal that by the end of their first year more specific signs of autism can be detected. In particular, these children are less likely than **typically developing** one-year-olds to respond to their own names, to look at other people's faces or to follow another person's direction of looking or pointing (Osterling & Dawson, 1994). They are also averse to social touch (Baranek, 1999).

By 18 months there may be a noticeable absence of play and a continuing absence of interest in other people including lack of **shared attention** behaviours such as protodeclarative pointing (illustrated in Figure 3.1). Speech may also be delayed. These specific signs can be sufficient for at least a tentative diagnosis of autism to be made (see Chapter 13). In practice, however, autism is usually diagnosed later than this, and in individuals with very high-functioning autism or PDD-NOS, diagnosis can be delayed until late childhood or even adulthood (see Box 4.1 for a description of a case of late but much-needed diagnosis).

BOX 4.1 From 'Peter' to 'PJ': Reflections on late diagnosis

I met Peter (as he was then) at the suggestion of a colleague in London who thought I might be able to help Peter overcome 'a communication problem'. At the time I was working at Sheffield University where Peter was studying, so I invited him to attend the speech and language therapy clinic in my department. His speech was slightly unclear, but nothing to worry about. However, it was evident to me after a couple of meetings that Peter was on the autistic spectrum, and that the lack of a diagnosis was causing problems both to him and to his relationships with his family. He was coming to the end of a Master's degree and seeking work, but was repeatedly rejected at interviews. He belonged to a unit of the Territorial Army and was ostensibly sociable. However he admitted to having no true friends, and told me his parents were impatient with his apparent lack of interest in finding a girlfriend. I introduced the words 'autism' and 'Asperger syndrome' cautiously, but found that Peter already had his suspicions about himself. As I am not qualified to make a diagnosis I asked Peter's GP to refer him to Digby Tantam, who was also working in Sheffield at the time. Peter's (PJ's) own words tell the rest of the story.

(Cont'd)

'On 13th July 1999 I was diagnosed with Asperger syndrome. I felt like I had woken up from a walking coma after 30 years. Up to the time I got a diagnosis, I felt I was living as somebody else. I felt a sense of relief because I had felt before that there was something there, but I did not know what it was; getting a diagnosis answered a lot of questions. It also felt as if my life had eventually turned the right way up. At the same time, I felt angry because I had not known earlier and was, therefore, unable to get the relevant support. I also effectively lost out on ten years or more of a suitable career. I really do have an overwhelming sense of anger and betrayal about this... somebody, somewhere must have realised that I am on the autistic spectrum.

'One of the most important aspects of receiving the diagnosis is that it helped me find who I truly was. Because not only did it answer many questions and turn my life the right way up, but it also gives me a chance to 'rebuild myself'. Since my diagnosis, my name is PJ because this is my new identity and, as such, Peter died the day I got diagnosed.'

(From PJ Hughes' book *Reflections: Me and Planet Weirdo*, London: Chipmunkapublishing, 2007, with the author's permission.)

In cases of early-onset autism, age of onset and age of diagnosis will always differ by a matter of months, and sometimes years. Moreover, if some precursors to autism have been present from birth it is somewhat misleading to use the word 'onset' at all. 'Age of onset' is, however, an important diagnostic criterion in DSM-IV and ICD-10 (see Box 1.4). Specifically, for autistic disorder to be diagnosed, onset must have been within the first three years of life. Onset later than this is one of the criteria for describing a child as having atypical autism, or PDD-NOS.

Acquired autism

'Age of onset' suggests that at some point in time a person does not have autism, but at a later time they do have autism, and occasionally this happens: in rare cases an older child or even an adult may develop all the behaviours associated with autism after an illness, usually **herpes simplex encephalitis**, that causes damage to certain areas of the brain (Gillberg, 1986; Ghaziuddin, Tsai, Eilers, & Ghaziuddin, 1992; see also Deonna, Ziegler, Moura-Serra, & Innocenti, 1993). Such individuals may be described as having 'acquired autism'. However, the symptoms of autism may subside after a time, in which case the description **quasi-autism** (or **pseudo-autism**) might be more appropriate.

Regressive autism

In less rare but nevertheless atypical cases, a child may develop the behaviours associated with autism in the preschool years after a period of ostensibly normal development. Individuals with this pattern of onset may be described as having **regressive autism** or late-onset autism.

Regressive autism has received a good deal of publicity because the hypothesis that the MMR can precipitate or cause autism is associated with the claim that there has been a significant increase in the incidence of late-onset, or regressive, autism. However, an increase in regressive autism has not been proven. Moreover, the causes of regressive autism are not well understood (Goldberg et al., 2003). Occasionally autism develops following an illness accompanied by fever and/or seizures; some parents report that their child became autistic after receiving the MMR injection; other parents report that regression followed a stressful event such as a death in the family or the birth of a sibling. However, in the majority of cases there is no identifiable cause of the regression. It is therefore an open question as to whether the regression is spontaneous – that is to say, it occurs as a result of developmental changes within the child; or whether it is triggered by some other factor in a genetically vulnerable child; or whether it is caused by illness, trauma or some other factor in a child who, until the time at which the illness or trauma occurred, was developing entirely normally.

The Developmental Trajectory: Continuities and Change

The **developmental trajectory** of each individual with an ASD is different, for all the reasons that were outlined in later sections of Chapter 3. Generalisations about people with ASDs must therefore always be tempered by recognition that not all individuals with an ASD conform to the common pattern, and that the range of variation within those that do to some extent conform will still be great. With that caveat in mind, some generalisations follow concerning the course of autism or some common patterns of lifetime development and change.

Continuities

In some important ways people do not change. This is true for everyone, not just for people with ASDs. The continuous, or unchanging, characteristics of an individual's physical make-up, personality or intellectual potential are important because they partly determine how a person develops. Some stable characteristics that are particularly important in considering how a person with an ASD may develop are discussed below.

First, in the majority of cases an individual who has been given an authoritative diagnosis of an autism-related condition at one age will meet the criteria for an ASD if assessed again at a later age (Lord, Risi, DiLavore, Shulman, Thurm, & Pickles, 2006), although the severity of the autism may have diminished (Seltzer, Krauss, Shattuck, Orsmond, Swe, & Lord, 2003; McGovern & Sigman, 2005). Rare cases of complete recovery have been reported (Sigman &

Capps, 1997: 141; see also Seltzer et al., 2003). In the large majority of cases, however, autism cannot currently be cured, nor does it spontaneously resolve.

In the second place, intellectual and linguistic potential remain fairly constant from early childhood, to adolescence, through to adulthood, and largely determine the long-term outlook for each individual (Lord & Schopler, 1989; Szatmari, Bartolucci, Bremner, Bond, & Rich, 1989). Thus, the intellectually able ASD child with above average language at age five years is likely to do well at school and progress to higher education, a job, and independent living. By contrast, the ASD child with an 18 months level of language at age five is likely to require special education, and to live (and possibly work) in sheltered settings in adulthood.

Other capacities that have been identified as stable across the lifespan of individuals with ASDs include the potential for emotional responsiveness (Dissanayake, Sigman, & Kasari, 1996). **Fluency**, also, in the sense of creative **generativity**, does not appear to change with age (Turner, 1999).

Positive change during development

Diminution of the severity of autistic behaviours The continuities that constrain the scope for normal development and normal life for people with ASDs might be seen as the bad news for any parent whose child has just received a diagnosis. Set against this is the good news that, with a combination of maturation and appropriate care and support, the majority of individuals can be expected to show fewer or milder signs of autism in adolescence and adulthood than they did when first diagnosed (Seltzer et al., 2003; McGovern & Sigman, 2005).

Examples of the progress in social behaviours that typically occurs in all but the most intellectually disabled individuals are given in Box 4.2.

BOX 4.2   Progress in social
behaviours from infancy to adulthood

✓ Children with ASDs generally become less aloof and withdrawn over time.
✓ Eye contact improves.
✓ Babies who do not want to be held and who do not reward their carers with looks, smiles, or other welcoming behaviours do, nevertheless, become needfully and rewardingly attached to their close carers at a later age, and will show this in their behaviour.
✓ Sharing behaviours such as protodeclarative pointing and shared ('joint') attention that are absent in infancy and often through early childhood may be taught or may spontaneously develop by middle childhood, and mindreading abilities can be acquired if language ability reaches a certain level.
✓ Young children who do not interact with their peers may seek to make friendships in adolescence or to have sexual relationships as adults.

Many other examples of gains in social development could be given. Equally, almost all individuals with ASDs progress to at least some extent in their ability to communicate, whether by spoken language, signing or other means. Repetitive behaviours and behavioural inflexibility also reduce and change in kind over the years, except in the lowest-functioning individuals. For example, motor stereotypies that are often prominent in young children with an ASD, are often less prominent in older children who may develop more 'normal' repetitive behaviours such as always putting on their clothes in the same order or asking repetitive questions. This in turn may give way to having a preferred activity or interest, such as playing computer games, drawing or listening to music. In some individuals, a preferred activity or interest may become an asset if it can be shared with others and form the basis of a friendship or if it can be utilised in some meaningful occupation or work in adult life.

Diminution of difficult or challenging behaviours   Behaviour problems generally reduce with age, as the individual becomes better able to communicate their wants and needs, and gains competencies and skills that help to reduce dependency and frustration. However, with the least able, and especially those with compulsions to self-injure, reductions in difficult behaviours are dependent on appropriate behaviour management, and sometimes medication (see Chapter 14). Within the general pattern of reductions in behaviour problems, there may also be fluctuations relating to periods of stress (see below).

Negative change that can sometimes occur

Adolescence constitutes a period of risk for children growing up with an ASD (Mesibov & Handlan, 1997). For a minority there may be a period of intellectual and behavioural deterioration for reasons that are not understood. The deterioration may be transient, but in some cases it marks a regression in development or a plateau beyond which little further development occurs. For a minority, also, epilepsy occurs for the first time during adolescence. It should be noted, however, that for some individuals (generally the more able), adolescence constitutes a period of improved social and intellectual functioning (Howlin, 2000).

There are other risk periods for people growing up with an ASD, several of which are associated with environmental changes involving novelty and/or loss of structure. The transitions from one school to another, for example, or from school to college or from the parental home to a residential setting can all precipitate deterioration in behaviour, as can the loss of a parent or other attachment figure or similar traumatic life event. Such deterioration is usually temporary, however, and can be minimised by careful management.

Cyclic changes can also cause unusually large variations in behaviour. Most commonly in women this is associated with menstruation (Kyrkou, 2005). However, seasonal changes or particular kinds of weather can also affect certain individuals for unknown reasons. If such cyclic changes in behaviour are recognised, they can be anticipated and catered for in ways appropriate to the individual.

Adult Outcomes

Parents of typically developing children generally hope that they will do reasonably well at school; move from school to college, university or other training or go straight into work; maybe travel a bit, have fun, change jobs a few times; experiment with relationships for a while before settling down with a life partner to make a home, have children, progress in a career, and eventually retire and enjoy reasonable health into old age.

Judged by these criteria for successful adult outcomes, people with ASDs do not as a group do well. For example, a study by Howlin, Goode, Hutton, and Rutter (2004) rated outcomes as 'Very good' in only 12 per cent of cases, 'Good' in 10 per cent, 'Fair' in 19 per cent, and 'Poor' or 'Very poor' in 58 per cent. Details of adult outcomes in key areas are given below.

Education

People with AS/HFA may be high academic achievers at school, who easily obtain a place at college or university. Some struggle to complete their courses, for a variety of reasons usually associated with social difficulties and/or problems of self-organisation in a relatively unstructured environment. Others, however, obtain their degree, and the most academically able may in fact excel within their year group (two out of 68 adults in the Howlin et al. study had obtained PhDs). People with what might be termed 'middle-functioning autism' frequently remain in education as young adults taking courses in colleges that offer learning support. This extension of education can be valuable in developing life skills, and it can also cushion the transition from school student to adult status. The least able individuals with ASDs may remain in school until the late teen years and have no further formal education, although they are likely to receive training to improve their self-care and daily living skills within care settings (see Chapter 15).

Employment/occupation

The same small minority of exceptionally able individuals who do well educationally may find paid employment that utilises their abilities and education, often in careers to do with computers, engineering, accountancy or academic research. However, entry into employment, or holding down a job, may not be easy because of social clumsiness or other autism-related behaviours (Hurlburt & Chalmers, 2004). Success in entering and maintaining employment is also dependent on cultural factors, including the amount of support provided by various agencies (Jordan, 2001, 2005a). Schemes designed to support higher-functioning individuals into work with the co-operation of employers are, however, proving successful and, once in work, people with ASDs are often viewed as particularly conscientious and reliable employees (Mawhood & Howlin, 1999; Howlin, Alcock, & Burkin, 2005).

A minority of middle-functioning people with ASDs also find paid employment in normal environments, tending to work in jobs that are routinised and require relatively little social interaction, such as gardener, kitchen assistant, assembly line worker or supermarket trolley collector. Here again, entry into work may be supported, and in some cases support may be maintained long term (Keel, Mesibov, & Woods, 1997). Some other middle- and lower-functioning individuals work as volunteers, for example in charity shops or for their local autism support group; or they work for pocket money on schemes run by their residential homes, for example growing and selling garden produce, recycling Christmas cards.

For the least able, paid work is rarely possible because of the level of sustained support required. Nevertheless it can be achieved, as illustrated in the account of Nancy, in Box 4.3. More usually, people with moderate or severe intellectual disability and autism will (if they have adequate motor skills) be occupied for a part of each day assisting with daily living chores such as shopping, cooking and cleaning within their regular residential settings.

BOX 4.3   Nancy: A successful example of supported work arrangements for a woman with low-functioning autism

Nancy is in her thirties with low-functioning autism. She is non-verbal and has some challenging behaviours. Despite this she works full-time in an office, for which she is paid at the standard rate for the job. This has been achieved over a period of several years during which Nancy was gradually introduced to the world of work by a support specialist/job coach, who also worked to help Nancy to control her challenging behaviours. With the help of her job coach, Nancy progressed from working one or two hours a day performing a simple repetitive task (collecting up library books from tables where they had been left) to full-time work including more complex tasks such as micro-filming and delivering mail between departments. She has slowly acquired good work habits and now carries out her tasks quickly and efficiently. She is also better able to control her own behaviour.

Nancy continues to need one-to-one supervision throughout the working day, and will always do so. However, she pays her support worker out of her own earnings, and with financial help from other sources and residential support she is able to live away from home and close to where she is employed. She is valued at work, and well known and well liked in the local area. Nancy is described by her parents as having 'excellent' quality of life.

(Recounted with permission from Joe and Marilyn Henn's article in the *Journal of Vocational Rehabilitation*, 2005)

Living arrangements

The small minority of highly able individuals who find salaried employment generally live independently in their own homes. A larger minority of people with ASDs continue to live with their parent(s) or in community-based accommodation where there is some degree of supervision and support. The majority (over 50 per cent in the study reported by Howlin et al., 2004) live in residential care homes of one kind or another. However, this situation is changing in response to policy initiatives designed to deliver more individualised care, supported by direct payments to families or guardians. Finally, a small minority of adults with ASDs are in long-term secure units for behavioural reasons (see below). A fuller account of living arrangements for adults is given in Chapter 15.

Relationships

Life partnerships   Very few individuals with an ASD (c. 4 per cent) enter into life partnerships, and an even smaller number enter into life partnerships that last. Relationships between a person with AS/HFA and someone who is not autistic are likely to break down because the partner who does not have an ASD finds the relationship too difficult to sustain. However, this is not always the case, given persistence and patience on both sides. Personal accounts by Maxine Aston (2001) and by Christopher and Ghisela Slater-Walker (2002) are illuminating concerning the difficulties that may be encountered – and sometimes overcome. Relationships between two individuals both of whom have an ASD appear to have a better chance of lasting. A couple described by Sacks (1995: 263–264), for example, both of whom have AS, report how they met at college and recognised each other's autism with a sense of 'affinity and delight'. This has kept them together, living out their autism with their two autistic children in the privacy of their home, and 'acting normal' in their public lives.

Life without a long-term partner, and effective celibacy, may reflect social inadequacy rather than a lack of interest in sexual relationships, especially in males (Ousley & Mesibov, 1991). Masturbation is common, and is supported in appropriate circumstances for those for whom a sexual relationship is not a realistic possibility. For a small proportion of individuals the lack of a 'girl-friend' or 'boyfriend', and sometimes specifically the lack of a sexual partner, is a source of distress and obsessive concern that can lead to inappropriate or even criminal behaviour, though this is rare (Stokes & Kaur, 2005).

Friendships   Some people with an ASD may become interested in having friends of their own age as they mature (Bauminger & Shulman, 2003). However, fewer than a quarter of adults with an ASD are reported to have friendships that have been made by the individuals themselves, as opposed to, for example 'befriending' relationships (Orsmond, Krauss, & Seltzer, 2004). The nature and quality of the friendships made are also somewhat limited, being typically based on a shared interest or hobby rather than on personal intimacy. Sometimes friendships are made with someone who has a disability of a different nature, where there can be mutual support. One such friendship that has lasted many years is described in Box 4.4.

BOX 4.4   Friendships that endure

David is now in his forties, living in his own flat, and working as he has done for several years in a university library, where his job is to fetch old books or documents from storage in the basement, when these are requested by readers. Although a superficially outgoing person, David is self-preoccupied and finds relationships difficult. He likes to stick to routines, and has obsessive and often anxious thoughts that dominate his conversation. He has never been diagnosed as having an ASD, though he knows that he is sometimes described as autistic; and it is doubtful whether a diagnosis would now have positive or negative effects on his life (it might be just one more thing to worry about).

David has a friend whom he has known for many years. This friend has well-controlled schizophrenia and lives locally. The pair generally meet twice a week, once at the friend's home and once at a local café for a drink and a snack. Occasionally they have a meal together or visit relations for a day out. David's practical competencies enable him to organise these trips, and to ensure his friend's wellbeing (for example, reminding him to take his medication). Equally, the young man with schizophrenia is socially undemanding and good-humouredly tolerant of David's obsessive behaviours and anxieties. They understand each other, and are understanding of each other's idiosyncrasies, as friends should be.

Other relationships Lower-functioning individuals with ASDs are likely to depend for their social relationships on family or other carers. These relationships are often close and central to the individual's sense of security and enjoyment of life. However, such relationships are dependent in nature, and reliant on the skills and commitment of the close carer. Looser relationships may also be formed within residential groups or within groups associated with work or leisure activities, as outlined next.

Leisure activities

Leisure activities tend to be predictable for any one individual with an ASD, and often solitary – or at least of a kind that can be enjoyed with or without the company of others. The most able, usually those who live and work without support, enjoy such activities as listening to music, travelling, photography, reading (though novels are almost never on the list), whilst finding informal socialising difficult and stressful.

In their study of social activities in a large group of mixed ability adolescents and adults with autism, Orsmond et al. (2004) found that three quarters of the group spent time walking or taking some other form of exercise each week;

nearly half spent at least some time on a particular hobby; a third took part in some group recreational activity, often organised for them by others. A third attended church on a weekly basis. This may reflect the fact that the study was carried out in the US where church attendance is high. However churches in the UK are also often involved in informal support. For example David, described in Box 4.4, regularly attends his local church and church-organised events.

The least able individuals, who may show little initiative in filling their own time, nevertheless usually have some preferred activity (for example rocking or leafing through a mail-order catalogue) and a preferred place to be (their own bedroom or a quiet corner of a sitting room or garden away from others). These times of 'doing their own thing' offer respite from the stresses of conforming to the expectations and directions of others, and deserve recognition as legitimate forms of leisure activity.

Hazards

Criminality The risk of an individual with an ASD committing a punishable offence is very low (Howlin, 2000). Nevertheless, a study of individuals in three secure hospitals in the UK found a slightly higher than expected prevalence of individuals on the autistic spectrum (Hare, Gould, Mills, & Wing, 1999). The majority of these individuals had additional problems, including severe intellectual disability or a mental health disorder. The crimes for which they were imprisoned involved violence against people or property, with an unusually high rate of arson and an unusually low rate of sexual violence. Several of the individuals studied had obsessive interests in violence of one kind or another, including wars, weaponry or Nazism.

Addiction and anti-social behaviour There is no evidence to suggest that individuals with ASDs are more likely than others to become addicted to drugs, alcohol or gambling. However, as Howlin (2000) remarks, given the rigidity of behaviour patterns in autism, such behaviours are likely to be difficult to modify, once established. Other anti-social behaviours are also rare, although inadvertent offence may be given by inappropriate behaviours (for example spitting or masturbating in public), and challenging behaviours may be misinterpreted as intentionally offensive when in fact resulting from stress or frustration. Acts that cause injury are more likely to be self-directed than other-directed, although this is not always the case (see the section on behavioural problems, in Chapter 3).

Accidents and illness are more common in people with ASDs than in the general population, especially in the less able (Shavelle, Strauss & Pickett, 2001). Occasional cases of suicide are reported, usually in those high-functioning individuals who are most prone to depression (Isager, Mouridsen, & Rich, 1999).

Life expectancy

Life expectancy is somewhat lower in people with ASDs than in the general population, most markedly in less able individuals, but to a less marked extent in more able individuals also. Lowered life expectancy does not appear to be associated with premature ageing or other deterioration, but rather with vulnerability to accidents, often in association with seizures, and also to certain illnesses at various life stages for reasons that are not understood (Isager et al., 1999; Shavelle et al., 2001).

Judging Long-term Outcomes

The kinds of hopes and expectations of parents of typically developing children outlined at the beginning of the section on adult outcomes are, of course, those that parents of children with ASDs might have had for their children in advance of discovering that their child has an ASD. Judged by these criteria, outcomes for people with ASDs may indeed be rated as 'Poor' or 'Very poor' in 58 per cent of cases (Howlin et al., 2004).

Judged by different criteria, for example 'the best possible outcome for that individual', outcomes might still be judged to fall far short of 'Very good' or 'Good' for the large majority of cases. However, the real-life cases of PJ, Nancy and David, outlined in Boxes 4.1, 4.3 and 4.4, illustrate how a reasonably good quality of life can be enjoyed by individuals with an ASD, including those such as Nancy who are quite low-functioning. This suggests that adult outcomes may be more meaningfully judged in terms of maximising the quality of life for individuals, rather than in terms of how 'normal' or 'successful' they are. Issues relating to appropriate goals of intervention, education and care for people with ASDs are discussed further in Chapters 14 and 15.

SUMMARY

The frequency of occurrence of autistic spectrum disorders is usually estimated in terms of the prevalence of individuals with an ASD at a particular point in time. Estimates of the prevalence of ASDs have risen since the 1980s, and continue to rise. If ASDs really have become more common, it will be of vital importance to search for the environmental factors underlying this increase. However, there are several reasons why the higher prevalence figures may be more apparent than real. These include the fact that definitions of what constitutes a clinically significant ASD have broadened; that public awareness of ASDs has increased; and that diagnostic services are more available, and also more sensitive than previously to the possibility of an ASD co-existing with some other developmental problem.

Males outnumber females across the spectrum, to a greater extent at the top end of the ability range than at the lower end. No reliable geographical or racial differences in the distribution and prevalence of ASDs have been reported, but evidence on this point is lacking. The early claim that autism occurred more often in families of middle or high socio-economic status has been largely disproved. However, some disparity between the social class distribution of high-functioning and low-functioning autism (as opposed to all ASDs) is a possibility that remains to be investigated.

Autism is almost certainly present, or incipiently present, within the first year of life in the majority of cases, even if not recognised until later – sometimes even in adulthood. Such 'early-onset' cases can be distinguished from the rarer cases of 'regressive autism', when a child develops normally (or appears to develop normally) during the first year or two of life before regressing into autistic behaviours. Early-onset autism is also easily distinguished from the very rare cases of 'acquired autism', when autistic behaviours result from brain disease, usually herpes encephalitis.

In some ways, people with ASDs do not change with development. In particular, autism itself rarely completely disappears, however much improvement is achieved through appropriate care and intervention. In addition, the individual's overall ability levels, including underlying capacities for language and learning, remain more or less constant, as they do in people without ASDs, significantly influencing life-long development. However, many positive changes do occur. In the majority of individuals the severity of the abnormalities and impairments associated with autism reduces, and behaviour becomes more 'normal' over the years. Exceptions to this can occur, however, particularly during adolescence when some temporary regression is not uncommon. Behaviour can also regress at times of stress, but such regression is usually transient if the sources of stress can be minimised.

Adult outcomes have been judged in various studies to be 'very good' in a small minority of cases, and 'poor' or 'very poor' in the majority, based on measures of academic success, employment, independent living, life relationships, friendships and leisure activities. There is a very slightly raised risk of being detained in a secure institution for a criminal offence (often related to a particular obsession); a slightly raised risk of accident and illness over the lifespan; and related to this a somewhat reduced life expectancy. However, if adult outcomes are judged in terms of maximising the quality of life for individuals, rather than in terms of how 'normal' or 'successful' an individual is, a more positive picture emerges, given appropriate care and support.

WHAT IS AUTISM? PERSONAL VIEW

AIMS

••••

INTRODUCTION

••••

SUGGESTIONS FOR CHANGE
Regrouping the Core Impairments
Adding to the Set of Behavioural Impairments that
Have to be Explained
Postscript

AIMS

The main aim of this chapter is to establish and justify the non-standard concept of autism/ASDs that forms the basis for some of the chapters in Part II. An underlying aim is to encourage student readers to think critically for themselves by dissenting from the standard models presented in Chapters 1 and 2, and suggesting ways in which concepts of autism may change in the future.

INTRODUCTION

This chapter is different in kind from the previous chapters in Part I in that it offers a personal opinion, whereas previous chapters have aimed to present generally accepted information as objectively as possible. Previous chapters contain the authoritative, majority view of autism/ASDs at the present time, as I understand it. This chapter offers my own view, and does not carry the same authority.

However, one of the themes of this book is that autism is a moving target: ways of describing and understanding this most complex and baffling mixture of abilities and impairments have shifted continuously over the years, and no final answer to the question 'What is autism?' has yet emerged. It is therefore legitimate and important to think critically about the definitions and descriptions that are current. Related themes are that current answers to the question 'What is autism?' may have things to learn from past attempts to answer that question; and that future answers will quite surely find our early twenty-first century attempts sadly wanting. Current definitions are not an end point, and are not sacrosanct.

The National Autistic Society (UK) used to have as its logo pieces of a jigsaw puzzle not quite fitting together. I have a similar but more complex image in my mind, of a mosaic made up of thousands of tiny pieces, all of which have to be fitted into place to provide the whole multi-dimensional picture of autism. The mosaic is filling up: Kanner and Asperger provided an outline, and each decade sees more fragments of the mosaic added. However, large areas of the mosaic remain incomplete or wrongly assembled.

In the present chapter I argue that some of the pieces of the mosaic that we already have are oddly grouped within the standard definitions of autism, and I suggest ways in which the core behavioural features of autism might be regrouped and also added to, to provide a more coherent and complete picture of behaviours that are integral components of autistic spectrum disorders. The behavioural features that I discuss are those described in Chapters 1 and 2, and in the earlier sections of Chapter 3. These behaviours supply the main headings and subheadings used in Chapters 8, 9, and 10 in Part II that are concerned with psychological explanations of autism-related behaviours. These headings, and the reasoning behind them, need some introduction and justification, as below.

SUGGESTIONS FOR CHANGE

Regrouping the Core Impairments

Uniting the social interaction and communication impairments: from triad to dyad?

Standard definitions of autism are based on a triad of behavioural impairments (see Chapters 1 and 2):

- social interaction impairments;
- communication impairments that may include impaired language;
- behavioural inflexibility (restricted and repetitive behaviour/lack of imagination).

However, as argued in Chapter 3, social interaction and communication are inextricably related: all successful communication involves social interaction, whether directly or indirectly; and all social interaction involves communication of some kind or another. Of course there are differences in the nuances of meaning between 'social interaction' and 'communication': if there were not, there would not be two distinct terms in the language. Communication can be one-sided or unsuccessful and fail to achieve interaction. For example, talking to a deaf person may not always achieve successful interaction; sending messages about humankind into the ether has not yet, so far as one can tell, achieved the aim of making social contact with aliens. In addition, not all interactions between people or between animals are social and therefore communicative. For example, a lion killing and eating a zebra is not engaging in a social interaction with, or communicating with, the zebra. However, the overlap and mutual dependencies between social interaction and communication are more compelling than the differences. Most importantly for the present argument, a social interaction impairment will always be reflected in a communication impairment, and vice versa. It is not possible to have one without the other: they are not **dissociable**.

Most writers on autism assume this. It is not, therefore, controversial to suggest that someone who has the social interaction impairments characteristic of ASDs will also have impaired communication. However, whereas I have argued on logical grounds, it is more usual to argue that social interaction and communication impairments are inextricably linked because they share a common psychological cause, namely impaired ability to understand other minds (see Chapter 8).

It is odd, therefore (though understandable in terms of the history of autism), that social interaction impairments and communication impairments are listed separately in the definitions of autism-related disorders in DSM-IV and ICD-10 and also in Wing's concept of a triad of core impairments. Separating them is not only logically and theoretically unjustified – it also causes problems in the allocation of certain types of impairments to these two members of the triad. For example, whereas DSM-IV places impaired use of non-verbal behaviours under the heading of social interaction impairments, Wing places them under the heading of communication impairments. For practical purposes such as diagnosis this does not matter, as was noted in Chapter 2: impaired use of non-verbal behaviours is indicative of an ASD regardless of whether theoreticians allocate it to a category of impaired social interaction or to a category of impaired communication. However, for theoretical purposes, and in particular for the purpose of explaining autism (as in Part II of this book), it matters a great deal. This is because impairments that are not dissociable do not require significantly different explanations: a single explanation, such as impaired ability to understand other minds, may explain both characteristics simultaneously, as has been repeatedly suggested. My personal view is, therefore, that, at least for the purposes of explaining ASDs, the social interaction and communication impairments should be combined into a single 'social-interaction-communication impairment'.

Separating out the communication impairment from the language impairment

That said, by no means everyone who has the socio-communication impairment characteristic of ASDs has impaired language. In fact people with AS/HFA sometimes have vocabulary and grammar that is superior to that of the average person in the general population. They have problems with the *use* of language in conversation, where it is essential to appreciate and take into account the other person's knowledge, point of view or state of mind. People with AS/HFA also have difficulties in comprehending and using non-verbal communication signals. Thus, these highly able people have autism-related *communication* impairments co-existing with excellent *language* ability. Communication and language are, therefore, dissociable, unlike communication and social interaction, which are not.

It is odd therefore, though again understandable in terms of the history of autism, that communication impairment and language impairment are listed together in both the subtypes and the spectrum definitions of ASDs. Again, this does not matter for the purpose of diagnosis, but it matters a great deal when it comes to explaining autism, because impairments that are dissociable require at least partly different explanations. For the purposes of explaining autism, therefore, it is logical to separate out the communication impairment from the language impairment.

The two suggestions I have made so far lead to a definition of autism in terms of a **dyad** of core impairments plus or minus additional language impairment. The shift from a triad to a dyad of core impairments would constitute a major change to current definitions of autism, but one that I would advocate for the reasons given above.

Classifying the lack of spontaneous pretend play under impaired imagination

The point made next is much less radical and concerns the issue of whether lack of spontaneous pretend play is more appropriately placed with the group of communication impairments, as in DSM-IV, or within the group of problems of imagination and creativity, as in Wing's descriptions. This issue is important for explaining impaired play, a point made in Chapter 2. Some of my own research with various colleagues, summarised in Box 5.1, leads me to side with Wing on this issue.

BOX 5.1   Lack of pretend play: A problem of symbolic representation or a problem of creativity?

Lewis and Boucher (1988) showed that children with ASDs can pretend if given appropriate play materials and asked: 'Show me what you can do with these – what could these be?' So, for example, given a playperson figure, a box, and a blue cloth, even low-functioning children did things like placing the box on the cloth and seating the doll in the box, saying 'boat'. This showed that children with ASDs have the capacity to pretend, in the sense of making one thing stand for another.

Jarrold, Boucher, and Smith (1996) (see also Lewis & Boucher, 1995) explored spontaneous pretend play further by testing whether or not children with ASDs have difficulty in generating ideas for pretence. In this study children with ASDs were given a set of props such as a football scarf, a plastic ruler, and a large metal cake tin, and asked to show the Tester all the different things they might pretend to do with them. The children with ASDs were much slower than children without ASDs in generating pretend play acts, and by the end of the allotted time they had produced approximately half as many ideas as the other children. This showed that impaired pretence in children with ASDs is caused in part by impaired generativity.

The conclusion from these studies is that lack of spontaneous pretend play fits better within the group of behaviours reflecting impaired creativity and imagination, than with impaired language. However, the ability to pretend is cognitively very complex, and impaired pretence in autism may have several contributory causes (see Lillard, 1994, Perner, Baker, & Hutton, 1994, and Harris, 1994; see also Bigham, 2008).

Adding to the Set of Behavioural Impairments that Have to be Explained

In Chapter 3 a brief account was given of those emotion processing impairments that are almost certainly universally experienced by people with ASDs, most notably a lack of empathy. It is increasingly commonly suggested in theories of the psychological causes of autism that impaired emotion processing, and in particular impaired empathy, is inextricably involved in the social interaction and communication impairments central to ASDs (see Chapter 8). If this is correct (and I personally believe it is), then emotion processing impairments are not dissociable from the socio-communication impairment that is an essential feature of all autism-related conditions.

It might seem odd, therefore, that although lack of emotional reciprocity is mentioned in DSM-IV as one of the behaviours that may be indicative of an autism-related social interaction impairment, impaired emotion processing is not identified in standard definitions as a necessary feature of autism. The lack of emphasis on (and until recently research interest in) impaired emotion processing in people with ASDs can, however, be explained in terms of what has been happening in mainstream psychology since autism was identified more than six decades ago. When Kanner and Asperger wrote their seminal papers, and for a decade or more following, psychoanalytic models were prominent in mainstream psychology. Within this period, also, Bowlby (1953) published his influential theory of maternal deprivation as a cause of emotional and mental health disorders. Not surprisingly, definitions and interpretations of autism focused then on disturbed mother–child relationships. When psychoanalysis ceased to be the dominant model in mainstream psychology and was superseded first by **behaviourism**, and then by an **information processing model**, which developed into a **cognitivist model** driven by computer analogies, the emotional elements of interpersonal relationships and social interactions in autism were marginalised. In fact when, at a conference in the early 1990s, I mentioned the importance of emotion processing for an understanding of autism, someone came up to me afterwards and congratulated me on having the temerity to use 'the E-word'!

Now that there is a greater willingness to recognise emotion processing impairments as a core feature of autism, it seems appropriate to identify emotion-related behaviours as an essential part of a 'social interaction, emotion processing, communication impairment'. Because it is cumbersome to include 'social', 'emotional', and 'communicative' within a single descriptive term, I will use the term 'interaction impairment' to include all these three inextricably related elements. However, from time to time I will include the full description of what is included in the simpler term, as a reminder of its three interrelated components.

Including intellectual impairment as a necessary feature of low-functioning autism

Intellectual impairment does not figure in the DSM-IV /ICD-10 definitions of autism except in so far as the *absence* of overall cognitive impairment is one of the criteria for diagnosing Asperger syndrome, as opposed to autistic disorder. The *presence* of intellectual impairment should by extension, however, form part of the definition of autistic disorder. It is odd, therefore, that the definition of autistic disorder in DSM-IV includes nothing about intellectual disability. Wing, on the other hand (Wing & Gould, 1979; Wing, 1988, 1996), gives full weight to intellectual ability as a dimension of behaviour that must be taken into account when considering different profiles within the autistic spectrum.

It is possible that intellectual disability is not included in the DSM-IV definition of autistic disorder because it is assumed that intellectual disability co-occurs with autism for reasons unconnected with autism itself. If so, intellectual disability need not be seen as an important component of the description of autistic disorder or LFA. However, the assumption is unwarranted, for the following related reasons:

- **verbal intelligence** is almost invariably lower than **non-verbal intelligence** in people with LFA (see Chapter 3);
- verbal intelligence is heavily dependent on language ability, in particular on verbal comprehension and meaning (which are particularly poor in people with LFA), and on the kinds of knowledge acquired via language, which contribute to crystallised intelligence;
- language impairment and intellectual disability in LFA are therefore related, and either both occur in association with autism by chance (which is improbable given how common the association is) or neither does.

The conclusion from this argument is that intellectual impairment as well as language impairment should be included as positive markers of lower-functioning autism (aka Kanner's syndrome, classic autism, autistic disorder, or, 'autism' in the emerging sense of 'not Asperger syndrome').

Further expansion of the behavioural criteria?

Other behavioural markers of autism might be included in future definitions and diagnostic descriptions of ASDs. The most obvious candidates are the sensory-perceptual impairments and anomalies and the uneven patterns of motor skills that are very commonly and possibly universally present, as discussed in Chapter 3. Sensory-perceptual and motor anomalies were identified in some of the early definitions of autism, outlined in Chapter 1; Mottron and Burack (2006) explicitly argue for the reinstatement of sensory-perceptual anomalies within the diagnostic criteria; and motor impairments are still regarded by some as essential for a diagnosis of Asperger syndrome. For these reasons, and because these impairments and anomalies may be important for understanding the nature and origins of autism, possible causes of these additional characteristics will be considered in Part II.

In sum, the chapter and section headings used in Part II, which reflect my personal view of the set of behaviours that have to be explained by psychological theories of autism, are as follows: Chapter 8 focuses on explaining the socio-emotional-communication impairments; Chapter 9 focuses on explaining the repetitive behaviours and lack of imaginative behaviour; and Chapter 10 focuses on explanations of the language and intellectual impairments, sensory-perceptual processing anomalies, and impaired motor skills. Spared abilities will be referred to wherever they consistently occur and help to narrow down the possible explanations of a particular impairment.

Postscript

If problems of emotion processing, and possibly also sensory-perceptual abnormalities, motor impairments, and spared abilities were to be recognised as universal features of autistic behaviour at some future date, this would bring the definition of autism very close to Creak's (1961) early diagnostic criteria, shown in Box 1.3. As pointed out in Chapter 1, there is not one of Creak's 'Nine Points' that would not be accepted today as descriptive of the problems of at least some individuals with autistic disorder. This is hardly surprising, because autism itself does not change. It does suggest, however, that there may be at least one facet of autism-typical, and probably autism-specific, behaviour that has been lost sight of in the last 50 years, namely the third of the nine points: 'Apparent unawareness of personal identity'. Problems of identity and sense of self are, however, coming back on to the research agenda, as is noted in Chapter 11 (see Box 11.1) and briefly again in Chapter 12.

PART II

WHAT CAUSES AUTISM?

A FRAMEWORK FOR
EXPLAINING AUTISM

AIMS

••••

WHY EXPLAINING AUTISM IS IMPORTANT

••••

COMPLICATIONS AND SIMPLIFICATIONS

Keeping the Explanatory Levels Apart and Putting Them Together

Identifying a Realistic Agenda

Simplifying the Search for Causes

Clarifying the Causal Routes to Autism

••••

ASSESSING THE MERITS OF CAUSAL THEORIES

Some Points to Bear in Mind

Some Criteria for Assessing the Merits of a Theory

••••

SUMMARY

WHY EXPLAINING AUTISM IS IMPORTANT

It is of considerable practical importance to understand the causes of ASDs in their various forms, so as to improve methods of treatment, and in the longer term to identify methods of prevention. Although far from complete, the process of unravelling the immediate psychological causes of autism has already contributed to establishing rationales for psychosocial and educational intervention (see Chapter 14). When the abnormalities of brain structure and function in autism are better understood, it is certain that pharmacological treatments will be developed that target specific aspects of behaviour, possibly in specific subgroups of individuals with ASDs. This process is already under way (see Chapter 14). Identification of environmental factors that may be contributory root causes of autism offers an even more urgent and exciting line of enquiry. This is because at least some environmental factors are potentially modifiable, offering the prospect of reducing the incidence of ASDs. Understanding the genetic abnormalities that can cause, or make an individual vulnerable to, autism may also contribute to prevention in the future, especially via informed genetic counselling.

There are also theoretical spin-offs from investigations into the causes of ASDs. In particular, research into the causes of autism will contribute to an eventual understanding of the functions of particular genes, **neurotypical** brain development, and the links between brain and behaviour in typical development, as well as in autism. These knowledge gains should have practical applications for the health and wellbeing of many groups of children.

COMPLICATIONS AND SIMPLIFICATIONS

Explaining autism is an exceedingly difficult and complicated undertaking, for the following reasons.

- There are three broad levels (and some subsidiary levels) at which accounts of the causes of autism may be pitched: the etiological or 'first causes' level, which attempts to identify the root causes or initial origins of ASDs; the neurobiological or 'brain bases' level, which attempts to identify brain structures, systems and functions that may be involved;

and the psychological level, which attempts to identify the psychological systems and processes that underlie autism-related behaviours (see Figure 6.1).

- Autism is a complex condition affecting very many aspects of behaviour. It is also very variable in the ways in which it is manifested in different individuals and at different stages of development, as emphasised in Part I.
- The causes of autism-related behaviours are certain to be complex, cumulative and interactive: there is no one-way causal route to any single facet of autistic behaviour.
- Even if one sets out to identify only the most important cause, or causes, of any one facet of autistic behaviour, the routes leading to any one significant causal factor may be many and various.

In the next four subsections more will be said about each of these sources of difficulty in turn, plus an explanation of the strategies to be used to simplify the material to be presented in subsequent chapters in Part II.

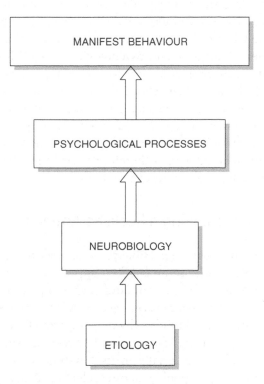

Figure 6.1 Levels of explanation

Keeping the Explanatory Levels Apart and Putting Them Together

Autism, like all neurodevelopmental disorders, can be explained at different levels, as illustrated in Figure 6.1. In the long term, the root causes of ASDs must be capable of explaining the brain abnormalities that give rise to the neuropsychological deficits that in turn cause the abnormalities of development and behaviour that define the various forms of autism. Identifying causal factors at any one level of explanation, and elucidating how these may be related to each other, is a daunting undertaking on its own. The need to relate all the causal factors at one level to those at other levels makes the task even more difficult and daunting. Figuratively speaking (and in terms of Figure 6.1), explanations have to make sense both 'horizontally', at a solely etiological, neurobiological or psychological level; they also have to make sense 'vertically', in terms of their fit with explanations at other levels.

The explanatory task can be simplified, at least for the time being, by first considering possible explanations at each level separately and only later considering how the explanations at each level may relate to each other. This is the strategy used here. Specifically, Chapter 7 provides brief reviews of what is known about, first, the etiology and then the neurobiology of autism; Chapters 8, 9, and 10 provide more detailed coverage of psychological theories of autism; and Chapter 11 reports attempts at synthesising explanations at the etiological, neurobiological, and psychological levels. Most space is given to explanation at the psychological level for two reasons. First, more is known about psychological causes than about the initial causes or brain bases of autism, although this situation is changing fast. Secondly, issues relating to root causes and brain bases involve specialised knowledge of genetics, embryology, and brain chemistry too detailed to include in this book. Only the most basic information about these subjects is therefore covered in Chapter 7, with references cited where fuller accounts can be found.

Identifying a Realistic Agenda

In the very long term it may be possible to explain all the myriad bits of the puzzle which is autism: why some children appear to be born with an ASD whereas others only show the signs of autism after a period of typical development; why more males than females have an ASD; why people with ASDs tend to have larger-than-usual heads; why they are often fussy eaters; why they so commonly develop epilepsy; the relation between autism and exceptional achievement; why autism (especially in its low-functioning forms) has not been removed from the gene pool by natural selection. And so on and so forth.

In the shorter term, however, it will be a great achievement to be able to explain those behavioural characteristics that occur in some form in all individuals with ASDs, from the least able to the most able. To recap Chapter 5, these are:

- the set of social interaction, emotion processing, communicative impairments;
- behavioural inflexibility (restricted and repetitive behaviours/lack of imaginative creativity);
- sensory-perceptual impairments and anomalies;
- uneven motor skills.

In Chapter 5 it was also argued that it is important to explain those behavioural characteristics that distinguish people with lower-functioning autism from those with high-functioning autism, namely:

- language abilities and impairments;
- intellectual abilities and impairments.

Finally, attempts to explain the above characteristics must be consistent with:

- the islets of spared ability, sometimes including strikingly superior abilities, that are characteristic of people with autism across the spectrum.

Chapters in Part II focus on this limited agenda.

Simplifying the Search for Causes

'Many-to-one'

Life would be easier for those seeking to understand the causes of ASDs if each of the defining features of behaviour had just one clear-cut explanation. Unfortunately this is not the case: for each set of defining behaviours, there are clearly numerous causal factors all contributing to that particular set of behaviours. For example, the interaction impairments may result mainly from problems of **primary intersubjectivity** (as argued in Chapter 8). However, obsessive interests, poor language comprehension (when present), and abnormalities of attention, perception, and memory may also contribute. Similarly, behavioural inflexibility (comprising restricted and repetitive behaviour, and lack of imaginative behaviour) may result mainly from problems to do with **executive functions** (see Chapter 9). However, anxiety, disorientation, habit, maladaptive learning or brain abnormality associated with compulsive, obsessive behaviour may also contribute (see Figure 6.2 (a)). Equally, language impairment, when it occurs, may result in part from impaired **mindreading** (see Chapter 10). However, many other factors may contribute, including intellectual disability, co-morbid hearing loss or co-morbid specific language impairment.

The phrase many-to-one (coined, I think, by Uta Frith) neatly captures the fact that the sets of behaviour most characteristic of autism have many contributory causes. There are no **single-factor explanations** of any of the common features of autistic behaviour.

'One-to-many'

Just as one set of autism-related behaviours can have many contributory causes, one causal factor, whether at the level of root cause, brain abnormality or

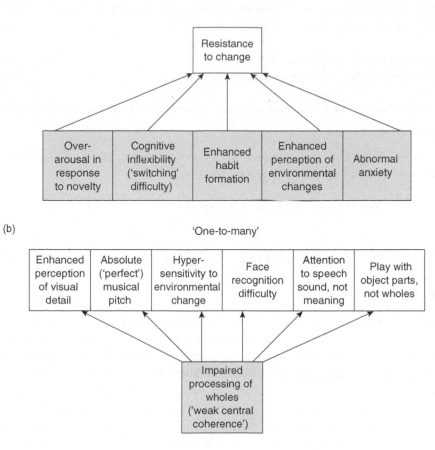

Figure 6.2 Examples of (a) 'many-to-one' and (b) 'one-to-many'

psychological deficit, can have multiple effects, as illustrated in Figure 6.2(b). At the level of root causes, one genetic abnormality (amongst the group that may contribute to autism) can have multiple effects, as in Down syndrome, for example. At the level of brain abnormality, one biochemical anomaly can also have multiple effects, as in, for example, the case of phenylketonuria. At the level of psychological deficits, a difficulty in understanding other minds will contribute to social interaction, communication, and language acquisition abnormalities, as has also already been pointed out. In sum, every significant causal factor contributing to autism-related behaviours has a cascade of divergent effects. Hence the phrase (also Frith's) one-to-many.

Causal interactions

It might be assumed that links in the chain of causes and effects always travel 'upwards' in terms of the vertical dimension of Figure 6.1: that is to say, from root causes to neurobiological effects, to psychological effects, to manifest behaviour. Unfortunately, yet again, the reality is not so simple: there are also backwards and sideways causal links.

For example, at the psychological level, impaired ability to recognise faces may contribute to a lack of attention to faces, which then feeds backwards into the original recognition impairment, making it worse than it originally was. Repetitive interests have the effect of making verbal communication egocentric and non-reciprocal, a 'sideways' effect from one diagnostic feature to another. Similarly, poor language comprehension can contribute to repetitive behaviour in the form of echolalia; another 'sideways' effect.

The causal linkages are just as complex at the level of brain growth and brain function. For example, a congenital abnormality in a subcortical structure that normally sends information to certain cortical structures during the first months of life, will interfere with the development of those cortical structures. Maldevelopment of these cortical structures may then have 'backwards' effects on the residual functions at subcortical level. Similarly, congenital abnormalities in two brain structures or systems may have 'sideways' effects on each other. For example, if two of the brain's chemical systems are malfunctioning, each may aggravate the malfunction in the other.

To take account of the backwards and sideways causal links in addition to the kinds of forwards links considered so far, one would have to draw a diagram representing a positive tangle of cause–effect links. The figurative terms 'causal pathways' or even 'a cascade of effects' that are often used when talking about causal routes to autism hardly seem adequate to describe the complexity of the actual situation. To understand and explain the causes of autism-related behaviours, it is necessary therefore to prioritise and to simplify, in ways that are described next.

The concept of critical causes

Although there are many contributory causes of each one of the defining impairments (many-to-one), it is likely that one or more causal factors are of critical importance, whereas other factors play a more minor contributory or optional role. Such critical factors may be said to be **necessary and/or sufficient** to cause a certain set of autism-related behaviours to develop. By 'necessary' is meant that a particular causal factor must be present for a particular effect to occur. For example, the measles virus is a necessary cause of measles: people do not develop measles unless exposed to the virus. It is also a sufficient cause, because nothing else is needed for measles to occur. By contrast, there is no necessary cause of an ailment such as toothache. Rather, toothache occurs for a number of reasons such as caries or an abcess, either of which are sufficient for it to occur, but neither of which are necessary causes.

In subsequent chapters in Part II, it will be assumed that there are certain necessary and/or sufficient causes of each of the defining impairments. These will be referred to as **critical causes**, and the next four chapters focus on identifying these critical causal factors, whether at the level of etiology, neurobiology or psychology. So, for example, in Chapter 8 impaired primary intersubjectivity will be identified as the likely critical cause of the particular set of interaction impairments characteristic of autism. The contributory role of such things as poor language comprehension or obsessive interests, which are neither necessary nor sufficient for these particular interaction impairments to occur, may be mentioned, but will not be explored.

This strategy involves ignoring the many additional contributory factors that may be operating in some or all individuals with an ASD diagnosis. Parents, teachers, therapists and others in day-to-day contact with specific individuals on the spectrum do not, of course, have the luxury of simplifying in this way. For them it will be necessary to unravel the whole complex of causes of a particular behavioural difficulty or stumbling block to learning in the individuals they work with or care for. Equally, discovering the route by which an individual has achieved something (so that that route may be used again) will be an important goal of practitioners' understandings of causes and effects in individuals. Nevertheless an understanding of the critical causes of autism should, in the long term, contribute to improving life for individuals and their families, as argued in the opening section of the chapter.

Clarifying the Causal Routes to Autism

Early attempts to explain autism focused on explanations implicating a single critical causal factor, or what came to be called a single **common pathway**. Some of these early theories are listed in Box 6.1. It is important to remember that all the theories described in Box 6.1 were formulated before the existence of Asperger syndrome was widely recognised. These early theorists were therefore attempting to understand and explain the origins of Kanner's syndrome (autistic disorder or LFA to use the current terms), that is to say, autism plus language impairment and intellectual disability. In addition, much less was known about autism (also about genetics and the brain) when these theories were formulated than is known today.

Theories such as Rimland's that suggested a genetic cause were particularly attractive because they proposed a single root cause and a single common pathway to all cases of autism, as illustrated in Figure 6.3(a). This type of theory was very plausible at the time, given that little was known about the genetic or brain bases of autism, whereas it was known that a wide range of physical and psychological consequences can stem from a single chromosomal abnormality, as in Down syndrome.

Theories such as Hutt et al.'s or Ornitz and Ritvo's that invoked a single common pathway to autism at the neurobiological level of explanation leave open the possibility that various different etiological factors might all lead to the same brain abnormality. This is illustrated in Figure 6.3(b). In this type of

At the etiological level
Genetically determined oversensitivity to oxygen administered at birth (Rimland, 1964).

At the neurobiological level
Abnormal function of the reticular activating system (Hutt, Hutt, Lee, & Ounsted, 1964).
Abnormal function of the vestibular system (Ornitz & Ritvo, 1968).
Basal ganglia and mesial frontal abnormalities (Damasio & Maurer, 1978).

At the psychological level
Lack of innate capacity for emotional relatedness (Kanner, 1943).
Faulty conditioning (Ferster, 1961).
Cold or neglectful parenting, especially by the mother (Bettelheim, 1967).
Severe language disorder (Churchill, 1972).
Defective understanding and use of symbols (Ricks & Wing, 1975).
Defective sequencing ability (Tanguay, 1984).

theory, the single common pathway is not, therefore, synonymous with a single underlying or more fundamental cause.

Theories concerning a single psychological cause of autism were commonly proposed in the past. For example, Churchill (1972) argued that a very severe language learning difficulty would lead to social isolation and withdrawal, and that behavioural inflexibility was a reaction to the frustration and confusion that would result from inability to communicate (a view that was widely held at the time). More recently, Baron-Cohen (1989a) argued that impaired **theory of mind** could explain all the diagnostic features (although he no longer holds this view). Single common pathway explanations at the psychological level leave open the possibility that a variety of neurobiological abnormalities, arising from a variety of etiological factors, might all converge on a single psychological explanation of all the diagnostic features of autistic behaviour. This is illustrated in Figure 6.3(c).

Less obviously, theories such as Churchill's, and also Baron-Cohen's theory of mind theory (but probably not Kanner's early theory listed in Box 6.1), leave open the possibility that a variety of factors at the *psychological* level might be needed to explain, for example, severe language impairment or impaired theory of mind. Thus, single common pathways at the psychological level of explanation are not necessarily synonymous with a single **fundamental cause** at the psychological level.

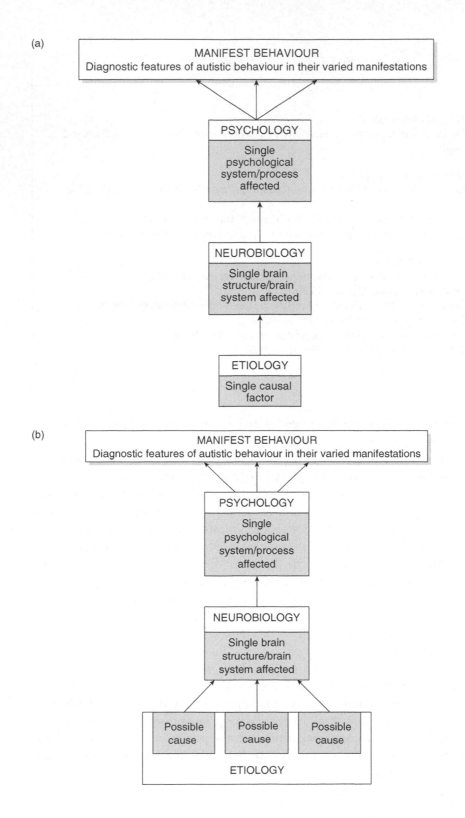

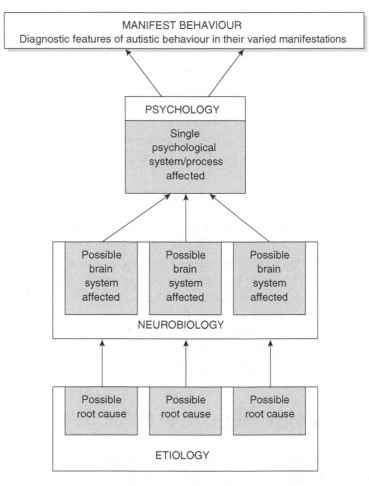

(c)

MANIFEST BEHAVIOUR
Diagnostic features of autistic behaviour in their varied manifestations

PSYCHOLOGY

Single psychological system/process affected

Possible brain system affected

Possible brain system affected

Possible brain system affected

NEUROBIOLOGY

Possible root cause

Possible root cause

Possible root cause

ETIOLOGY

Figure 6.3 Schematic representation of three types of 'single common pathway' explanations of ASDs: (a) at the etiological, or first causes, level and thereon; (b) at the brain bases level and thereon; (c) at the psychological level, only

In Part II, and especially in Chapters 8, 9, and 10 in which psychological explanations of autism-related behaviours are considered, the distinction between *common pathways* and *fundamental causes* is reiterated at various points, to avoid a common source of confusion.

Unfortunately (for those who would prefer a simple explanation), there is unlikely to be any single common pathway to autism at any level of explanation, let alone any single fundamental cause. Instead, evidence from the broader autism phenotype suggests that each of the three major behavioural strands that contribute to the spectrum of autism-related disorders can occur in isolation in individuals who do not warrant a diagnosis of an ASD. So, for example, some people whose behaviour places them within the broader phenotype have the interaction impairment (social, emotional, and communicative) typical of autism, but not the repetitive and uncreative behaviours or any impairment of language or intellectual ability (Murphy, Bolton, Fombonne, Pickles, Piven, Rutter, 2000). Others have obsessive tendencies or are inflexible and routine-bound in their behaviour, but they do not have interaction impairments, nor any impairment of language and intellectual ability (Hollander, King, Delaney, Smith, & Silverman, 2003). A third group report that they had language acquisition or literacy problems in childhood, in the absence of interaction impairment or behavioural flexibility problems (Folstein et al., 1999). In other words, the defining features of ASDs are dissociable: any one of them can occur without the others.

It follows that the three groups of impairments that currently define the spectrum of autistic disorders cannot result from a single common pathway, let alone a single fundamental cause at any level of explanation. If they shared a single common pathway, however caused, all three behaviours would occur. If it takes some additional factor to trigger a behaviour in one individual but not another, then that behaviour has a two-factor, not a single-factor, explanation.

This is not a new argument (Bishop, 1989; Goodman, 1989; Boucher, 1996b; Coltheart & Langdon, 1998). However, it is an argument that has proved remarkably resistant to universal acceptance (Boucher, 2006; see also Happé, Ronald, & Plomin, 2006), perhaps because explaining autism would be so much simpler if some single common pathway were involved.

ASSESSING THE MERITS OF CAUSAL THEORIES

At present no one knows what causes autism, whether in terms of root causes, brain bases or fundamental psychological deficits. It is essential, therefore, to keep an open mind, but at the same time to be critical in the best sense of that word, when considering possible causes of autism. In what follows, some points to bear in mind when critically appraising the merits of any particular theory are suggested. Some criteria for assessing the adequacy of particular theories are then outlined. These criteria are used in the 'Critique' sections of subsequent chapters.

Some Points to Bear in Mind

Recent does not necessarily mean right

A glance at the contents of Box 6.1 is enough to show that explanatory theories come and then usually go, and are superseded by other theories, which are superseded in their turn. Each of these theories was amongst the most recent at the time at which it was presented, but each left centre stage and retreated to the wings. There is no reason to suppose that this process has ceased.

Old does not necessarily mean wrong

The contents of Box 6.1 also demonstrate that older theories should not be entirely discounted. Most strikingly, Kanner's (1943) original explanation of autism at the brain–behaviour levels has stood the test of time, at least as an explanation of the interaction impairments in autism. Kanner's theory was superseded temporarily by theories based on psychoanalytic models or on behaviourist models; and then by a series of linguistic, cognitive–linguistic, and finally information-processing and then cognitivist theories, in line with changes in the **prevailing models** in mainstream psychology. However, in the last couple of decades Kanner's original hypothesis has been revived and is now seen as consistent with mainstream contemporary theories, as will become clear in Chapter 8.

It is also important to recognise that theories receiving even temporary recognition, such as those shown in Box 6.1, are not plucked out of thin air: they are all based at the very least on observation and experience, and usually also on evidence from research. The large majority of older theories may be unsatisfactory as final explanations of any aspect of autism (let alone as explanations of the whole of autism, as was claimed in each case). However, the evidence that gave rise to them usually remains to challenge future understandings of autism.

So, for example, one may ask on what evidence psychoanalytic theories such as Bettelheim's (Box 6.1) were based. The answer almost certainly is that mothers' relationships with their young autistic children *are* abnormal, and many mothers *do* need understanding, support and guidance to help them to establish a mutually satisfying relationship with their children; and psychotherapeutic methods *may* benefit some individuals with ASDs themselves, as will be argued in Chapter 14. However, mother–child relationships are not abnormal because these mothers are cold and uncaring, as was suggested by the early theories. Rather, it is because it is difficult, often unrewarding, and sometimes distressing to try to establish a loving, interactive relationship with a young child with an ASD, especially if the nature of the child's problem is not at first understood.

Who says?

The people who know about autism in vivid detail are people who are themselves autistic, their families, carers, and others in day-to-day contact with them, and any theory that is not informed by, and consistent with, the experience of the majority of those closely involved with autism is not likely to be correct. Research findings generally confirm what parents, teachers, and high-functioning people themselves know. Research may clarify or extend what 'insiders' know, whilst rarely conflicting with it (and when it does it is generally the research that needs to be looked at again). Equally, anecdotes or observations from insiders' accounts are often the seed corn for a particular theoretical hypothesis. For example, the first study of pretend play with which I was involved, carried out at a time when it was commonly said that children with autism cannot pretend, was motivated by a teacher telling me that a not very able girl with autism had returned from a visit to a stately home and trailed a coloured scarf behind her, saying 'bird': she had seen peacocks on her day out!

People with ASDs, and those who care for and work with them, may not, however, be in a good position to see the bigger picture: they see some of the trees in vivid detail, but are not in a position to see the whole wood made up of many and diverse trees. Researchers and theoreticians have their eyes on the wood as a whole. Reliable evidence about ASDs *in general* must therefore come from research studies, and these must be properly conducted and properly interpreted.

In Chapter 14, the topic of which is intervention, some criteria for well-conducted **efficacy studies** are presented (see Boxes 14.2 and 14.3). Equally rigorous criteria apply to other kinds of research studies, such as will be referred to throughout subsequent chapters. For example, the participants in any study must be fully and clearly described with documented evidence of their diagnostic status. In quantitative studies there must be sufficient numbers of participants to ensure that a statistically meaningful result will emerge, whether positive or negative. A comparison group, or groups, should generally be included in quantitative studies, selected according to stated criteria and equated with the ASD group under investigation for characteristics that are not under investigation but which might influence the findings from the study. These characteristics commonly include gender, age, language level or intellectual ability, and sometimes more specific characteristics such as family background (for example in a test of reading ability) or the presence of epilepsy (in a study of brain function). In qualitative or single-case studies the data presented should be systematically collected and, if there is any element of subjectivity associated with data collection, more than one person should be involved to reduce inaccuracy or bias. Where an argument for a particular theory is made it is important that the evidence cited should come from more than one research group, and not solely from the authors proposing the theory (who may be biased in their interpretation of their own findings).

Well-conducted, appropriately interpreted research studies are most likely to be found in journals that use the vetting process of **peer review**. Research reports that are published without peer review constitute what is known as the **grey literature**. It is wise to be aware of the theories and evidence being discussed in the grey literature: there is rarely smoke without fire, and much of the grey literature is written by parents or clinicians who have detailed experience of autism. However, the more reliable source of evidence and theories concerning the causes of autism is the peer-reviewed journals. Essentially all the research studies referred to in subsequent chapters are published in journals with a high standard of peer review. Although this by no means ensures that every study referred to was rigorously carried out and reported to the highest standards, it is assumed that at least reasonably high standards have been adhered to. For this reason, the methodology of studies cited is rarely commented on in subsequent chapters. Readers interested in a more critical assessment of the evidence relating to the theories reviewed should consult more detailed texts such as, for example, chapters in the *Handbook of Autism and Pervasive Developmental Disorders* (Volkmar, Paul, Klin, & Cohen, 2005).

Some Criteria for Assessing the Merits of a Theory

Criteria for judging the adequacy of theories

When judging the adequacy of explanatory theories relating to autism, it is useful to bear in mind the following criteria.

Specificity criterion   If a theory proposes that critical factor x is *necessary and sufficient* to cause a particular facet of autism, then factor x must be specific to, that is to say, unique to, individuals with ASDs (or with a named form or subtype of autism). If factor x is not specific to individuals with ASDs there is a problem of explaining why other individuals to whom factor x applies do not show autistic behaviours. For example, it was proposed for a time that impaired theory of mind, ascertained in terms of inability to pass certain specific tests (see Chapter 8), causes the social and communicative impairments diagnostic of autism. However, some individuals who are not autistic also fail to pass these tests at the expected age. Impaired theory of mind cannot, therefore, be both necessary and sufficient to cause the interaction impairments in autism. It is important to note, however, that factor x (e.g., impaired theory of mind, even if masked by 'hacking out') could be a *necessary* cause of social interaction impairments in ASDs, though not *by itself sufficient* to cause any facet of autism: additional factor y might be needed for autism to result.

Universality criterion   The **universality criterion** states that if a theory proposes that critical factor x is a *necessary* (even if not sufficient) cause of a particular facet of autism, then factor x must be shown to occur universally in all individuals with ASDs or with the form or subtype of autism to which the hypothesis applies. If factor x does not occur in all members of the relevant group/subgroup, there is a problem of explaining what causes the autism-related behaviour in individuals in whom factor x is not present. For example, if it is proposed that impaired theory of mind is a necessary (if not sufficient) cause of interaction impairments in autism, then it must be shown that impaired mindreading occurs in all people with ASDs (which is almost certainly the case, even though well compensated for by high-functioning individuals).

The primacy, or causal precedence, criterion   This criterion requires that factor x must occur at an earlier developmental stage than the brain or behavioural abnormality factor x is supposed to explain. The 'impaired theory of mind' explanation of the social and communicative impairments diagnostic of autism fails on this criterion: the ability to pass standard theory of mind tests does not mature in typically developing children until around the age of four years, whereas at least some autism-related social and communicative impairments are present within the first three years of life.

The **primacy criterion** applies most sharply to theories of the fundamental causes of a particular facet of autism-related behaviour. So, for example, if inability to pass theory of mind tests is ascribed to an underlying, fundamental problem of **metarepresentation** (see Chapter 8), then it must be shown that the ability to metarepresent is present in typically developing children before the age of one year, by which age most infants who will later be diagnosed with an ASD are already showing early signs of impaired social interaction.

The moral of this section on assessing the merits of causal theories is to be cautious about being persuaded that any particular contemporary theory has the final answer to the question 'What causes autism?' Given the complexities and difficulties outlined in this chapter it seems highly unlikely that a complete answer to this question will be found for several years. Meanwhile, all the contemporary theories to be outlined in Part II should be assessed critically but also constructively: no theory is likely to be completely wrong, nor completely right. The aim must be to reconcile well-supported, well-argued but competing theories, if this can be done in ways consistent with the evidence.

SUMMARY

It is important to understand the causes of autism in order to progress towards better treatments and possible prevention at some future time. Understanding the causes of autism will also contribute to understanding brain development and brain–behaviour relations in typically developing children.

However, explaining autism is difficult, for numerous reasons. These include the fact that a full explanation of autism will involve understanding the root causes, linking these to abnormalities of brain development and function, and linking these to psychological deficits that in turn cause the kinds of behaviour that are characteristic of people with ASDs. In other words, there are at least three levels of explanation that have to be causally linked to each other. Tempting as it may be to try to explain the whole of autism in terms of a single causal factor, this is not a logically justifiable approach. The root causes of ASDs are likely to be different, at least in detail, in different individuals. Moreover, genetic or other initial abnormalities are likely to have complex and cumulative effects on brain development that will differ between individuals. A further source of difficulty for explanations of autism is that each of the defining sets of behaviour has multiple causes ('many-to-one') and most causal factors have at least some effect on more than one set of autism-related behaviours ('one-to-many'). In addition, causal linkages do not operate only 'forwards': some effects feed 'backwards' or 'sideways', creating a tangle of causes and effects.

Some ways of simplifying the explanatory task are suggested. These include not trying to explain everything about ASDs in all their forms and individual manifestations, focusing instead on the universal or most common behavioural characteristics, then identifying causal factors at each level of explanation separately first, and attempting to relate the levels only at a later stage. The focus can be further narrowed by seeking to identify the major, or critical, cause(s) of each of the defining or universal behavioural impairments separately, following the argument that there is no single cause of autism as a whole. This involves ignoring, at least for the time being, the complexities introduced by the phenomena of 'many-to-one', 'one-to-many', and the tangle of causal links.

It is important to maintain a critical attitude when considering the relative merits of particular theories of the causes of autism. The most recent theory is unlikely at this stage of knowledge to be completely correct; equally, older theories should not be automatically discounted. The research evidence cited in support of a particular theory should be carefully considered before being accepted, and the explanatory adequacy of each theory judged on the criteria of specificity, primacy, and universality.

7

FIRST CAUSES AND BRAIN BASES

AIMS

••••

FIRST CAUSES
Introduction
Evidence that both Genetic and Environmental Factors Contribute
to Autism
Genetic Risk Factors for Autism
Environmental Risk Factors for Autism

••••

BRAIN BASES
Brain Structure and Function in Typical Development
Methods Used to Study Brain Structure, Chemistry, and Function
Findings Concerning the Brain Bases of Autism
Implications of Findings Concerning the Brain Bases of Autism
Comment

••••

SUMMARY

AIMS

The main aim of this chapter is to provide a minimal account of what is currently known about the first causes and brain bases of autism. However, to understand the material presented it is necessary to have some understanding of basic concepts and terms, and also of commonly used methods of research. A secondary aim of the chapter is to provide this basic information for readers with no prior specialist knowledge.

FIRST CAUSES

Introduction

Idiopathic and 'non-idiopathic' autism

The causes of most cases of autism are unknown. The medical term for conditions that apparently arise from within an individual for unclear reasons is **idiopathic**. This chapter will be mainly concerned with what is known about the causes of idiopathic autism, first at the level of root causes (etiology), then at the level of brain bases (neurobiology). In a minority of cases autism is 'non-idiopathic' in the sense that it occurs co-morbidly with a known medical condition that provides clues as to causes. Cases of non-idiopathic autism, and the clues they provide about causes of idiopathic autism, will be considered at points throughout the chapter.

Various causal factors; various combinations

There is no single cause of autism, as pointed out in the previous chapter. Rather, it is likely that there are several factors that are not by themselves sufficient to cause autism, but which, if occurring together in certain combinations, become sufficient.

Causal factors at the first causes level fall into two groups, genetic and environmental. Genetic factors are those associated with the chromosomes inherited from biological parents, the genes that make up the chromosomes, and the chemical constituents of genes and gene products. This genetic inheritance is referred to as a **genotype**. Individual genotypes are unique except in the case of identical (or **monozygotic (MZ)**) twins, who develop from the same fertilised egg. Twins who develop from different fertilised eggs do not share identical genotypes and are referred to as **dizygotic (DZ)** twins. The genotypes of dizygotic twins are no more and no less alike than those of non-twin siblings.

The human **genome**, unlike the genomes for very simple organisms, does not provide a blueprint for development. Instead, it sets constraints on development ensuring, for example, that the genome produces a human baby rather than a baby of another species, and that lifetime changes involving growth, maturation, and ageing occur in species-predictable ways. Within these constraints the genes and their products generally have regulatory and mutually interactive roles rather than prescriptive roles. This allows for environmental factors to interact with gene products and influence development.

Environmental factors include those operating prenatally with affect on the developing **embryo** and **fetus**, as well as those operating post-natally. Environmental factors include those impinging on the individual from the outside, and also those constituted by internal bodily states. So, for example, each gene operates in an environment created by the activities of other genes; each **neurochemical** involved in building a brain operates in the environment created by other neurochemicals; each **brain system** in the developing child is affected by the state and activities of other brain systems. It is important, therefore, not to equate environmental factors only with things such as diet, parenting, illnesses or vaccinations post-natally: environmental factors are much broader than this. However because more is known about external than internal environmental factors and their effects, more is said about external than internal factors in what follows.

Environmental factors operating from the moment of conception interact with the given genotype to produce a **phenotype**. 'Phenotype' can refer to the genotype × environmental factors outcome for any one individual. However, the term can also be used to refer to outcomes characteristic of a particular group. Thus reference is made to an **autism phenotype**, which describes people with typical autism, or to the 'broader autism phenotype', which refers to people with mild autism-related behavioural traits (see Chapters 2 and 6).

Evidence that both Genetic and Environmental Factors Contribute to Autism

Evidence for the role of genetic factors

Evidence that genetic factors contribute to idiopathic autism comes from studies of twins (Folstein & Rutter, 1977; Bailey et al., 1995). These studies show that in monozygotic twins one of whom has an ASD, an ASD also occurs in the second twin in approximately 60 per cent of cases. Moreover, in a further 30 per cent of cases the second twin has some autism-related behaviours. In dizygotic twins, however, approximately 90 per cent of second twins show no signs of autism, with autism or isolated autistic traits occurring in the remaining 10 per cent, as illustrated in Figure 7.1.

The high rate of **concordance** in monozygotic twins, contrasted with the high rate of **discordance** in dizygotic twins, provides irrefutable evidence that genetic factors strongly predispose individuals towards developing an ASD.

This conclusion is reinforced by evidence from studies of relatives of people with autism. These family studies show that the chance of an individual with

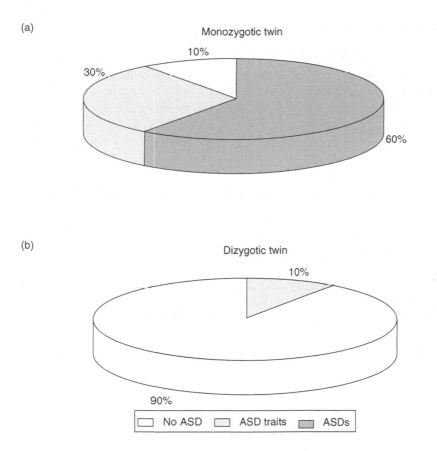

Figure 7.1 For monozygotic and dizygotic twin pairs in which one twin has an ASD: the chances that the second twin will have an ASD, ASD-related behaviour traits or no such traits

an ASD having a brother or sister with full-blown autism is between 2 per cent and 6 per cent (Rutter, Silberg, & Simonoff, 1999), far higher than the incidence of ASDs in the general population (1 per cent according to the highest estimate). Parents and other close relatives are also unusually likely to have some slight behaviour anomaly, either past or present, that places them within the broader autism phenotype (Piven, Palmer, Jacobi, Childress, & Arndt, 1997; Pickles et al., 2000; Dawson et al., 2007).

The fact that ASDs tend to run in families not only provides evidence of the role of genetic factors in the etiology of autism but also demonstrates that the genetic factors underlying ASDs are **familial**. This contrasts with, for example, Down syndrome or **Williams syndrome**, disorders where there is rarely another person similarly affected within the same family because the disorders are caused by some **sporadic,** or chance, abnormality or variation of genetic material within the egg or sperm.

Evidence for the role of environmental factors

The findings from twin studies summarised above rule out environmental factors as the main cause of idiopathic autism: if environmental factors were the main cause of idiopathic autism, then concordance rates in monozygotic twins would be no more than those in dizygotic twins, which is not the case.

At the same time, the findings from twin studies *rule in* environmental factors as *contributory* to idiopathic autism, because the following facts have to be explained.

- In 10 per cent of monozygotic twin pairs one has autism and one does not have autism in any form.
- In the 60 per cent of cases in which both twins have an ASD, learning ability and the severity and pattern of autism-related behaviours varies considerably, and to no lesser extent than in dizygotic twins both of whom have autism (Le Couteur et al., 1996).
- In 30 per cent of monozygotic twin pairs one has autism in its full form but the other has only some features of autism-related behaviour, and this is reflected in differences in brain structure and function (Kates et al., 2004; Belmonte & Carper, 2006).

Shared genes cannot explain these differences, which must be explained by environmental factors, broadly interpreted.

Genetic Risk Factors for Autism

Research studies designed to identify the genes that contribute to autism utilise a range of methods, as summarised in Box 7.1.

The results of studies using the methods shown in Box 7.1 suggest that idiopathic autism is unlikely to be caused by a single gene, although this possibility has not been completely ruled out (Bauman & Kemper, 2005a). More probably, autism is a **polygenic** disorder with different sets of genes contributing to different forms of ASDs as well as to the different forms of the broader autism phenotype. Rutter (2005b) suggests that the results of twin and family studies indicate that there are somewhere between 3 and 12 **susceptibility genes** that interact to produce autism.

There is, however, a lack of consensus concerning the identity of the susceptibility genes involved. **Candidate genes** have been identified at numerous different sites on at least 12 different chromosomes in different research studies (Rutter, 2005b). However, the results of any one study are rarely replicated in other studies. This is partly because of methodological variations across studies (Wassink et al., 2004). It is also partly because any one gene may only weakly effect susceptibility to autism and may not be involved in all individuals.

BOX 7.1 Methods used in research into the genetic bases of autism

Genetic Screening
Genetic screening involves the analysis of DNA samples. The genetic material is analysed using various strategies, as below.

Genome-wide screening may be carried out in a search for genetic anomalies in a particular population.

Candidate genes may be specifically investigated. For example it is known that certain neurochemical system abnormalities are frequently found in people with ASDs, and the genes involved in the normal development of these systems constitute candidate genes.

Linkage studies involve analysing genetic samples from two or more affected relatives in the same family to see if there are genetic anomalies held in common. Genome-wide screening or candidate gene assessment may be used in linkage studies.

Association studies involve analysing genetic samples from individuals with a clear diagnosis of an ASD and comparing the results with samples from individuals who are not autistic. Genome-wide screening or candidate gene assessment may be used in association studies.

Quantitative trait loci (QTL) studies are similar to association studies but more precise in that, instead of looking for gene abnormalities that are associated with autism as a whole, they look for gene abnormalities that may be associated with specific behaviours that occur in autism, such as 'desire for sameness' or 'age of speech onset'.

Animal Models
Animal models are used to study the behavioural consequences of eliminating or 'knocking out' a particular gene post-conception. Rodents are the animals most commonly used. For example, the gene responsible for establishing a neurochemical mediator of social reward is known, and it has been claimed that 'knock-out mice' lacking this gene also lack the kinds of social behaviour that might be dependent on social reward.

Nevertheless there is some convergence in the evidence, the most frequently identified candidate genes being on chromosomes 2, 7 and 15 (Santangelo & Tsatsanis, 2005). Some direct evidence of abnormalities on chromosomes 2 and 7 (e.g., Bartlett et al., 2004) is strengthened by indirect evidence concerning the genetic basis of specific language impairment (SLI). Certain genes on chromosomes 2 and 7 are known to relate to speech and language development, and may be implicated in the etiology of SLI (O'Brien, Shang, Nishimura, Tomblin, & Murray, 2003). Autism and SLI sometimes co-occur, and this could suggest that they share some genetic susceptibility factors (but see Williams, Botting, & Boucher (in press) for a critique of the evidence).

The direct evidence of abnormality on chromosome 15 is similarly strengthened by indirect evidence concerning the genetic basis of a behaviourally overlapping and sometimes co-morbid intellectual disability condition, **Prader-Willi syndrome.** This syndrome is caused in part by a genetic variation on chromosome 15 that has been identified as linked to 'insistence on sameness' resembling that which occurs in autism (Shao et al., 2003); also to anomalously superior visual–spatial constructional skills, again similar to those characteristic of autism (Dykens, 2002). This behavioural overlap and occasional co-morbidity could suggest that autism and Prader-Willi syndrome share some genetic susceptibility factors (Dykens, Sutcliffe, & Levitt, 2005; DeLong, 2007; but see Ma et al., 2005 for some negative evidence). Candidate genes on chromosome 15 contribute to the formation and function of the **gamma-amino-butyric acid (GABA)**ergic neurochemical system during gestation and post-natally (Blatt, 2005). GABA is a brain substance with inhibitory functions post-natally (see below). It is plausible to suggest, therefore, that at least some elements of repetitive behaviours in autism can be caused by abnormalities on chromosome 15 (a first cause) that result in malfunction of the GABAergic system (a cause at the level of brain bases). This has not, however, been proved.

Other candidate genes that have been investigated include the **oxytocin** gene, and genes on the **sex-linked** X-chromosome. The oxytocin gene is responsible for the formation and function of oxytocin and **vasopressin neuropeptide systems** that are involved in the mediation of social affiliation and social reward (Wassink, Brzustowicz, Bartlett, & Szatmari, 2004). A study by Lim, Bielsky, and Young (2005) using an animal model (see Box 7.1) produced evidence that mice lacking this gene have impaired species-typical social behaviours.

It has been suggested that evidence from **Turner's syndrome** (Skuse et al., 1997; Skuse, 2005) and from Fragile-X syndrome (Vincent et al., 2005), both of which occur co-morbidly with autism more often than would be predicted by chance, supports the hypothesis that sites on the sex-linked X-chromosome contribute to susceptibility to autism. This suggestion is attractive because it could in theory explain the preponderance of males with autism. This is because females with one healthy and one absent or abnormal X-chromosome develop relatively normally, because the healthy chromosome provides protection from the effects of the absent or abnormal chromosome. In males, however, an abnormality affecting their single X-chromosome will always have adverse effects because they lack the protection provided by a second (healthy) X-chromosome. Involvement of the X-chromosome in the etiology of autism is, however, controversial, and it seems more likely that co-morbidity between autism and both Turner's syndrome and Fragile-X syndrome is better explained by shared brain abnormalities than by shared genetic etiologies, as suggested later in the chapter.

In sum, genetic susceptibility factors remain to be identified. However, there are several promising lines of research and it is certain that at least some of the genetic susceptibility factors will be identified within the next decade or so. Reviews of this complex area of research, with more detailed information about methodologies and individual studies, can be found in Muhle, Trentacoste, and Rapin (2004), Bespalova, Reichert, and Buxbaum (2005), and DiCicco-Bloom et al. (2006).

Environmental Risk Factors for Autism

There is such strong evidence that genetic factors are implicated as contributory causes of autism that it is easy to forget that, for a time, autism was thought to be caused solely by factors within the home environment. That claim now strikes most people as badly misguided. However, it would be equally misguided to go to the other extreme and assume that autism is caused solely and in all cases by genetic factors. There are as many 'candidate environmental factors' as there are candidate genes for autism. Nor should it be assumed that a single environmental factor contributes to autism, nor that the same environmental factors are involved in all cases of autism. As with susceptibility genes, different combinations of environmental factors may contribute to ASDs across the spectrum. Rarely, a single environmental factor may be capable of causing autism in an individual with no genetic susceptibility. However, environmental factors more probably act as 'triggers' in genetically susceptible individuals, as will be suggested below.

Prenatal risk factors

There is evidence that prenatal environmental factors are particularly important for understanding the root causes of autism. Specifically:

- various **teratogens** (toxic substances to which an embryo or fetus is exposed) are known to cause autism if present early in pregnancy. These include maternal rubella (a risk factor for mild or atypical autism – Chess, 1977); **thalidomide** (a drug prescribed for morning sickness until its effects became known – Miller et al., 2005); and **valproic acid** (an anticonvulsant medication) (Arndt, Stodgell, & Rodier, 2005);
- people with ASDs are unusually likely to have the kinds of minor physical malformations (for example, unusually shaped ears) seen in children known to have been exposed to teratogens early in pregnancy (Wier, Yoshida, Odouli, Grether, & Croen, 2006);
- subtle signs of autism frequently occur too early after birth to be easily explained in terms of post-natal factors: many parents report that, looking back, they realise that their child was different from the start;
- brain regions most reliably affected in people with ASDs are those known to develop early post-conception.

So what might these prenatal risk factors be, apart from those already known to be capable of causing non-idiopathic autism (maternal rubella, etc.)? Risk factors that have been discussed include the following, although none has been definitely proven.

1　**Cytomegaloviral (CMV) infections** in the mother during pregnancy. Cytomegalovirus is a type of herpes virus that is present in most people, usually in latent form. However, when a woman has a clinically significant CMV infection during pregnancy, this infection is passed to the unborn child and can lead to birth defects or developmental anomalies including, occasionally, autism (Sweeten, Posey, & McDougle, 2004). The degree of risk for autism posed by such infections is, however, uncertain (Libby, Sweeten, McMahon, & Fujinami, 2005).

2　Stress during pregnancy is known to produce chemicals circulating in the mother's bloodstream that put the developing fetus at risk for a range of neurodevelopmental and mental health disorders in childhood and thereafter (Huizink, Mulder, & Buitelaar, 2004). There is some evidence suggesting that exposure to stress during the first three months of pregnancy may be a risk factor for autism (Beversdorf et al., 2005).

3　Heavy smoking or alcohol abuse (Fombonne, 2002; Miles, Takahashi, Haber, & Hadden, 2003) in early pregnancy may constitute risk factors for autism in the child, as well as predisposing towards other known disorders (Hultman, Sparen, & Cnattingius, 2002).

4　Abnormally high levels of the male hormone testosterone during fetal development is central to Baron-Cohen's **extreme male brain (EMB)** theory of autism (Baron-Cohen, Knickmeyer, & Belmonte, 2005), which will be more fully described in later chapters. Baron-Cohen et al. cite some indirect evidence of raised levels of testosterone in people with ASDs, and are in the process of testing their hypothesis that raised levels will be found in the **amniotic fluid** of women who give birth to children later diagnosed with autism. Raised levels of testosterone in utero could, however, be secondary to genetic abnormalities or some other primary cause. If this were the case, high levels of male hormones might just be a link in the causal chain, rather than a fundamental etiological factor.

All the above environmental factors impinge on the developing embryo or fetus from the external environment provided by the mother's body. The internal environment within which specific bodily organs or brain structures are developing is certain to influence development at least as much as the external environment, as noted above. So, for example, it may be the case that monozygotic twin pairs differ from each other because some small difference in **embryogenesis** alters the internal environment within which subsequent development takes place, with cascading effects. If, for example, abnormalities of the GABAergic system (as described above) or of the protein **reelin** (see below) alter the course of brain development early in gestation, this would create an abnormal environment for subsequent brain growth.

Perinatal risk factors

Obstetric complications are unusually common in cases where the child later develops autism. The consensus is that these complications result from existing abnormalities of the fetus rather than being a critical first cause of autism. However, a prolonged or difficult birth may increase the risk of later development of an ASD (Bolton, Murphy, Macdonald, Whitlock, Pickles, & Rutter,

1997; Rutter, 2005b). Perinatal factors may also increase the risk of later language impairment (Stromswold, 2006).

Risk factors in childhood

The following possible risk factors in childhood have been identified.

1 *Viral infections* can affect the **central nervous system (CNS)** causing irreversible brain damage, and it is known that the herpes simplex virus can cause autism, or transient autism-related behaviours, in previously normal individuals (Ghaziuddin et al., 1992). Other indirect evidence suggesting that viral infection in early infancy could cause or contribute to autism comes from experiments in which neonatal rats were injected with the **Borna virus** with results suggestive of autism (Pletnikov & Carbone, 2005). It must be stressed, however, that the Borna virus is not thought to affect humans. The direct evidence of early viral infections as a risk factor for autism is ambiguous, with some studies showing positive relations between, for example, measles infection and autism, and some studies showing no relation (Libby et al., 2005). It has been suggested that viral infections are only a risk factor if the infection is persistent or if there is a cumulative effect of successive infections.

2 *Immune system abnormalities* of various kinds (already considered in the section on co-morbid disorders in Chapter 3) have also been proposed as risk factors. Some studies have shown an increased family history of autoimmune diseases, which could relate to a genetic susceptibility. Other studies have shown abnormally high levels of **autoantibodies** of kinds that would attack tissues in the brain. These could have resulted from repeated infections or from a single viral infection in a child with a genetic susceptibility to autoimmune disease. However, the evidence relating to either a familial susceptibility or an environmentally triggered reaction is inconclusive (see the review by Ashwood & Van de Water, 2004).

3 *The triple measles, mumps, and rubella (MMR) vaccine* has been hotly debated as a possible environmental trigger for autism. Two suggestions have been made concerning ways in which the MMR vaccine might be implicated in autism. The first is that the measles component of the vaccine causes a gut disorder that produces chemicals that are carried in the bloodstream to the brain causing regressive autism in previously typically developing children. The second is that brief exposure to a substance used to preserve vaccines, **thimerosal**, can cause or precipitate autism. Thimerosal contains mercury, which is known to have toxic effects on the brain. Its use as a preservative in the MMR vaccine was discontinued once the possible risk was recognised.

There is now an accumulation of evidence from numerous large and careful studies carried out in several different countries, showing that MMR vaccination is not significantly implicated as a causal factor in autism (Chen, Landau, Sham, & Fombonne, 2004; Klein & Diehl, 2004; Doja & Roberts, 2006; Richler et al., 2006; Uchiyama, Kurosawa, & Inaba, 2007). For example, Uchiyama et al. looked at the incidence of regressive autism in the period before the MMR was used in Japan (from 1989 to 1993, only), during the period of its use, and after use of the MMR had been terminated, and found no differences in the incidence across these three periods. They also compared the incidence of regressive autism in children who were, as opposed to children who were not, given the triple vaccination in the period from 1989 to 1993, and again found no difference in the incidence. It follows from results such as these that neither an autoimmune reaction to the measles component, nor exposure to thimerosal, can explain any (as yet unproven) rise in the prevalence of autism.

However, as many reviews of the evidence point out, the lack of a *statistically significant* relation between the MMR and regressive autism does not rule out the possibility that in *very rare cases* the MMR is, figuratively speaking, the straw that breaks the camel's back. In other words, in a child with a strong genetic susceptibility to autism it might be that the addition of just one further risk factor, conceivably the MMR, could precipitate brain changes leading to the onset of an ASD. Families who have seen their child deteriorate following vaccination may be very rare indeed but they have, most understandably, wanted to make their voices heard. One family known to me had this experience, as described in Box 7.2.

BOX 7.2   Robert: One in a million?

Robert was a normally developing baby for the first 14 months of his life: healthy, sociable, playful, and communicative. He was a second child, so his parents knew what to expect in terms of normal development, and they had no concerns about him during this first year.

Following the MMR vaccination at 14 months, however, Robert became extremely ill, running a high temperature and falling into what his parents describe as a coma for 24 hours or more. When he came round he was drowsy for several days and 'very poorly', as if recovering from a bad bout of flu. He was unresponsive, and did not seem to recognise his parents or his older brother.

As he recovered physically Robert remained much more passive than he had been before, and although he clearly knew members of the close family he did not approach them or solicit their attention as he had done previously. He seemed content to sit and play repetitively with bricks or a favourite musical box, which he held close to his ear. Most distressingly for the family he no longer attempted to speak, and only communicated with them when he wanted to be fed or picked up or have some other need provided for. He was diagnosed with an ASD before he entered school, and he attended special schools throughout his childhood.

Robert has in fact done remarkably well with the help of his family, speech and language therapists, teachers and others. He has near-normal language and has recently gained proficiency in IT skills at college. He spends a great deal of time on the computer, but does also have friends whom he sees on a regular basis. However, he remains mildly to moderately autistic, living at home and unlikely to be able to achieve full independence.

Several members on both sides of the family have, or have had, autism-related traits in their behaviour, such as late talking, marked social reserve or a preference for routines and dislike of change. This has not stopped any of them from living full and successful lives. However, Robert was almost certainly genetically vulnerable to developing autism.

(With thanks to 'Robert's' parents for their permission to base this account on their son.)

If the MMR did in fact trigger Robert's autism (which is neither proved nor disproved) he is probably one case in a million. Whereas the vast majority of children receive the MMR with all its benefits and no ill effects, it appears from his parents' account that for this genetically vulnerable child the MMR just may have contributed.

A great deal of confusion has been generated by the failure of the media to distinguish between what may be a *statistically significant* risk factor for autism, capable of explaining a rise in prevalance (if a real rise has in fact occurred), as opposed to the possibility that the MMR might be an *extremely rare* contributory factor that could not possibly explain any real rise in prevalence. The MMR is definitely not the former; which is why autism investigators want to move their research to investigating what may be the significant causes of ASDs, rather than carrying out yet more studies showing that the MMR is not significantly involved, if at all.

In sum, although a small group of teratogens are known to be capable of causing or contributing to the development of autism, other environmental risk factors for autism are as yet unknown or unproven.

BRAIN BASES

Brain Structure and Function in Typical Development

In this introductory section some basic facts concerning first the **neuroanatomy**, or structure, of the brain and then the **neurophysiology**, or functions, of the brain will be presented, followed by a section on brain development. The material is highly selective, covering only information most relevant to the brief account of brain bases of autism that follows. A full account of neurotypical brain structure, function and development can be found in Carlson (2007), with simpler accounts in primers of child development such as Bee and Boyd (2007) or Berk and Ashkenaz (2006).

Brain structure

The major structural divisions of the brain are shown in Figure 7.2. Some distinctions at more detailed levels of description are as follows.

- **Neurons** are cells involved in transmitting information in the form of electrical impulses, whereas **glial cells** protect, support, and maintain neurons, including forming the **myelin sheaths** around **axons**. Clusters of neurons all of which are involved in transmitting and receiving the same information are called **nuclei** (singular: **nucleus**).
- Axons are nerve fibres that carry information from one neuron to another, whereas **dendrites** are nerve fibres that act like antennae, receiving the information carried by axons

from neighbouring cells. The point at which an axon from one neuron junctions with the dendrites of another is called a **synapse**.

- **Grey matter** refers to the cell bodies of neurons, which are greyish-brown coloured, whereas **white matter** refers to the glial cells, which are whiteish.
- **Neurotransmitters** are substances released by one neuron to stimulate or inhibit activity in other neurons, whereas **neuroreceptors** are molecules within neurons that are selectively responsive to particular neurotransmitters. **Neurotrophins** are substances that influence the growth of neurons and their connections.

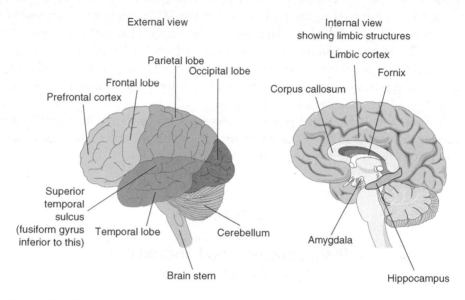

Figure 7.2 Major structural divisions of the brain, indicating the positioning of structures that may be involved in the brain bases of ASDs

Brain function

The whole brain functions as a hierarchy of nested systems referred to as **neural circuits** or **networks**. Each network consists of interconnected nuclei that operate together to subserve a particular function. Those circuits that involve relatively few nuclei situated close together in the brain are referred to as **local networks**. These carry out highly specific functions, such as registering the colour or the shape of an object. To register all salient aspects of an object simultaneously and as a whole (for example the colour, shape, size and movement of a bird) activity in several local networks must be co-ordinated in a **global network**. Even more extended networks, or brain systems, can be identified in terms of brain areas or structures that are all involved in one large field of activity. For example, hearing is mediated by the auditory nerves that connect mechanisms in the inner ear to various nuclei in the brain stem, which connect to the primary auditory **cortex** in the left and right temporal lobes; and thereon to adjacent auditory association cortex in each temporal lobe. For local, global or structure-based networks to operate efficiently, **connectivity** between neurons, nuclei, and specific brain structures is important. This can be physical, i.e., tissue-based, or functional, as described next.

Brain systems, or circuits, can also be identified in terms of the neurotransmitters and neuroreceptors subserving particular functions. Of the many different neurotransmitter–neuroreceptor systems, two are crucially important and operate throughout the brain. **Glutamate** and its receptors convey information by stimulating neural activity. GABA and its receptors (referred to earlier in the chapter) ensure that information is conveyed efficiently by inhibiting irrelevant or unwanted neural activity. Thus the balance between these two neurotransmitter systems is important for efficient and focused information transmission.

Other neurotransmitter–receptor systems operate within specific brain circuits rather than across the whole brain. These include **serotonin, dopamine**, and **norepinephrine** (sometimes called **noradrenalin**), all of which will be commented on below. These neurotransmitters modulate activity across a whole circuit, either stimulating or inhibiting it. There are many of these **neuromodulator** substances operating within brain circuits with particular psychological or behavioural functions. For example, various **peptides** including the **opioid peptides** oxytocin and vasopressin, mentioned earlier, modulate activity within brain circuits mediating pain perception, emotion, appetite, and social and sexual behaviours.

Brain development

Prenatal development The brain starts to develop within the first month after conception, with the formation of the neural tube within which the central nervous system will grow. Within the first four months of gestation, the neural tube has differentiated into a recognisable brain shape within the head, on a long stalk within the spinal column. Most of the neurons an individual will have over a lifetime develop during these first four months. Neurons develop in the base of the brain and then migrate to other sections of the brain to form specialised structures and systems. Amongst the earliest neurons to develop are the clusters of cells forming nuclei in the **brain stem**; also a particular type of cell called **Purkinje cells** that are found in the **cerebellar vermis** (see Figure 7.2). The first axons and dendrites begin to develop in the last two months before birth.

Post-natal development At birth the most developed parts of the brain are the evolutionarily old parts that regulate vital functions such as respiration, sleeping, eating, and eliminating waste products. The least developed part of the brain is the evolutionarily new **cerebral cortex**, which subserves higher-order functions.

During the first 18 months of life this situation changes, as multiple new connections are established between neurons in the process of **synaptogenesis**. Synaptogenesis involves the growth of axons and dendrites that meet up with each other at new synapses. The process occurs throughout the brain, but especially in the previously underdeveloped cerebral cortex. It is mainly driven by the infant's experiences, and in the first months of life involves establishing neural connectivity in those parts of the cortex that register bodily sensations, perceptions and emotions, and that control movement. The proliferation of new nerve fibres is accompanied by increases in protective and supportive glial cells, or white matter, and as a result of these combined growth processes the weight of the brain doubles between birth and 18 months.

Thereafter, a process of **synaptic pruning** occurs, in which the less-used axonal pathways are eliminated and only the most-used pathways are retained. In addition, space for the proliferating axons and dendrites is made by the **programmed cell death**, or **apoptosis**, of some of the surrounding neurons (the prenatally formed neuron 'bank' allows for this). The combination of synaptogenesis followed by synaptic pruning and programmed cell death is sometimes referred to as a process of 'sculpting' the brain into a functionally efficient form.

Spurts in brain growth, with ensuing processes of synaptic pruning and cell death, occur at roughly predictable ages from infancy through childhood and adolescence. These growth spurts are selective, building and sculpting specific brain systems in turn. The earliest spurt in brain growth occurs within the first few months of life, when the cortical components of the auditory and visual systems are developed. Another growth spurt occurs at around two years of age, accompanied by gains in language development, and another around four years of age, accompanied by a step change in the ability to think about one's own thoughts and those of other people, an ability that is important for understanding autism (see Chapter 8). Further spurts of brain growth, mainly involving increased connectivity between neurons in the **frontal lobes** and neurons in relatively distant parts of the brain, continue through middle childhood to the late teenage years, each accompanied by stepwise improvements in increasingly sophisticated and human-specific abilities such as abstract reasoning and mathematical ability.

Another aspect of brain development that begins prenatally and continues from infancy is **lateralisation**. Much of the brain is divided into roughly symmetrical halves. Thus there is a left and a right **cerebral hemisphere** communicating with each other via an extended band of nerve fibres called the **corpus callosum** (see Figure 7.2). Each cerebral hemisphere contains an **occipital, parietal, temporal** and frontal lobe. The **cerebellum**, like the cerebral cortex, is divided into two symmetrical halves. **Subcortical** structures in the **limbic system** are also paired. The left and right members of a pair of structures often subserve different functions that are complementary in nature. So, for example, the auditory cortex in the right hemisphere receives sound coming predominantly from the left ear, whereas the auditory cortex in the left hemisphere receives sound coming predominantly from the right ear; speech production is generally carried out in the left hemisphere, whereas prosody (the emotion-bearing patterns of pitch and intonation) is generally carried out in the right hemisphere. Rather confusingly, paired structures are often referred to using singular rather than plural terms, for example, 'the temporal lobe', 'the **amygdala**', 'the **hippocampus**'. Unless otherwise stated, therefore, the singular terms should be taken to refer to paired structures.

What drives brain development   Brain development is ultimately controlled by the activities of *genes* and their products, including many of the neurochemicals mentioned in a previous section. However, *environmental factors* also influence both pre- and post-natal brain development. For example, synaptogenesis occurs in response to experience that stimulates the growth of axons and dendrites, increasing brain connectivity and building the brain circuits that will subserve an increasingly wide repertoire of abilities and behaviours. The chemical processes involved in synaptogenesis are, however, mediated by *gene* products. Moreover, the processes of pruning and programmed cell death are also *genetically* controlled. However, because experience determines which neuronal connections are well established (and hence not pruned) as opposed to those that are poorly established (and hence pruned) *environmental factors* also have a role in brain sculpting. This kind of interplay between genetic and environmental factors is typical of the processes of brain development and change throughout the lifespan, ensuring that every individual is unique.

In sum, genetic and environmental factors involved in neurotypical brain development are interdependent. There is, however, some disagreement concerning the balance between the contributions of nature and nurture, particularly concerning the extent to which the genes control exactly what circuits are built, and whereabouts in the brain. So-called **modularists** (such as Frith & Happé, 1998) argue for a much greater degree of genetic control than the **constructivists** (e.g., Elman, Bates, Johnson, Karmiloff-Smith, Parisi, & Plunkett, 1996), who emphasise instead the **plasticity** of the brain. This dispute is relevant to the kinds of theories proposed as explanations of autism and is referred to at greater length in Chapter 11.

Methods Used to Study Brain Structure, Chemistry, and Function

Methods used in studies of brain structure, brain chemistry, and brain function in people with ASDs are summarised in Boxes 7.3, 7.4, and 7.5 respectively.

> ## BOX 7.3 Methods of assessing brain structure
>
> *Autopsies/postmortem studies* Useful for detailed examination at both macro and micro levels of analysis, and has the advantage that examination can be extended over time. Disadvantages: small numbers of cases available, tending to be older individuals or individuals with multiple disorders that may have affected the brain.
>
> *Computerised (axial) tomography (CT/CAT scan)* Uses X-Rays; useful for examining bony tissue, but undesirable because of radiation risks.
>
> *Structural magnetic resonance imaging (sMRI/MRIs)* Uses a machine-generated magnetic field that is reflected back in specific ways and can be used to build up a detailed three-dimensional image of brain structure. There are different kinds of sMR imaging methods in use, which can be used for different assessment purposes. Advantages are in the scope for very detailed examination of brain tissue, and in the noninvasive nature of the procedure. Disadvantages: the machine is claustrophobic and noisy, and the individual being examined has to keep still for significant periods of time; also use of the machines is expensive. For all these reasons, studies tend to include small numbers of participants, and few studies include very young or low - functioning individuals.

> ## BOX 7.4 Methods of assessing brain chemistry
>
> *Magnetic resonance spectroscopy imaging (MRSI/ MRS)* This noninvasive procedure (similar to sMRI as described in Box 7.3) provides information about the chemical constituents of specific brain regions.
>
> *Positron emission tomography (PET scan)* Uses a radioactive 'tracer' injected into the bloodstream, the progress of which can be monitored by the scanner. Measures changes in blood flow, indicating levels of activity in specific neurochemical systems. Used clinically, but undesirable for research because of radiation risks.
>
> *Lumbar puncture* May be used to draw off a sample of cerebro-spinal fluid for analysis. However, this is an invasive procedure and its use for non-clinical purposes is controversial.
>
> *Blood or urine samples* Can be informative about the by-products of brain metabolism.
>
> *Efficacy studies* Studies of the effects of medications known to have their effects on particular neurotransmitters or neuromodulators provide an indirect method of assessing brain neurochemistry.

Positron emission tomography (PET scan) (see Box 7.4)   Can be used to measure levels of activity in specific brain regions during specific activities (but contraindicated for research as opposed to clinical purposes because uses radioactive material as a 'tracer').

Single photon emission computed tomography (SPECT)   Similar to PET scan method: assesses blood flow using a radioactive 'tracer', from which to infer relations between brain activity and specific behavioural functions.

Functional magnetic resonance imaging (fMRI)   Similar to sMRI (see Box 7.3), but measures levels of ongoing brain activity rather than brain structure. The person being scanned is generally asked to undertake a particular task designed to involve a particular function such as reading aloud, or counting, or watching an emotion-arousing video.

Electroencephalography (EEG)   Involves placing electrodes on the skull and measuring brain electrical activity in response to certain stimuli (evoked response potentials, or ERPs) or in resting situations. Somewhat invasive, but can be used with very young or vulnerable individuals, given careful preparation.

Magnetoencephalography (MEG)   Measures magnetic fields produced by electrical activity in the brain to assess the brain's response to particular stimuli. For technical reasons it is more sensitive than EEG. It is also less invasive than EEG: the person being assessed sits in a comfortable chair with their head in what looks like a hair dryer of the kind used in hairdressing salons.

In addition to the methods described in Box 7.5 for assessing brain function directly, two indirect methods have been used to study brain function in ASDs. Both of these involve **modelling**. **Animal models** involve **lesioning** specific brain areas and assessing subsequent effects on the animal's behaviour (compare the use of animal models in genetic research, Box 7.1). Computer-inspired **computational models** simulate ways in which neural networks operate in the brain, and are generally used to study processes involved in learning.

Findings Concerning the Brain Bases of Autism

All the methods outlined in Boxes 7.3–7.5 above have specific uses, and each has particular advantages and disadvantages. Many of the methods are relatively new and the technologies of data collection and analysis are developing all the time. As a result, studies of brain structure and function in people with ASDs have used a variety of methodologies (as well as participants of differing ages and ability), making their results difficult to compare. In addition, many reported findings are unconfirmed or controversial, and there are huge gaps in current knowledge, not least concerning brain development.

For these reasons, only those findings that are reasonably secure, or which are of particular interest though in need of confirmation, will be reported here. More information can be found in reviews by Dawson, Webb et al. (2002), DiCicco-Bloom et al. (2006), and in the more advanced accounts in Bauman and Kemper (2005b) and chapters in Volkmar et al. (2005). However, because this is a rapidly developing field, which is certain to yield increasingly informative results within the next decade, interested readers should look for new reviews as these become available.

Early studies

Many of the methods of assessing brain structure, neurochemistry, and function that were described in Boxes 7.3–7.5 were used to study autism from the 1950s onwards, and numerous hypotheses were proposed that aimed to identify the brain bases of autism as it was understood in the 1960s and 1970s (see Box 6.1 for examples). Brain stem abnormalities were most commonly cited as basic to abnormal brain development and function in autism. Limbic structures, especially the hippocampus, which is involved in memory and learning, were cited in some theories, and a number of theories focused on abnormal lateralisation of functions in the cerebral hemispheres. The roles of various neurochemical systems were extensively investigated in the hope of identifying effective medications or dietary treatments. Schopler and Mesibov's (1987) edited volume *The Neurobiology of Autism*, also chapters in Dawson (1989), demonstrate the progress being made by that time.

Brain anatomy

Abnormalities of brain size   Abnormal brain size is now the most reliably established finding concerning brain anatomy in people with ASDs (see Nelson & Nelson, 2005; Redcay & Courchesne, 2005 for reviews of the evidence). Brain size can be measured using head circumference as an indicator; it can also be assessed in postmortem studies and using **structural magnetic resonance imaging (sMRI)**. Brain size is normal in newborns who later develop an ASD. However, within the first two years of life brain size increases abnormally rapidly and is significantly larger than average by the end of the second year (Courchesne, 2004). Thereafter the rate of brain growth slows down, but at age three to four years brain size is still approximately 10 per cent greater than average. By adolescence, brain size in groups of people with ASDs may be greater than in typically developing individuals, but the difference is not significant in all studies (Palmen, van Engeland, Hof, & Schmitz, 2004).

Increased amounts of both grey matter (neurons) and white matter (glial cells) in specific brain areas are responsible for increased brain size in young children with ASDs. This suggests either that synaptogenesis, including the growth and myelinisation of nerve fibres, has occurred to excess; or that the genetically programmed processes of synaptic pruning and cell death have not taken place normally; or that both these abnormalities of brain growth have occurred. However, the precise nature of the excessive brain growth, and reasons why it occurs unchecked by the usual processes of brain reduction, are not understood. It can only be concluded that the chemical processes regulating the balance between growth and reduction are not operating as they should.

The fact that increased brain size is less marked in adolescents with ASDs than in toddlers reflects the fact that excessive brain growth in early infancy is followed by a lack of normal brain growth in middle childhood. In typically developing children, those parts of the temporal and frontal lobes that subserve higher-order social and intellectual functions grow by up to 20 per cent between the preschool years and adolescence, an increase in size that is not matched in children with ASDs.

Abnormalities of specific brain structures　Postmortem and sMRI studies have identified numerous structural abnormalities both at the level of brain structures and regions, and at the level of cell types and organisation. Findings tend to be inconsistent across studies, no doubt because of differences in study methods, and differences in the brain development, age and ability of the individuals studied. The fact that a particular structure or area is not named in what follows does not therefore mean that it may not be involved in all or some cases of autism, merely that the evidence is inconsistent or lacking.

The best-established abnormalities are in the brain stem (Rodier & Arndt, 2005), and in the closely related cerebellum where a lack of Purkinje cells has been observed in postmortem studies (Ritvo, Freeman, & Scheibel 1986; Bailey et al., 1998).

Malformations of the cerebral cortex have been reported in some but not all postmortem studies. However, very detailed examination of the organisation of nerve cells in the cerebral cortex using other methods of investigation, indicates that subtle but potentially important abnormalities do exist (Courchesne & Pierce, 2005; Casanova et al., 2006). **Neural network modelling** confirms that abnormalities at the level of cellular organisation and function in the cortex could lead to abnormal learning of kinds seen in autism (McClelland, 2000; Gustafsson & Papliński, 2004). Lateralisation at the level of the cerebral cortex has been shown to be abnormal in some studies. In particular, certain areas of the frontal cortex that are larger in the right than in the left hemisphere in most people, show **reversed asymmetry** in children with ASDs (de Fossé et al., 2004) and also in adults (Boucher et al., 2005). There is some evidence of decreased grey matter in that part of the cerebral cortex identified with the **mirror neuron system (MNS)** (Hadjikhani, Joseph, Snyder, & Tager-Flusberg, 2006). This finding is consistent with those from **functional MRI (fMRI)** reviewed below. Finally, the corpus callosum (the band of fibres connecting the two cerebral hemispheres) is reduced in size (Boger-Megiddo et al., 2006; Vidal et al., 2006).

Studies of two key structures in the limbic system, the amygdala (which is involved in social and emotional behaviour) and hippocampus (which mediates memory and learning), have produced somewhat inconsistent findings. However, a majority of studies have found abnormalities, both at the level of overall size (sometimes oversized, sometimes undersized) and also at the cellular level.

There is, in addition, some indirect evidence of the likely involvement of limbic system structures in the temporal lobes more generally. This evidence comes from what is known about some causes of non-idiopathic autism. Most strikingly, tuberous sclerosis (described in Chapter 3) frequently involves fibrous growths in the temporal lobes, and when growths are present in this brain region, full-blown or partial forms of autism commonly occur (Steyn & Le Couteur, 2003). Turner's syndrome and Fragile-X syndrome, both of which can occur co-morbidly with ASDs, have been mentioned above in connection with the hypothesis that vulnerability to autism involves genes on the X-chromosome. However, both these syndromes involve abnormalities of the hippocampus (Murphy et al., 1993; Jäkälä et al., 1997). It might be the case that sex-linked syndromes (including autism, according to some theorists) have some association with hippocampal abnormalities. However, a more cautious interpretation of the behavioural overlap and occasional co-morbidity between autism, Turner's syndrome, and Fragile-X is that some of the same brain regions are affected, but for different reasons in each case. In other words there is a common pathway, but not a shared root cause.

In sum, research into brain anatomy in people with ASDs has produced some reliable findings and many less consistent findings that require further investigation. An authoritative review of findings on brain anatomy in autism can be found in Palmen et al. (2004).

Brain chemistry

The literature on neurochemical abnormalities in autism is large and expanding. Most research has used indirect methods of study such as the analysis of urine, blood or spinal fluid, or the results of efficacy studies of pharmacological interventions (see Box 7.4). Recently however, studies using the direct method of MRSI have been reported, and this offers a promising line of research that has already demonstrated some abnormalities in the chemical constituents of brain tissue in situ (Zeegers, van der Grond, van Daalen, Buitelaar, & van Engeland, 2007).

The most striking aspect of this field of research is the number of studies that have shown no differences between people with ASDs and people in the general population. In addition, there is as yet no consensus concerning neurochemical abnormalities in people with ASDs, findings being highly variable across studies. The most widely investigated systems are identified below, with comments on the strength of the evidence of abnormalities in people with autism.

Serotonin (5-hydroxytryptamine, or 5-HT) is an important neurotransmitter involved in sleep, eating, mood, and arousal. Serotonin also plays a vital role in the development of brain cells and their connections, and in the organisation of brain growth (Anderson, 2005; Whitaker-Azmitia, 2001). Abnormalities associated with serotonin levels and processes have been observed in people with ASDs for many years, leading to numerous drug treatment studies, none of which have had unambiguously successful results (see Chapter 14). There is, however, an increasing amount of evidence that low levels of serotonin synthesis in autism contribute to abnormal brain development (Chugani, 2002; Chandana et al., 2005).

Dopamine is a neurotransmitter involved in motor functions (people with Parkinson's disease have dopamine abnormality) and also in the mediation of reward value, or 'feel good' factors (most recreational drugs act via dopaminergic reward systems), and thus is also important for attention and learning. Direct evidence for abnormalities of the dopamine system in autism is controversial, some researchers rating it as quite strong, others as less so.

Some indirect evidence is, however, supportive. This evidence again comes from cases of autism that result, at least in part, from a known medical condition, in this instance phenylketonuria (PKU). PKU is a single gene disorder that leads to a specific metabolic abnormality. The condition can be detected at birth and successfully treated. Untreated cases, however, have intellectual disabilities, autistic behavioural traits and, more rarely, full-blown autism; and the behavioural abnormalities in PKU are known to be associated with frontal lobe dysfunction and brain dopamine deficiency. The association with autism is unlikely to be explained by a shared genetic cause and is more likely to be mediated by shared abnormalities of frontal lobe dysfunction and possibly dopamine deficiency. In other words there may be a common pathway, rather than a shared root cause.

Norepinephrine (noradrenalin) is a neurotransmitter involved in **autonomic nervous system (ANS)** functions including the neurochemical **correlates** of fear and anxiety, such as sweating and increased heart rate. It is synthesised from dopamine and therefore dependent on that system. There is some evidence to suggest that some individuals with ASDs are over-responsive to stress, which could imply overactivity in this system. However, over-reactivity to stress might also involve the **hypothalamic-pituitary-adrenal axis (HPA)**, which is importantly involved in control of autonomic functions (Marinović, Terzić, Petković, Zekan, Terzić, & Šušnjara, 2003; Corbett, Mendoza, Abdullah, Wegelin, & Levine, 2006).

GABA has been mentioned already in connection with possible abnormalities of prenatal brain development, when it has an excitatory function. In the developed brain, GABA acts as the major inhibitory neurotransmitter, and has been mentioned above in connection with repetitive behaviour and desire for sameness. Blatt (2005) argues that the close relationship between GABA and the Purkinje cells in the cerebellum (which are sparse in the brains of people with ASDs), and also between GABA and cells in the limbic system (which also show abnormalities), is significant for an understanding of brain–behaviour links in autism.

The opiod peptides oxytocin and vasopressin are neuromodulators involved in social behaviours, as has been mentioned above. The potential explanatory value of abnormalities of these neuromodulators has aroused research interest in the past (e.g., Gillberg, 1995). They are sex-related, and more recently it has been suggested that an imbalance between the two might help to explain the predominance of males with autism (Carter, 2007). However, clear evidence of their involvement is currently sparse.

Reelin is a recently discovered protein that has a critical role in brain development. It could have explanatory value for autism (and other neurodevelopmental disorders), and is therefore an important area for research as argued by Fatemi (2005). However, direct evidence of the involvement of reelin in abnormal brain development in autism is currently lacking (Bonara et al., 2003).

Brain-derived neurotrophic factor (BDNF) is a neurochemical that is also increasingly mentioned as having possible relevance for brain development and function in autism (see various chapters in Bauman & Kemper, 2005b).

In sum, brain chemistry in autism is currently poorly understood, but may hold the key to understanding the brain bases of autism (which is why it has been given space here, despite all the uncertainties in the evidence). A review of relevant theories and evidence can be found in Anderson and Hoshino (2005) and more detailed information about some key neurochemical systems can be found in chapters in Bauman and Kemper (2005b).

Brain function

Autism researchers have been particularly interested to examine which brain areas are active when individuals carry out tasks relating to their autism-specific behavioural impairments. Only the social impairments have been extensively investigated, with scattered findings relating to other impairments, as reported next.

Abnormal activation in the 'social brain'   Brothers (1990, 1997) coined the term **social brain** to refer to the brain system that enables humans 'to perceive the intentions and dispositions of others', sometimes equated with 'social cognition'. This has clear relevance for the problems of theory of mind or mindreading, about which much more is said in the next chapter. However, the social brain is also involved in perceiving, interpreting, and probably sharing the emotional expressions of others. Use of the term social cognition to refer to the functions of the social brain will therefore be avoided here, although widely used in the literature (see comments on usage of 'cognition', in the Glossary).

The social brain includes several widely distributed structures most of which are shown in Figure 7.2, earlier. These include the amygdala, which is involved in processing emotion; the **fusiform gyrus**, which has a specialised role in face processing; the **superior temporal sulcus**, which is involved in processing biological motion; the **ventromedial prefrontal cortex**, which may have a role in representing the self; and **orbitofrontal cortex**, thought to be implicated in mediating social reward. Each of these areas can be reliably activated in people in the general population by asking them to carry out tasks such as recognising a familiar face, interpreting intentions from movement or reasoning about another person's knowledge or intentions. Numerous studies have now demonstrated a relative lack of the expected activity in these structures when people with ASDs are asked to carry out these same tasks. There is also ample evidence of structural (neuroanatomical) abnormalities of the amygdala in particular (e.g., Baron-Cohen, Ring, Wheelwright, Ashwin, & Williams, 2000; Howard et al., 2000). Reviews of the relevant literature can be found in Dawson, Webb et al. (2002), Pelphrey, Adolphs, and Morris (2004), and Schultz (2005).

There is also some fMRI evidence that suggests the mirror neuron system functions abnormally in people with ASDs (Dapretto et al., 2006; Williams, Waiter, Gilchrist, Perrett, Murray, & Whiten, 2006). An EEG study also found evidence of abnormal activity of mirror neurons (Oberman, Hubbard, McCleery, Altschuler, Ramachandran, & Pineda, 2005). However, these findings are newer and less secure than those mentioned in the previous paragraph.

Abnormal activation of brain areas involved in executive functions Impaired executive function is thought to be an important cause of behavioural inflexibility in autism (see Chapter 9). Executive functions are those that are involved in starting, stopping, and maintaining control of ongoing behavioural actions, including **working memory**. They are subserved by various regions of the frontal lobes in combination with the cerebellum and intervening structures making up an 'executive circuit'. A small number of fMRI studies have shown abnormal activity within this circuit in people with ASDs as they carry out executive function tasks involving **spatial working memory** (Koshino, Carpenter, Minshew, Cherkassky, Keller, & Just, 2005), planning (Just, Cherkassky, Keller, Kana, & Minshew, 2007), **response inhibition** (Anagnostou, Soorya, Stamper, & Hollander, 2006), and **attention switching** (Gomot et al., 2006). Koshino et al. and Just et al. interpret their findings in terms of impaired connectivity between the several areas involved in any one executive function task, rather than in terms of abnormality within any single brain structure (for further discussion of connectivity see Chapter 11).

Abnormal activation of brain areas involved in motor skills There is some evidence of abnormal activation, especially in the cerebellum, when carrying out a motor task (Allen & Courchesne, 2003).

Abnormal activation of brain areas involved in speech and language A small number of studies using EEG and **evoked response potentials (ERPs)** to investigate auditory processes in people with ASDs at the level of the brain stem have shown abnormalities in response to heard speech (see Minshew, Sweeney, Bauman, & Webb, 2005, for a review of research into brain stem ERP studies). Other studies using fMRI show abnormal activation in temporal and frontal lobe areas known to subserve language (Just, Cherkassky, Keller, & Minshew, 2004; Harris et al., 2006). Interestingly, the people with ASDs who took part in these studies were high-functioning, and would not have had clinically significant language impairments. Just et al.'s findings are again interpreted in terms of impaired connectivity.

Implications of Findings Concerning the Brain Bases of Autism

Evidence relating to the brain bases of autism is on the whole too inconsistent and too sparse to yield firm conclusions. However, some tentative conclusions and promising avenues for further research are beginning to emerge.

Implications of the findings on brain anatomy

The fact that nuclei in the brain stem and Purkinje cells in the cerebellum have been found to be abnormal in most studies is widely interpreted as evidence that brain development in people with ASDs is generally abnormal from an early stage in gestation. This is because these particular nuclei and cells are amongst the first to develop after the neural tube has formed. The brain stem is thought to be involved in low-level behaviours to do with associative learning, attention and motor skills (Rodier & Arndt, 2005). The cerebellum is critically involved in the control of posture and movement, but is also involved in attention, cognition, language and possibly also emotion (Schmahmann & Caplan, 2006). Early abnormalities of the cerebellum might therefore have numerous secondary effects on those aspects of brain development normally stimulated by input from cerebellar regions (this possibility is discussed in Chapter 11).

Failure to eliminate unwanted grey and white matter in the second and third years of life (leading to increased brain size) is likely to impair brain connectivity and information transmission, in that there would be too much brain wiring and too many neurons firing. Conversely, the relative lack of growth in connectivity in later childhood would result in poorer information transmission across widely disparate brain regions, with a reduction in top-down control (Frith, 2003).

Structural abnormalities of the amygdala are consistent with evidence from studies indicating abnormal function of the set of structures that make up the social brain. Structural abnormalities of other limbic structures, and especially the hippocampus, may contribute to abnormalities of memory and learning (Bachevalier, 2008; Loveland, Bachevalier, Pearson, & Lane, 2007; see also Chapters 11 and 12).

Implications of the findings on brain chemistry

No clear implications emerge from these findings because of uncertainties in the evidence. However the findings relating to norepinephrine and the hypothalamic-pituitary-adrenal axis may help to explain the high levels of anxiety in individuals with ASDs, although more research into this needs to be done. The dual role of GABA in prenatal brain development and subsequently as a major neurotransmitter makes it another likely growth area for research. The similar dual roles of serotonin and its known involvement in autism are also of considerable potential interest. Further research on the sex-linked neuropeptides oxytocin and vasopressin is also likely, not only in view of the need to explain the preponderance of males with ASDs, but also because of possible links with Baron-Cohen's extreme male brain theory, mentioned above.

Implications of the findings on brain function

The implications of findings on brain function are easily identified because the research is always hypothesis-driven. That is to say, each study is designed to test a specific hypothesis concerning the neural activity that occurs when the person being tested is carrying out a specific task. Thus, there is evidence that all the structures in the social brain are implicated in the social impairments associated with autism, with weaker evidence concerning the possible brain bases of impaired executive functions, impaired language, and impaired motor skills.

Comment

It is important to remember that high-functioning individuals with ASDs are often extremely able and always very much more 'normal' than 'abnormal'. The challenge for explanations of autism at the level of brain bases is, therefore, not to explain too much: in most ways the brains of people with AS/HFA are operating effectively though probably differently from the brains of people without autism. The anatomical and functional evidence tends to suggest that almost every region and every structure-based system of the brain in people with ASDs can be shown to be structurally or functionally atypical in one way or another. This impression partly results from the fact that **negative findings** (those that do not demonstrate differences between people with autism and people without autism) are less likely to be published than those that produce **positive findings**. However, it also undoubtedly reflects the fact that in people with ASDs the brain develops and functions in ways that are different from the norm, but nevertheless often efficient and sometimes super-efficient.

The evidence from studies of brain chemistry in people with ASDs, unlike the evidence from anatomical and functional studies, reveals relatively few differences between people with and without autism. The combined evidence suggests that intact chemical systems may be operating within different neural circuits and different brain structures from those of people without autism, but operating to produce normal or superior achievement in many spheres of behaviour. This suggests that a goal of research in the future might be to understand how this efficiency is achieved instead of, or in addition to, understanding how autism-related impairments arise. The important issue of 'difference' as opposed to 'deficit' was discussed in the section headed Terminology in Chapter 2, and is referred to again in Chapter 15.

SUMMARY

The etiology of autism is discussed in terms of genetic and environmental factors that may constitute the first, or root, causes of autism. First causes are not the same in all cases. Moreover, it is rare for an ASD to result from a single root cause. Usually several causal factors are involved that, in varying combinations, cause autism to occur in one of its forms from the least to the most complex and severe. Evidence that genetic factors frequently contribute to autism comes from the fact that ASDs tend to run in families; also from the fact that, in genetically identical twins one of whom has an ASD, the other is quite likely also to be autistic or to have autism-related behavioural traits. However, the fact that the second identical twin does not invariably have an ASD shows that environmental factors must also be involved.

In a minority of cases the cause of autism is known or partly known. For example, the morning sickness drug thalidomide caused some cases of autism before being withdrawn. When autism co-occurs with some known medical condition, for example phenylketonuria, it can sometimes be inferred that whatever causes the other medical condition can also be a risk factor for autism. In a majority of cases, however, autism is described as 'idiopathic,' meaning that first causes are unknown. Idiopathic autism is being intensively studied by geneticists and numerous genes that may contribute to autism have been tentatively but not definitively identified. Less is known about environmental susceptibility or 'risk' factors, except that prenatal exposure to toxic substances such as thalidomide can cause or contribute to autism. Vaccination has been proposed as a cause of regressive autism, but intensive study shows that vaccination is not a significant risk factor for autism.

The brain bases of autism are also being intensively studied using increasingly sophisticated methods of assessment. Here again, however, few definite conclusions have been reached, with the following exceptions. Brain size is normal at birth but abnormally large by age three to four years, reflecting failure to prune excess grey and white matter following the normal spurt of brain growth in the first two years of life. Less than normal brain growth occurs during the school-age years, causing brain size to return towards the average.

Structural abnormalities have been fairly reliably found in the brain stem and cerebellum, and less consistently in the cerebral cortex, corpus callosum, amygdala and hippocampus. Neurochemical abnormalities have proved difficult to identify, although abnormalities associated with the neurotransmitter serotonin have frequently been shown. Dopamine, norepinephrine, GABA and certain neuropeptides are thought by some theorists to be abnormal in autism, but there is no agreement. Functional abnormalities have been reliably found in structures that make up the social brain, abnormal brain activity occurring during face-processing and mindreading tasks in particular. A few studies have shown abnormal brain function when people with ASDs are carrying out executive function tasks, speech-processing tasks, and motor tasks.

In the future it will be important to investigate ways in which the brains of people with ASDs have developed to function as efficiently as they do: it will be important to investigate differences rather than focusing exclusively on deficits.

EXPLAINING THE SOCIAL, EMOTIONAL, AND COMMUNICATION IMPAIRMENTS

AIMS
••••
INTRODUCTION
What Has to be Explained
Early Theories
••••
THE IMPAIRED THEORY OF MIND AND MINDBLINDNESS
THEORIES
The Impaired Theory of Mind Theory
Other Theories of the Origins of Impaired Theory of Mind
The Mindblindness Theory
••••
PRIMARY INTERSUBJECTIVITY DEFICIT THEORIES
The Concept of Primary Intersubjectivity
Theories Emphasising Emotion Processing
Theories Emphasising Imitation
Theories Emphasising the Centrality of Social Stimuli
Theories Emphasising Timing
Critique of Primary Intersubjectivity Deficit Theories
••••
SUMMARY

AIMS

The major aims are to provide basic information about a range of theories; to give full recognition to impaired theory of mind as the immediate cause of the social and communicative impairments of autism (but not the major emotion processing impairments); but to emphasise that more recent theories provide a more fundamental and complete explanation of socio-emotional-communicative impairments in autism than those focusing on impaired theory of mind.

INTRODUCTION

What Has to be Explained

The socio-communicative impairments listed in the DSM-IV criteria are as follows.

- Marked impairments in the use of non-verbal behaviours such as eye-to-eye gaze, facial expression, body postures, and gestures to regulate social interaction.
- Failure to develop peer relationships appropriate to developmental level.
- Lack of spontaneous seeking to share enjoyment, interests or achievements with other people (for example, by a lack of showing, bringing or pointing out objects of interest).
- Lack of social or emotional reciprocity.
- Marked impairment in the ability to initiate or sustain a conversation with others.
- Stereotyped and repetitive use of language or idiosyncratic language.

Problems of emotion processing, which will also be considered in this chapter, were described in Chapter 3 as including the following.

- Spared emotion contagion and spared experience of basic emotions such as sorrow or fear.
- Impaired ability to understand others' non-verbal expressions of emotion.
- Impaired empathy in the sense of knowing what another person's emotion is about or knowing what one's own experienced emotion is about.
- Impaired experience and understanding of complex emotions such as pride or guilt.

Fuller accounts of social, emotional and communicative impairments, and of islets of spared ability within these broad groups of behaviour, can be found in Chapters 2 and 3.

Early Theories

Brain-based theories

Kanner (1943) suggested that autism derives from 'an innate inability to form the usual biologically provided affective contact with people'. Kanner's suggestion is remarkable for two reasons. First it proposed a biological basis for autism in the face of what was then the prevailing tendency to explain mental health problems in children in terms of abnormal mothering (a trend to which Kanner himself briefly succumbed, but from which he quickly retreated). Secondly, in identifying affective (emotional) problems as fundamental to autism, Kanner proposed a type of theory that largely disappeared from the mainstream literature for several decades but which has returned to prominence.

From the 1980s onwards, however, occasional journal articles began to appear suggesting that social and communication impairments in autism result from brain-based problems in processing emotions (e.g., Hetzler & Griffin, 1981). Fotheringham (1991) specifically suggested that abnormalities affecting the amygdala result in loss of the emotional significance of incoming stimuli. This suggestion, like Kanner's, prefigures some of the explanations of social impairments in autism that are now prominent (see below). However, Fotheringham's hypothesis attracted little attention at the time.

Psychodynamic theories

Despite Kanner's early insight, the more usual explanation of autism in the mid-twentieth century was that it was caused by disturbed mother–child relationships (Mahler, 1952; Bettelheim, 1967). Some psychoanalysts and psychotherapists continued to claim that disturbed mother–child relationships (Welch, 1988), or abnormal personality development (Tustin, 1981, 1991), are the fundamental causes of autism, at least in cases of what Tustin calls **psychogenic autism**.

Although Tustin's psychoanalytic theory represents very much a minority view, her concept of psychogenic autism, defined as autism resulting from adverse early experience, receives support from studies of Romanian orphans, some of whom have autism or autistic traits even after adoption into good homes (Rutter, Anderson-Wood et al., 1999; Hoksbergen, ter Laak, Rijk, van Dijkum, & Stoutjesdik, 2005), and also from studies of blind children, a higher than expected proportion of whom also have autism or some autistic-like behaviours (Hobson, 2002; Pring, 2005). An inference from these studies is that sensory deprivation by itself (as in blind children) or more pervasive deprivation (as in institutionalised orphans) may cause or contribute to the development of autism-related behaviours. More is said about these studies in Chapter 10.

THE IMPAIRED THEORY OF MIND AND MINDBLINDNESS THEORIES

The Impaired Theory of Mind Theory

Baron-Cohen, Leslie, and Frith's seminal paper

In 1985, Baron-Cohen, Leslie, and Frith published a paper that radically altered the focus and direction of research into the causes of autism, with long-lasting effects on the understanding of autism, and on theories of typical development. In this paper, Baron-Cohen et al. reported a test of the hypothesis that children with autism lack a theory of mind. The test used was the 'Sally and the marble' task that has become a classic in child development research. This test utilises the following scenario acted out for the child:

> A doll-sized box and a basket, both with lids/covers, are placed side by side, a small distance apart.
> A doll, 'Sally', enters, holding a marble.
> Sally puts the marble into the basket, and exits.
> A second doll, 'Ann', enters; goes to the basket; takes out the marble and places it in the box; then exits.
> Sally returns.
> The Tester asks the child: 'Where will Sally look for her marble?'

When asked 'Where will Sally look for her marble?' most of the typically developing children and the Down syndrome children tested by Baron-Cohen et al. responded correctly 'In the basket'. They were able to work out that Sally had not seen the marble being moved, and that she would therefore act on the false belief that the marble remained in the basket. Most of the children with autism, by contrast, responded incorrectly 'In the box'. Baron-Cohen et al. interpreted this failure as 'an inability to impute beliefs to others and to predict their behaviour', or 'impaired theory of mind', and argued that this is the main cause of social interaction and communication impairments in autism. Specifically, someone who lacks understanding of other people's knowledge and beliefs will be socially at a loss and communicatively egocentric.

Baron-Cohen et al. ascribed impaired theory of mind to defective metarepresentation as defined in a model of cognitive development that one of the authors, Leslie, was developing at the time. The precise definition of the term 'metarepresentation' has been much discussed – even Leslie changed his original views about how the term should be used (Leslie, 1987; Leslie & Roth, 1993). Box 8.1 contains a simplified account of how metarepresentation may be understood. Full description, analysis and argument can be found in Perner (1991) or Karmiloff-Smith (1992).

BOX 8.1   Representation and metarepresentation: A minimal account

Representations The contents of the mind – what we think about – can be referred to as consisting of 'representations'. Representations in the mind must in reality consist of patterns of neural activity in the brain, but it is convenient to think of them as images or symbols.

Primary representations represent things in the world as they are (sounds, smells, sights), and are acquired from a late stage of prenatal development onwards. Primary representations enable infants to react appropriately to familiar real-world things: for example, a proffered banana evokes a primary representation and the knowledge associated with it (good to eat, etc.), and the infant opens her mouth.

Secondary representations are mental copies, or re-representations, of primary representations, which develop during the second year. Secondary representations can be used in ways that are not constrained by real-world knowledge, and are used to imagine, plan, etc. For example, a proffered banana evokes a primary representation (good to eat, etc.), but a secondary representation may also be evoked that can be used to imagine a banana is a telephone or a long nose.

Metarepresentations are representations of the relationship between something that is known/believed/imagined, etc. and the mental state of knowing/believing/imagining, etc. Only when young children have metarepresentations (at around the age of four years) are they able to represent in their own mind someone else's false belief as distinct from their own true belief; or someone else's ignorance (of a particular fact or happening) as distinct from their own knowledge (of the fact or happening).

Frith's modification of the original theory

Frith (1989) argued against using the term 'theory of mind', describing it as 'cumbersome and misleading' – misleading because 'theory' suggests conscious reasoning, whereas human understanding of other minds is generally unconscious and instantaneous. Frith also pointed out that typically developing infants show some mind-sharing abilities three or more years before they succeed on tests of false belief such as the 'Sally and the marble' task. In particular, by the end of their first year infants will turn their heads to look where someone else is looking, a response known as **gaze following**, as illustrated in Figure 8.1. A little later, infants will turn back to check where the other person is looking, demonstrating awareness that something in the environment can be the object of shared or **joint attention**. In the first half of their second year they start to use protodeclarative pointing (as described and illustrated in

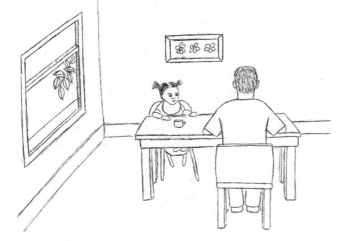

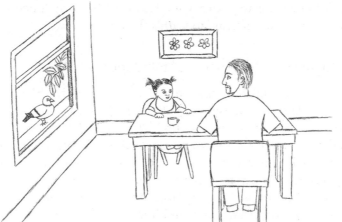

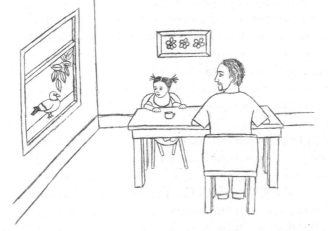

Figure 8.1 Gaze following: the little girl is looking at her father; he turns to look at the bird that has appeared at the window; the little girl follows the direction of his gaze and sees the bird

Chapter 3). Children with ASDs, by contrast, had long been known to lack these early mind-sharing behaviours (Curcio, 1978; Loveland & Landry, 1986; Mundy, Sigman, Ungerer, & Sherman, 1986).

For these reasons Frith (1989) introduced the term **mentalising** in place of 'theory of mind' and suggested that defective mentalising might explain not only failure on false belief tasks, but also the earlier mind-sharing impairments. Frith ascribed mentalising ability to the ability to metarepresent (as in the original Baron-Cohen et al. paper). However, she argued that impaired metarepresentation resulted from **weak central coherence** such as would affect development from infancy onwards (see Chapter 10).

In this book, 'theory of mind' and the acronym 'ToM' will be used to refer to the relatively high-level understanding of other minds that normally develops at around the age of four years. 'Mentalising' will be used to refer to all manifestations of mind-sharing and mind-understanding from infancy onwards when referring to Frith's work. However, the term 'mindreading' will be preferred when not referring to Frith's theoretical views.

Support for the impaired theory of mind theory

Numerous studies confirmed that most individuals with ASDs either never acquire, or are late in acquiring, the ability to pass what became known as 'ToM tasks' (see review by Yirmiya, Erel, Shaked, & Solomonica-Levi, 1998). Some studies used versions of the original **false belief task**; others used the now standard **false appearances test** (sometimes called the 'smarties task'), or the **appearance–reality test**, which typically developing children pass at approximately the same age as they succeed on false belief tasks. Baron-Cohen (1989b), also Ozonoff, Pennington, and Rogers (1991), reported impairments on tests of **second-order belief** ('John thinks that Mary thinks that…').

Further evidence tended to confirm Baron-Cohen et al.'s (1985) claim of a selective impairment in the ability to think about *mental*, as opposed to physical, states. This evidence came from studies in which a Polaroid camera was used to take a picture of one situation (for example, a doll in a red dress); the situation was then changed (to a doll in a blue dress); and children were asked what colour dress the doll is wearing in the picture that will come out of the camera. This is roughly analogous to the standard false belief task, except that instead of the child's answer being dependent on their understanding of Sally's mind, it depends on what picture they think is in the camera. Children with ASDs who failed on standard false belief tasks were nevertheless able to succeed on this **false photographs** task (Leekam & Perner, 1991; Leslie & Thaiss, 1992). This suggested that children with ASDs have a selective problem in understanding *mental* representations, which does not extend to a problem in understanding physical representations. (However, see Bowler, Briskman, Gurvidi, & Fornells-Ambrojo, 2005 for evidence against this conclusion.)

Critique of the theory

Pluses   The original Baron-Cohen et al. (1985) findings were ground-breaking, in that they identified for the first time the difficulty people with ASDs have in knowing what is going on in someone else's mind. Impaired ToM goes a long way towards explaining the social interaction and communication impairments of autism, as the authors originally argued.

In addition, impaired theory of mind is almost certainly a universal characteristic of people with ASDs. This did not at first appear to be the case: not every child with autism failed the ToM tests reported by Baron-Cohen et al. (1985) in their original paper, nor in the tests they and others carried out in the years immediately following. However, it is now generally considered that those high-functioning individuals who can pass false belief tasks have learned how to **hack out**, or effortfully *work out*, what other people might falsely believe (Happé, 1994). These able people still lack the usual *intuitive* understanding of other minds. Thus an impairment of intuitive mentalising, to use Frith's preferred term, is universal.

Problems   There were, however, some significant limitations and problems with the theory.

1   Many groups of people fail ToM tests but do not socially interact and communicate in ways that suggest autism. Most obviously, typically developing children below the age of three and a half years rarely pass false belief tasks and may therefore be described as lacking theory of mind; but they are not autistic. Similarly, deaf children often have delayed ability to pass false belief tasks (Peterson & Siegal, 1995) as do individuals with intellectual disability, some of whom never acquire theory of mind (Yirmiya et al., 1998; Zelazo, Burack, Benedetto, & Frye, 1996). Few deaf children, and only a minority of individuals with intellectual disability are, however, autistic. Thus impaired ToM as an explanation of autism-related socio-communication impairments fails to meet the **specificity criterion**.

    Impaired ToM cannot, therefore, by itself explain the social interaction and communication impairments diagnostic of autism. Something else must be involved that affects people with ASDs, but not very young children or people with hearing impairment or (generally speaking) people with intellectual disability. Impaired ToM may therefore be a *necessary* contributory cause of the socio-communicative impairments characteristic of autism. However, it is not by itself *sufficient* to cause them.

2   The claim that impaired ToM results from a fundamental inability to metarepresent is untenable because it does not satisfy the primacy criterion (see Chapter 6). Metarepresentational ability as understood in Leslie's original theory is not observed in typically developing children until, approximately, age four years. Many of the social interaction impairments typical of autism, however, including lack of gaze following, joint attention, and protodeclarative pointing, are apparent in children with ASDs much earlier than this, as noted by Frith (1989). Impaired metarepresentational ability has no power, therefore, to explain these early occurring impairments. Frith initially avoided this difficulty by suggesting that weak central coherence (WCC) (which would be present from birth) might explain the whole gamut of social impairments. However, she later moved away from this suggestion, seeing impaired metarepresentation (and mentalising ability) and

weak central coherence as independent causes of the social and non-social impairments in autism, respectively (Frith, 2003).

3 The impaired ToM theory cannot explain the emotion processing impairments that are inextricably associated with the social and communicative impairments in autism, except in as far as complex emotions such as embarrassment or guilt require some understanding of how others perceive us.

In sum, impaired ToM may well be a common pathway or convergence point on the causal route leading to autism. However, something additional, earlier occurring and more fundamental, must also be involved.

Other Theories of the Origins of Impaired Theory of Mind

Although it was widely accepted that impaired theory of mind is central to the impairments of social interaction and communication in autism, several theorists argued against the suggestion that impaired ToM results from defective metarepresentation. Some attempts to explain impaired ToM in people with ASDs in terms of cognitive deficits other than defective metarepresentation are outlined below.

Harris (1989, 1991) suggested that the poor performance of people with ASDs on ToM tasks could be explained in terms of a fundamental deficit in the ability to **simulate** or imagine other people's mental states. Most importantly, from the outset of the discussion of the origins of impaired ToM in people with ASDs, Harris stressed the importance of simulating emotional and **volitional** states (feelings and desires) as well as **epistemic** states (to do with knowledge and beliefs). He wrote:

> An inability to understand people's beliefs would render their mistaken actions quite puzzling: 'Why on earth is she looking for her toys in that cupboard if it's empty?' An inability to grasp their desires, on the other hand, would make their actions completely incomprehensible…. 'Why is she moving toward that cupboard; why is she now pulling at its door; why is she now looking inside?' (Harris, 1989: 203).

Such meaninglessness of others' actions could well explain the social indifference and social avoidance so often characteristic of young children with autism.

Russell (1997) suggested that the poor performance of people with ASDs on ToM tasks resulted from a lack of executive control. He pointed out that to succeed on the 'Sally and the marbles' test the child being tested has to inhibit the **prepotent response** of stating where the marble actually is in favour of stating where Sally erroneously believes it to be. A somewhat similar suggestion was made in Peterson and Bowler's (2000) impaired **counterfactual reasoning** theory. Executive dysfunctions, including evidence for impaired inhibition of prepotent responses in people with ASDs, are described in more detail in Chapter 9.

Others proposed more language-related explanations. In particular, it was suggested by De Villiers (2000) and by Frye et al. (Frye, Zelazo, & Palfai, 1995; Zelazo, Jacques, Burack, & Frye, 2002) that the ability to pass false belief tasks is dependent on forms of reasoning that involve complex grammatical constructions. Frye et al., for example, argued that the ability to pass false belief tasks involves the use of **embedded rules**. Embedded rules are rules within rules, as in the following example, in which the embedded rules are shown in square brackets:

> If the lights at the crossing are flashing on amber, then [if no pedestrian at the crossing, drive on]; but [if pedestrian attempting to cross, stop].

In the 'Sally and the marble' task the embedded rules are:

> If searching for the marble, then [if me, look in the box]; but [if Sally, look in the basket].

These authors' **cognitive complexity and control (CCC)** theory grew out of a model of cognitive development in which the typically developing preschool child's increasing powers of reasoning are explained in terms of successive increases in consciousness resembling the stages of representational development outlined in Box 8.1 (Zelazo & Zelazo, 1998; compare Perner, 1991; Karmiloff-Smith, 1992; Leslie, & Roth, 1993). Frye et al.'s explanation of impaired ToM in autism therefore resembles the impaired metarepresentation theory in that both theories propose that people with ASDs have problems of **metacognition**, or, 'thinking about thinking'.

Critique of other explanations

Pluses The diverse set of alternative explanations of the failure of children with ASDs on ToM tasks illustrates both the complexity of the issues and the inevitable complexity of the eventual explanation of impaired ToM. Thus, Harris is almost certainly correct in identifying the ability to *comprehend and share others' emotions* as important for the development of theory of mind. Equally, it is now widely accepted that *executive control* is necessary for passing false belief tasks, as suggested in several of the theories outlined above, although controversy remains concerning relationships between ToM, metarepresentation, and executive function (Perner & Lang, 1999; Leslie, Friedman, & German, 2004). There is also ample evidence to show that performance on ToM tasks is related to *language ability* in neurotypical individuals as well as in individuals with autism, although here again the nature of the relationship is controversial (Tager-Flusberg, 2000; Fisher, Happé, & Dunn, 2005; Slade & Ruffman, 2005).

Problems None of the alternative explanations of impaired ToM outlined above has been shown to meet the specificity criterion. Executive functions, in particular, are well known to be impaired in several developmental disorders other than autism (see Chapter 9). Nor is there sufficient evidence to show which, if any, of the proposed deficits occur universally in people with ASDs.

With regard to the primacy or causal precedence criterion, all the hypothesised impairments (of simulation, response inhibition, a capacity for counterfactual thinking or use of embedded rules) may well meet the primacy criterion as explanations of failure on ToM tasks. However, as Frith pointed out in 1989, it is more important to explain the earlier signs of impaired mindsharing. Any attempt to explain these impairments in terms of defective counterfactual reasoning or inability to use embedded rules would undoubtedly fail the primacy criterion. An attempt to explain the earliest signs of autism in terms of defective simulation or impaired inhibition might satisfy the primacy criterion. However, none of these theories were in fact proposed as explanations of those signs of autism that are apparent within the first and second years of life. By contrast, the **mindblindness** theory, considered next, was explicitly proposed as an explanation of those mind-sharing abilities that precede theory of mind in normal development.

The Mindblindness Theory

Mindreading and mindblindness

The term 'mindblindness' offers a striking metaphor of an inability to understand what minds are, to 'read' the minds of others or to introspect about one's own mind. This is not the same as not having a mind: a dog clearly *has* a mind, but it does not *know* it has a mind; it does not understand what a mind is; and it cannot reflect on the contents of the mind of another dog (their thoughts or feelings) or on the contents of its own mind. A dog may read another animal's *behaviour*, but it cannot read *minds*. Baron-Cohen's central claim, spelled out in his book *Mindblindness* (1995), is that this is true, also, for people with autism: not only do they fail at the stage of acquiring a theory of mind, but also at an earlier, critical stage in the incremental process of becoming a mindreader. This process is described next, according to Baron-Cohen's model.

Baron-Cohen's mindreading model

Baron-Cohen (1995) proposed a model of the abilities that underlie typically developing children's mindreading ability. The model is shown in Figure 8.2 (adapted from Baron-Cohen, 1995: 32).

The **intention detector** and the **eye direction detector** enable neonates and babies to acquire knowledge of **mental states** from **dyadic interactions** (two-way, face-to-face interactions) between themselves and another person. The **shared attention mechanism**, however, comes on stream towards the end of the first year, enabling the infant to engage in **triadic** (three-way)

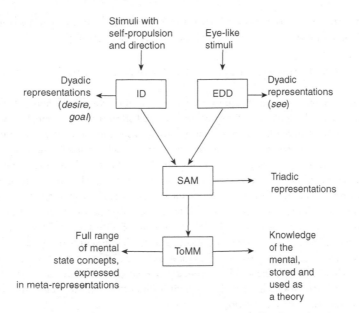

Figure 8.2 Baron-Cohen's model of 'the mindreading system'. ID = intention detector; EDD = eye direction detector; SAM = shared attention mechanism; ToMM = theory of mind mechanism (from Baron-Cohen, 1995: 32 with permission of MIT Press)

interactions in which two people knowingly share a mental state that relates to a third focus of interest (as illustrated in Figure 3.1). (Note that use of the terms dyadic and triadic to refer to two-way as compared to three-way social interactions is distinct from use of the terms to identify a dyad (pair) or triad (trio) of autism-diagnostic behaviours.)

According to Baron-Cohen's 1995 account, the fundamental psychological cause of impaired social interaction and communication in autism is a defective shared attention mechanism. Baron-Cohen supported his claim with reference to numerous experimental findings, a summary of which can be found in Baron-Cohen (1999).

Critique of the mindblindness theory

Pluses The mindblindness theory was an advance on the impaired ToM theory in that it was capable of explaining some of the early occurring social abnormalities in autism, including the impairments of joint attention and protodeclarative pointing.

Research has shown that early occurring impairments of shared (or joint) attention are *specific* to autism (Baird et al., 2000). In practical terms this means that if a toddler is observed to lack these abilities at around 18–20 months, it is highly likely that a full diagnostic assessment at some later stage will show them to have an ASD. Impaired triadic relating in early childhood is also *universal* in autism (Leekam, Lopez, & Moore, 2000).

Problems   Despite the gains made by the theory, some problems remain.

1   The explanation is circular because it explains impaired triadic relating (which includes impaired shared attention) in terms of an impaired shared attention mechanism.
2   The impaired shared attention mechanism hypothesis meets the primacy or causal precedence criterion in so far as it can explain impairments of triadic relating. However, dyadic (one-to-one) relating is not unimpaired in infants with incipient autism, as is implied by the theory. Home videos of infants aged 9–12 months who were subsequently diagnosed as autistic show that these children were less likely than typically developing infants to respond to their own names or to look at other people's faces; they were also averse to social touch (Adrien et al., 1993; Osterling & Dawson, 1994; Baranek, 1999). These are all behaviours involving dyadic relating. Impairments of dyadic relating persist into later infancy and beyond in children with ASDs (Charman, Swettenham, Baron-Cohen, Cox, Baird, & Drew, 1997; Leekam & Ramsden, 2006). As an explanation of the earliest manifestations of incipient autism, therefore, the mindblindness hypothesis fails to meet the primacy criterion.
3   The model says almost nothing about emotions, although by 1995 there was plenty of evidence of specific problems of emotion recognition and of impaired empathic responsiveness in children with ASDs (Sigman et al., 1992; Yirmiya, Sigman, Kasari, & Mundy, 1992). Baron-Cohen was, however, aware of this gap in his model, stating that 'future models of mindreading will need to give a full account of the role of emotion in this domain' (Baron-Cohen, 1995: 136). In his latest theory, the extreme male brain theory, defective empathy figures prominently as a cause of the social impairments associated with autism, as explained later in the chapter.

PRIMARY INTERSUBJECTIVITY DEFICIT THEORIES

The Concept of Primary Intersubjectivity

The term **primary intersubjectivity** was coined by Trevarthen (1980) to refer to the kind of face-to-face interaction referred to above as 'dyadic relating'. Trevarthen used the term **secondary intersubjectivity** synonymously with what was referred to above as 'triadic relating' (Trevarthen & Hubley, 1978; see Trevarthen & Aitken, 2001, for a review of research relating to intersubjectivity). The terms 'primary intersubjectivity' and 'secondary intersubjectivity' will generally be preferred to 'dyadic relating' and 'triadic relating', to avoid potential confusion between 'triadic relating' and a 'triad' of autism-related impairments.

Primary intersubjectivity between infants and carers involves behaviours such as eye-to-eye gazing, looking and smiling, imitation of facial postures (such as mouth opening, lip pursing), imitative noise-making, and face-to-face lap play involving shared affect. The dynamic characteristics of these behaviours are identified in Box 8.2 using quotes from a review of early infant behaviours and their relevance for autism.

BOX 8.2   Characteristics of primary intersubjectivity between very young infants and carers

Temporal co-ordination of mothers' and infants' expressions and movements
'By six months mothers and [typically developing] infants have well-established patterns for synchrony and attunement: they know each other intimately and are able to predict each other's [emotional] expressions in time.'

The protoconversational character of mother–infant interactions 'Studies of the vocal expressions of mothers and infants in face-to-face interaction have highlighted the precise temporal and prosodic organisation of their utterances and their use of protoconversational rules such as turn-taking.... Between two and six months infants are particularly expressive in the vocal register; they actively respond to and initiate vocal engagement with interactive partners and they spontaneously imitate or mirror their mothers' expressions.'

Perceptual abilities supporting protoconversational interactions 'The timing of vocal interaction is organized around the close matching and monitoring of affect by mother and infant, as expressed through acoustic cues such as pitch, loudness, and timbre. The overall temporal structure of vocal interaction has been found to present a high degree of regularity with clear rhythmic features... From the first six months of life, infants are sensitive to temporal structure in both the auditory and visual modalities, and are particularly attuned to the perception of subtle temporal changes in linguistic and musical stimuli... [and] can discriminate between different visual rhythms.'

(Extracts from Sigman, Dijamco, Gratier, & Rozga, 2004: 223)

The quotes in Box 8.2 emphasise the following points.

- The importance of affect, or emotion, in the interactions between mothers and very young infants.
- The role of imitation.
- The centrality of faces and voices – pre-eminently social stimuli – as the vehicles of the interactions.
- The importance of timing and rhythm.

The next four subsections describe groups of primary intersubjectivity deficit theories, each group relating particularly to one of the four characteristics listed above. All the theories described would cause impaired secondary intersubjectivity (including impaired joint attention and impaired protodeclarative pointing), and thereafter impaired theory of mind.

Theories Emphasising Emotion Processing

Hobson's impaired interpersonal relatedness theory

Hobson's (1993) book *Autism and the Development of Mind* is as important in the search for the causes of autism as was Baron-Cohen, Leslie, and Frith's (1985) paper on impaired theory of mind, because it anticipated the kind of primary intersubjectivity deficit explanations now increasingly argued for. Hobson fully accepted the evidence of impaired ToM in autism. However, he argued against Baron-Cohen et al.'s explanation of these findings in terms of a fundamental deficit of metarepresentation. He proposed instead an explanation rooted in the earliest forms of dyadic social interaction between babies and their carers, emphasising the role of emotional relatedness and reciprocity.

Hobson proposed that typically developing infants are biologically prewired to relate to people in ways that are special to people, and that it is this innate readiness to relate *emotionally* to people that is lacking in autism. In other words, Hobson reiterated Kanner's early hypothesis of 'an innate inability to form the usual biologically provided affective contact with people'. However, Hobson elaborated the hypothesis and extended it to explain the recently demonstrated problems in understanding other minds. He was also able to cite a great deal of evidence from both typical development and the study of emotion processing in children with autism, evidence unavailable to Kanner.

Hobson summarised the core of his argument as follows:

> It is through the experience of reciprocal, affectively patterned interpersonal contact that a young child comes to apprehend and eventually to conceptualise the nature of persons with mental life. (Hobson, 1993: 104)

An example he gave of 'reciprocal, affectively patterned interpersonal contact' is the common human experience of 'You smile (and feel happy): I smile (and feel happy)'; 'You look sad (and feel sad): I look sad (and feel sad)'. He then argued that a problem in *experiencing* another person's emotions responsively (feeling happy when they smile, sad when they look sad) would impair the ability to *perceive* another person's emotions. This, Hobson suggested, amounts to **affective agnosia**, or, **emotion blindness**.

Emotion blindness would diminish the very young infant's desire for social interaction because there would be no shared pleasure in it, only a self-centred pleasure from the sensations provided by, for example, being rocked or tickled. More importantly, the lack of co-experience of emotion would impair the ability to realise (unconsciously, of course) that other people have emotions like the child's own: that Daddy can feel happy or sad, *like me*. Thus the infant misses out on the first stage of understanding about others' (and their own) mental states. They also fail to appreciate the essential difference between people and objects: namely that people have experiences and feelings, unlike tables and chairs.

A little later in development, when the typically developing infant under-stands that Daddy wants (and I want) the cake, the infant with an ASD will have no understanding of the shared 'wanting', and the shared attention to, the cake. Protodeclarative communication, such as bringing and showing or point-ing at something interesting, will not occur because the child has no awareness of the possibility of sharing mental states.

Baron-Cohen's impaired empathising system theory

Ten years after the original model of a mindreading system was presented, Baron-Cohen (2005) published an updated and extended model of the route into mindreading, which he renamed the **empathising system**. The empathis-ing system is contrasted with the **systemising mechanism** (Baron-Cohen, 2006), the latter being generally better developed in males and the former generally better developed in females. According to this theory, people with ASDs have an extreme form of the typical male brain and this renders their empathising system defective (Baron-Cohen et al., 2005). The focus on impaired empathy as the main cause of socio-communication impairments in autism builds on a similar suggestion by Brothers (1997), whose identification of systems within 'the social brain' was referred to in Chapter 7.

Like the original mindreading system, the empathising system is seen as an innate psychological system, or module, made up of dissociable subsystems, or, minimodules. Thus, added to the original mindreading model are two minimod-ules named, respectively, the **emotion detector** and the empathising system. Baron-Cohen has not, at the time of writing, proposed a definitive hypothesis as to which component of the empathising system is malfunctioning in infants with incipient autism. If it is the emotion detector, this would bring his theory into line with other primary intersubjectivity deficit theories that place the origins of the social impairments of autism within the very young infant's two-way interaction abilities, and specifically those involved in emotion processing.

Defective integration theories

This group of theories revolves around the fact that normal experience, whether social or not, almost always involves affective (emotion-related) as well as perceptual and cognitive content, and these components are experi-enced as integrally related.

Hermelin and O'Connor (1985) were the first to suggest that in autism there is a problem in the integration of the affective and cognitive components of experience. This problem would lead to questions such as 'Did I like it when I went on the bouncy castle?' (see the section on empathy in Chapter 3). Ben Shalom (2000a; Faran & Ben Shalom, 2008) has proposed the more specific hypothesis that people with ASDs experience the physiological components of emotion but fail to associate this experience with whatever stimulated the emotion. Thus someone with an ASD might see a snake and experience a cold sweat without automatically connecting the sweat with the snake. Equally, an infant with an ASD would experience the physical pleasure of being stroked or tickled, but they would not associate the pleasurable feelings with the person stroking or tickling. This theory fits well with the observation that, whilst emotion contagion and the raw experience of basic emotions is intact in people with ASDs, understanding of what other people's or one's own emotion *is about* (that is to say, the cognitive as opposed to the affective component of any experience) is not integrated with the raw feel.

Other theorists see the integration failure as specific to social, as opposed to non-social, experience (Sigman & Capps, 1997; Sigman et al., 2004). Mundy (1995, 2003) focuses on the possible neurobiological basis of such a failure. He identifies specific regions within the social brain that normally mediate social reward, but which function anomalously in people with ASDs. Mundy's detailed arguments and evidence thus constitute a development of Fotheringham's (1991) theory, mentioned in the section 'Early Theories' at the beginning of this chapter.

Loveland (2001) has a somewhat different perception from other integration theorists concerning what constitutes 'reward value' within a social interaction. Whereas Ben Shalom emphasises the physiological phenomena associated with emotion – the raw 'feel' of the different emotions – and Mundy emphasises a 'social reward' system in the brain, Loveland hypothesises that there is a failure to connect social stimuli such as faces and voices to their learned **affordances** such as would imbue them with pleasurable associations. Affordances are defined rather charmingly as the 'invitational' quality of something. Some of the invitational qualities that a parent might have for a young child are illustrated in Figure 8.3.

Theories Emphasising Imitation

As with so many theories about the causes of autism, the suggestion that defective imitation might help to explain at least some aspects of autism was made by some early theorists (DeMyer et al., 1972; Jones & Prior, 1985). It was not until 1991, however, that a paper by Rogers and Pennington brought this hypothesis into prominence. Basing their theory on the work of Trevarthen and also Stern (1985), Rogers and Pennington argued that a fundamental deficit in imitation would have a cascade of effects on emotion sharing, secondary intersubjectivity, and theory of mind.

Meltzoff and Gopnik (1993) extended the suggestions made by Rogers and Pennington. Meltzoff and Gopnik suggested that, whereas typically developing infants have an innate ability to associate others' movements that they *see* with their own imitative movements that they *feel* (in the sense of experiencing them kinaesthetically), infants who will develop autism do not make this association. Meltzoff and Gopnik suggested that the first step along the route to acquiring a theory of mind occurs when babies imitate the facial postures or hand gestures of another person and understand that 'Here is something

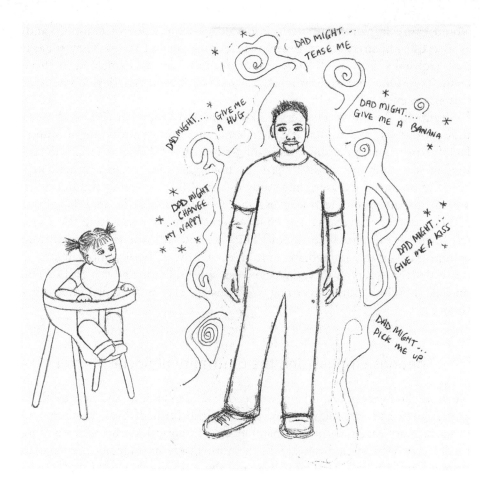

Figure 8.3 Examples of some of the 'affordances' a father might have for a young child, according to Loveland's (2001) theory

like me'. Subsequent studies of young children with early signs of autism reported by Gopnik, Capps, and Meltzoff (2001) and by Rogers, Hepburn, Stackhouse, and Wehner (2003) have confirmed the prediction that defective imitation and impaired mindreading abilities are related in children with ASDs.

Williams, Whiten, Suddendorf, and Perrett (2001) took this argument a step further. These authors argue that both imitation and the ability to simulate or imagine the mental states of others (as suggested by Harris, quoted earlier in this chapter) are ultimately dependent on mirror neurons (Gallese, Keysers, & Rizzolatti, 2004). Mirror neurons have the unique double role of being activated when an individual carries out an action themselves, and also being activated (below threshold levels) when seeing someone else carrying out that action. Williams et al. hypothesise that dysfunctional mirror neurons would cause impaired imitation, impaired co-experience of emotion, and, as a result, impaired ability to simulate others' mental states. They suggest that Hobson's 'lack of affective responsiveness' can be explained in these terms (see Oberman & Ramachandran, 2007, for further development of this argument).

McIntosh, Reichman-Decker, Winkielman, and Wilbarger (2006) showed that adolescents and adults lack the normal involuntary imitation of others' facial expressions, providing interesting support for Williams et al.'s defective mirror neurons theory. There is, however, some contrary evidence, albeit of an anecdotal kind. In a study of the ability of young children with autism to interpret facial expressions, Gepner, Deruelle, and Grynfeltt (2001) observed several of the children spontaneously imitating the facial expressions presented to them. This is not an isolated observation: **echopraxia**, or the immediate imitation of others' bodily movements, is quite widely observed in younger or less able individuals with ASDs. The jury is therefore out concerning Williams et al.'s potentially interesting theory.

Theories Emphasising the Centrality of Social Stimuli

Newborn and very young infants are needy and demanding, and new mothers are fatigued and sometimes depressed after the birth. If birth mothers and other primary carers are not to abandon their infants, the process of **bonding** must occur reliably and quickly. Birth mothers are hormonally prepared to respond preferentially to their babies, and there is some evidence that fathers who are closely involved with the birth and earliest care of their newborn babies may also experience hormonal changes that facilitate bonding (Storey, Walsh, Quinton, & Wynne-Edwards, 2000).

In addition, evolution has ensured that babies are rewarding in that they respond preferentially and engagingly to their primary carer(s) from the moment they are born. Some examples of neonates' and very young infants' people-oriented behaviours are described in Box 8.3.

These innate, or **hardwired**, responses make the people around them, and especially those most familiar to them, feel rewarded and special, helping to cement the bonding process from the first days of life. Emotion sharing and imitation are, of course, part of this. However, the perception and discrimination of social stimuli, and **selective attention** to this class of stimuli, are necessary if emotion sharing and imitation are to take place. The hypotheses to be considered in this section converge on the suggestion that infants who will become autistic lack one or other of the required attentional or perceptual mechanisms. However, the theories differ as to where the fundamental problem(s) might lie.

BOX 8.3   Examples of typically developing infants' preferential social responsiveness

Neonates

- already know their mother's voice and prefer it to any other;
- recognise their mother's smell and the taste of her breast milk within a day, and preferentially seek it out;
- attend to human faces in preference to other visual stimuli, and are attentive to faces to the extent that they attempt to imitate facial postures (e.g., mouth opening; tongue protrusion);
- prefer human voices, especially female voices, to other auditory stimuli;
- reflexively turn their heads towards a touch on the cheek; grasp a proffered finger.

Week-old babies

- prefer their mother's face to any other face (if she is their main carer).

Six–ten-week-old babies

- hold another's face-to-face gaze as if entranced, and smile in response to a smiling face.

(Supporting references can be found in Berk & Ashkenaz, 2006)

Problems of preferential attention and social orienting?

Dawson and her colleagues coined the term **social orienting**, now widely used to refer to the innate bias of neonates and very young babies to attend preferentially to faces and voices and to respond accordingly (see for example Dawson, 1991; Dawson, Meltzoff, Osterling, & Rinaldi, 1998a; Dawson et al., 2004). Klin (1991) showed that young children with ASDs do not attend preferentially to their mother's voice. Dawson et al., also Leekam et al. (2000) extended this observation by showing that young children with ASDs turn to look at non-social sounds such as the noise of a rattle, or non-social visual stimuli such as the appearance of an interesting toy, whereas they do not respond to the sounds made by people or turn to look at people. Dawson et al. (2004) have also shown that a lack of social orienting is a useful way of distinguishing young children with ASDs from other children: in other words, it is specific to young children with ASDs.

Dawson and her colleagues suggest that impaired social orienting results from failure to associate social stimuli with emotional reward. Although their emphasis is on the lack of preferential responsiveness to social stimuli, Dawson et al.'s theoretical position is therefore close to that of the 'impaired integration' theorists, whose views were outlined in the previous section.

Leekam (2005) agrees that impaired social orienting is likely to be related to motivational and affective factors. However, she points out that the direction of cause and effect could go either way: a fundamental deficit in social orienting might cause impaired affective responsiveness; equally, a lack of affective responsiveness might cause impaired social orienting. Tager-Flusberg and Sullivan (2000), however, suggest that impaired social orienting could result from a face- and voice-specific perceptual impairment, rather than either an attentional or motivational impairment. This hypothesis is consistent with evidence of anomalous face and voice processing in older children and adults with ASDs, including evidence of abnormalities in the brain systems involved (for reviews see Dawson et al., 2005, or Jemel et al., 2006, on face processing; Gervais et al., 2004, on voice processing). However, there have been no studies of face and voice perception and discrimination in very young children with autism, such as would be required to confirm the hypothesis.

Theories Emphasising Timing

We live in a four-dimensional universe, and just as all animals have inbuilt mechanisms for perceiving, learning about, and acting in space, they also have inbuilt mechanisms for perceiving, learning about, and acting through time (Gallistel, 1993). Social stimuli, notably faces, voices, and body movements, are essentially dynamic in the sense of moving through time. Voices are temporal, non-spatial stimuli, and a static voice is a contradiction in terms. The kinds of movement and touch that babies respond to, such as rocking and jiggling, tickling and stroking, are temporally patterned, rhythmical, and predictable through repetition. It has been argued that interactive timing is crucial for the normal development of primary intersubjectivity, and thereafter secondary intersubjectivity, communication and language (Newson & Newson, 1975; Trevarthen & Aitken, 2001; Feldman, 2007).

People with ASDs have a poor sense of the passage of time, as commonly reported in first-hand accounts, and by parents, teachers, and other carers (Wing, 1996; Peeters & Gillberg, 1999). These observations have led a few clinician-theorists to suggest that defective timing mechanisms may underlie the failure to engage in normal two-way social interaction, with a cascade of effects on secondary intersubjectivity, theory of mind, social interaction and communication. Newson (1984) and Trevarthen (1989) were the first to propose a defective timing explanation of the socio-communicative impairments in autism. Wimpory, Nicholas, & Nash (2002) also proposed this hypothesis, later supporting their theory with evidence that the **clock genes** involved in the development of brain mechanisms for timing are abnormal in people with ASDs (Nicholas, Rudrasingham, Nash, Kirov, Owen, & Wimpory, 2007). More is said about possible time-processing deficits in autism in Chapter 12.

Critique of Primary Intersubjectivity Deficit Theories

Pluses

1 The main strength of this group of theories is they identify problems that would affect development from the earliest weeks and months of life. They have the potential, therefore, to explain those manifestations of social, emotional and communicative abnormality that are apparent in infants younger than one year old who are subsequently diagnosed with an ASD, as well as the later-occurring impairments of secondary intersubjectivity (triadic relating) and theory of mind. These theories therefore meet the primacy criterion.

2 Evidence to date suggests that social orienting and emotion responsiveness are *always* impaired in young children with ASDs, but *not impaired* (or not impaired in the same ways) in young children with other developmental delays and difficulties. It seems likely, therefore, that primary intersubjectivity deficit theories also meet the specificity criterion. However, more evidence is needed.

3 Abnormalities of affect are stressed within all the theories, several of which suggest ways in which emotion processing deficits might be fundamental, rather than occurring only as a secondary effect of impaired ToM.

4 Explanation of spared socio-communicative abilities is attempted by at least some of the theories: see for example the sections on attachment and on protoimperative pointing in Hobson (1993).

5 The theories are **grounded** in established knowledge concerning the basic building blocks of primary intersubjectivity in typically developing infants, such as innate reflexes, pre-set sensitivity to certain sensory stimuli and thereby **attentional biases**, and conditionability leading to rapid learning. These are all well-established genetically determined mechanisms that set typically developing babies on the road to normal social, emotional and communicative development. To the extent that these building blocks may be psychologically primitive and irreducible, they are at least the *kinds* of processes that must figure in fundamental explanations of autism at the psychological level.

6 Some of the theories go further and suggest brain mechanisms that might be involved in some of these processes, for example specific impairments within the social brain (Mundy); defective mirror neurons underlying infant imitation and emotion contagion (Williams et al.); or abnormal brain waves (oscillations) subserving fine-grained timing (Wimpory et al.). In the long term, psychological explanations of autism must interface with neurobiological explanations: in other words they must be neuropsychological. Explanation in terms of neuropsychological processes avoids the use of **place-holder** terms such as 'the empathy detector' that have unproven neuropsychological reality. Here again, therefore, the right *kind* of explanation is being proposed – even if the actual theories are unproven.

7 Finally, the convergence of opinion is noteworthy. Although the precise mechanisms underlying impaired primary intersubjectivity in infants with incipient autism are not fully agreed, the various theories outlined above are potentially consistent with each other. And it may well be the case that different mechanisms underlie impaired primary intersubjectivity in different children, though all go on to have problems of secondary intersubjectivity, theory of mind, and anomalous social, emotional, and communicative behaviours.

Problems

1 Contrary evidence. All the theories reviewed in this section imply that impairments of primary intersubjectivity will be detectable from birth or very soon afterwards: certainly the mechanisms invoked are those known to be present in typically developing neonates and

infants in the first months of life. However, there is at least one research report of a child studied from birth who showed relatively normal social responsiveness during the first six months of life, with gradual deterioration during the second half of the first year to the point at which a diagnosis of autism was made in the child's second year (Dawson, Osterling, Meltzoff, & Kuhl, 2000). Moreover, normal early development with subsequent deterioration is quite commonly reported by parents (see the section 'Age of Onset' in Chapter 4). This kind of evidence is quite difficult for the defective primary intersubjectivity theories to explain, at least in their present form.

2 Alternative non-social explanations have not been ruled out. The problems of primary intersubjectivity that have been considered in this section could, in theory at least, be caused by fundamental deficits that are not specifically to do with social functioning, but which affect both social and non-social aspects of development equally. For example, it might be argued that problems of primary intersubjectivity result from impairments of early occurring components of executive function, such as attention switching, or from the kind of fragmented perceptual processing identified in weak central coherence theory. Executive dysfunctions in autism are discussed at some length in Chapter 9, and weak central coherence in Chapter 10. Relations between social impairments, executive function, and central coherence in people with ASDs are discussed in Chapter 11.

SUMMARY

There is robust evidence that people with ASDs across the spectrum have persistent problems with what has been variously called theory of mind (ToM), mentalising, and mindreading ability. This evidence has made a significant contribution towards explaining the social and communication impairments in older children and adults with ASDs. However, impaired ToM is not a sufficient explanation of these impairments because other groups of individuals, such as young children, lack ToM but are not autistic. Nor can impaired ToM explain the socio-communicative impairments that occur in very young children with incipient autism, because typically developing children do not succeed on ToM tasks until around the age of four years. The ToM theory also fails to explain most of the emotion processing impairments that are part of the social interaction impairment in autism.

Numerous explanations of the ToM impairment itself were proposed in the 1990s. These explanations included defective metarepresentation, impaired simulation, executive dysfunction, language-related deficits, and malfunction of a shared attention mechanism. However, none of these hypothetical explanations offers an adequate explanation of the abnormalities of social interaction seen in infants with incipient autism within the first year of life.

Primary intersubjectivity and dyadic relating are interchangeable terms that refer to the very young infant's two-way, face-to-face interactions with another person. Secondary intersubjectivity and triadic relating are interchangeable terms referring to three-way interactions in which two people knowingly share an interest in, or focus on, a third object, person or event. Several current theories propose that deficits in one or other aspect of primary intersubjectivity cause impairments of secondary intersubjectivity, such as a lack of shared attention, and thereafter impaired theory of mind. Many of these theories stress problems of emotion processing or the integration of emotional feeling with social experience. Other theories hypothesise that defective imitation constitutes the primary deficit, possibly associated with dysfunctional mirror neurons. Another group of theories identifies deficits in social orienting (preferential attention and responsiveness to social stimuli) as primary. Finally, a few clinician-theorists have hypothesised that autism derives from a fundamental deficit in the timing mechanisms that co-ordinate the dyadic interactions essential for learning about people.

Theories implicating primary intersubjectivity deficits as fundamental to the social and communication impairments of autism are attractive for several reasons. In particular, they have the potential to satisfy the primacy criterion in that they identify very early occurring social interaction problems, which may well be universal in infants who are later diagnosed with an ASD; the role of emotion processing abnormalities is assumed (in contrast to the almost exclusively cognitivist earlier theories); some of the theories attempt to explain why certain aspects of social interaction and communication are not affected in people with ASDs, as well as explaining why other aspects of social interaction are affected; and the theories are grounded in basic processes that it is well-known are present in typically developing infants, thereby avoiding the circularity of invoking special mechanisms with doubtful neuropsychological status. However, primary intersubjectivity deficit theories may find it difficult to accommodate the evidence that a proportion of individuals subsequently diagnosed with an ASD have apparently entirely normal social interactions in early infancy. In addition, it may be the case that impairments of primary intersubjectivity derive from fundamental deficits that affect both social and non-social behaviours equally, such as weak central coherence or executive dysfunctions.

EXPLAINING THE REPETITIVE BEHAVIOURS AND LACK OF IMAGINATIVE CREATIVITY

AIMS

••••

INTRODUCTION
What Has to be Explained
Contributory Causes that are not Specific to Autism

••••

EXECUTIVE FUNCTIONS: DESCRIPTION AND DEFINITIONS
Broad Usage: An Umbrella Term
Narrow Usage: The Central Executive in Working Memory

••••

EXECUTIVE FUNCTIONS IN PEOPLE WITH AUTISM
Problems of Stopping
Problems of Shifting: Mental Inflexibility
Problems of Starting
Problems of Organisation and Monitoring
Limitations of Research into Executive Functions in People with ASDs

••••

LOCATING EXECUTIVE FUNCTION IMPAIRMENTS WITHIN THE
CAUSAL CHAIN
'Upwards' Links: Do Impaired Executive Functions Cause Behavioural
Inflexibility?
'Downwards' Links: What Causes Executive Function Impairments
in Autism?
Critique of Executive Dysfunction Explanations of Behavioural Inflexibility

••••

OTHER 'CRITICAL CAUSE' THEORIES
Hypersystemising as a Critical Cause of Behavioural Inflexibility
Overuse of Spared Abilities as a Critical Cause of Behavioural Inflexibility

••••

SUMMARY

INTRODUCTION

What Has to be Explained

The behaviours brought together under the headings of restricted and repetitive behaviours (DSM-IV) and lack of imaginative creativity (Wing) are diverse. Behaviours that fall under these descriptions and are mentioned in the DSM-IV criteria (though not always under the heading of restricted and repetitive behaviours) are as follows.

- Encompassing preoccupation with one or more stereotyped and restricted patterns of interest that are abnormal either in intensity or focus.
- Apparently inflexible adherence to specific, non-functional routines or rituals.
- Stereotyped and repetitive motor mannerisms (for example, hand flapping, rocking).
- Persistent preoccupation with parts of objects.
- Stereotyped and repetitive use of language.
- Lack of varied, spontaneous make-believe play or social imitative play appropriate to developmental level.

Other repetitive behaviours that are common include the following.

- Insistence on sameness (this was included in earlier definitions of autism).
- Obsessions or compulsions (such as hair pulling or eating non-food substances).
- Self-injury (for example, biting the hands, or poking fingers into eyes).

Other aspects of lack of imaginative creativity that are extremely common are:

- impaired planning;
- impaired initiation of novel actions.

Not all of these kinds of behaviour occur in every individual with an ASD. In addition, an individual may have one form of restricted or repetitive behaviour as a young child, which is replaced with other forms with increasing age. So, for example, hand flapping and toe-walking are common in young children with an ASD but less common in adults, except those who are very low-functioning. Similarly, echolalia is quite common in young children or adults with poor language comprehension, but as comprehension improves, echolalia may be replaced by repetitive use of **formulaic** phrases and monologuing on a preferred topic. So the repetitiveness remains, but is manifested in different ways.

In addition to the kinds of restricted, repetitive behaviours and lack of imaginative creativity identified in diagnostic descriptions and widely observed in people with ASDs, the outstanding creativity of some autistic savants must also be explained, for example musical improvisation or poetry composition (Hermelin, 2001).

Contributory Causes that are not Specific to Autism

Chapter 6 included a section headed 'Many-to-one' in which it was stated that, for any set of behaviours such as 'social interaction impairments', there are numerous contributory causes. The set of restricted repetitive and uncreative behaviours (summarised here as 'behavioural inflexibility') was used to illustrate this point precisely because this set of behaviours is so diverse and has so many contributory causes.

The majority of these contributory causes are, however, neither specific to, nor universally present in, people with ASDs: that is to say, they commonly cause forms of repetitive behaviours and behavioural rigidity in people who are not autistic, as well as contributing to this set of behaviours in some (but not all) people who are autistic.

So, for example, anxiety or stress may contribute to a preference for familiar routines, to stereotyped movements, and to insistence on sameness and dislike of novelty. These are normal reactions: at times of stress many people will pace or rock; and when particularly anxious about something, most people take comfort from those things that feel familiar and 'safe'. High levels of anxiety are so common in people with autism (see Chapter 4), and anxiety is such a likely contributor to behavioural inflexibility in autism, that for many years this set of behaviours was generally explained *only* in terms of an attempt to create and maintain predictability in an otherwise confusing and anxiety-provoking environment (Rimland, 1964; Churchill, 1972; Baron-Cohen, 1989a).

Another non-specific, non-universal, but common, cause of behavioural inflexibility, and especially repetitive behaviour, is maladaptive learning. This is most likely to occur in those individuals least able to express themselves linguistically or to exercise control over events in more overt and conscious ways. As pointed out in Chapter 3, an individual who finds the close proximity of other people stressful and unpleasant may learn (unconsciously) that spitting tends to make people move away, so spitting becomes for that individual a habit that is reinforced because gaining space lowers the individual's anxiety. Some socially 'active but odd' individuals discover that enquiring what someone's name is or the make of car they drive almost always achieves a friendly response. This is reinforcing, so the question becomes that individual's habitual way of opening up an interaction; and because they cannot sustain a conversation, the same question may be repeated, sometimes over and over again, to the same person.

A third contributory cause of repetitive and especially compulsive, behaviour in some individuals with ASDs is abnormal brain function of kinds known to cause repetitive behaviours in disorders such as Tourette's syndrome or obsessive-compulsive disorder. Some of the most intractable repetitive behaviours in a proportion of individuals with ASDs probably reflect co-morbidity or overlap with one or other of these conditions.

A fourth contributory cause of repetitive behaviours in some individuals with ASDs may be sensory understimulation, as suggested by studies of blind children and Romanian orphans described in previous chapters. These studies show that a lack of normal sensory stimulation and experience can cause autistic-like behaviours such as rocking and head banging in young children. Absence of pretend play was also noted. In children of primary school age intense circumscribed interests and abnormal preoccupations were characteristic (Rutter et al., 1999; Hobson, 2002). Individuals with ASDs who do not readily engage in novel and varied forms of activity may effectively lack sensory stimulation, even if sensorily intact and not suffering environmental deprivation.

None of the above causal factors is, however, specific to autism, nor is any one factor likely to be operative in all individuals with ASDs. Subsequent sections of this chapter are, therefore, concerned only with theories that attempt to identify psychological deficits *specific* to people with ASDs and which may be *universal* in people with ASDs – the kind of problems that were described in Chapter 6 as the critical causes of a particular set of behaviours.

Over the last couple of decades the major candidate(s) for the critical cause(s) of behavioural inflexibility in autism have implicated executive function impairments. In the next three main sections of this chapter an outline of what is meant by 'executive functions' is first presented, followed by an account of the evidence concerning executive functions in autism, and finishing with a section discussing, first, the links between executive dysfunctions and behavioural inflexibility in autism and, secondly, the possible causes of executive dysfunctions.

In the final section of the chapter, some alternative theories concerning possible critical causes of behavioural inflexibility in autism are considered.

EXECUTIVE FUNCTIONS: DESCRIPTION AND DEFINITIONS

Broad Usage: An Umbrella Term

The notion of an executive system in the brain derives from an analogy with computers in which a master programme controls and directs all the software programmes on the machine. Based on this analogy, the term 'executive functions' as used in psychology generally covers the set of cognitive processes that are involved in the organisation and control of mental and physical activity. At the minimum, executive functions enable an individual to:

STOP doing one thing: this involves *inhibitory control* and the ability to *disengage attention* from a current stimulus, ongoing thought process or action;

SWITCH to something else: this involves *mental flexibility*; not just stopping doing one thing, but shifting attention to a new stimulus or shifting **mental set**;

START on something else (for example, a new topic of thought or a different physical action): this involves *generating* a new focus of attention such as a topic or goal, *planning* how to achieve the goal, and *initiating* the selected behaviour.

Executive functions are also involved in:

ORGANISING ongoing behaviour;

MONITORING ongoing behaviour;

TROUBLESHOOTING or MAKING CORRECTIONS, if required.

These additional components may involve *strategy generation, decision making,* **self-monitoring** and **action–outcome monitoring**, and *working memory*.

All the terms in upper case, italic or in bold type above appear in accounts of executive functions, plus others not included here. Not surprisingly, 'executive function' is often described as an umbrella term, covering multiple processes.

Narrow Usage: The Central Executive in Working Memory

A narrower meaning of executive function occurs in Baddeley and Hitch's model of working memory (Baddeley, 1986). This model as originally formulated has three components: two **slave systems**, known as the **phonological loop** and the **visuospatial sketchpad**, in which linguistic and visual-spatial information, respectively, can be held and manipulated; plus a control system, known as the

central executive. Later, the central executive component of working memory was identified with the **supervisory attentional system (SAS)** as described by Norman and Shallice (1986). The supervisory attentional system identifies the roles of the central executive as including the generation of goals, the maintenance of these goals in working memory, and the guidance of behaviour towards the achievement of particular goals.

The term 'executive functions' will be used here in its broad sense unless it is explicitly stated that what is being considered is the central executive system in working memory.

EXECUTIVE FUNCTIONS IN PEOPLE WITH AUTISM

There is now a great deal of evidence concerning executive functions in individuals with ASDs (see Hill, 2004 for a comprehensive review). Some key findings from this evidence are outlined below.

Problems of Stopping

Response inhibition

It is intuitively appealing to ascribe behavioural inflexibility in individuals with ASDs to a problem of response inhibition in situations in which it is necessary to stop doing one thing (such as turning the pages of a catalogue or asking the same question repeatedly) before doing something different. Response inhibition in children with ASDs was assessed within a study by Russell, Mauthner, Sharpe, and Tidswell (1991) using a test that became known as the 'windows task'. In this task, as first carried out, the child being tested had to win a chocolate, or other desired treat, by pointing to the one of two containers that did *not* contain the treat. If they pointed to the container with the treat, the tester 'won' it. The child was able to see into the containers, and typically developing children quickly learned to point to the empty container.

Astonishingly, the majority of the children with autism whom Russell et al. tested were completely unable to succeed on the windows task, making the wrong response as many as 20 times in succession. This striking finding could suggest that children with ASDs have impaired response inhibition: they simply cannot stop themselves from pointing to the chocolate. However, there are in fact many other ways of explaining the finding, and Russell and various colleagues proceeded to investigate alternative explanations in a series of experiments summarised in Box 9.1.

Is the underlying problem related to the element of deception? No: children with
autism still perform poorly when there is no 'opponent' to be deceived (Hughes
& Russell, 1993).

*Is there a problem with working memory impairing the ability to hold an arbitrary
rule in mind?* Probably not: verbal working memory is unimpaired (Russell, Jarrold,
& Henry, 1996).

Is there an impairment of self-monitoring and action–outcome monitoring? No:
children with ASDs know the difference between an intended and an
unintended outcome of an action; and between an effect they are
controlling and an effect someone else is controlling (Russell & Hill, 2001).

Is there a problem disengaging attention from the desired object? No: even when
the desired object remains visible, children with autism can shift their
attention to a knob that can be turned to obtain it (Hughes & Russell, 1993).

Is the required response critical? Quite probably: although a naming response (for
example, 'The blue one') in place of pointing does not improve the
performance of children with ASDs, an automated response such as pressing a
lever or turning a knob, does improve performance (Hughes & Russell, 1993;
Russell, Hala, & Hill, 2003).

*Is there a problem in formulating and using an arbitrary rule or strategy for obtaining
the desired object?* Yes, probably: children with autism can learn to use a
strategy that operates in a way they can understand (for example, the knob
operates a paddle that sends the desired object down a shute), but not one
which appears arbitrary (for example, turning over a cup opens up access to the
desired object via an unseen manipulation by the tester) (Hughes & Russell,
1993; Biro & Russell, 2001).

Is the involvement of another person, the tester, important? The social element
provided by the role of a tester may, just possibly, be part of the problem:
children with autism do better when only engaging with a machine (Russell
et al., 2003).

Box 9.1 illustrates that many different factors may influence performance in
what may look like a simple task, and shows why it would be wrong to conclude that children with ASDs' poor performance in this task results from
impaired response inhibition. In fact this interpretation was explicitly ruled
out, not just in work carried out by Russell and colleagues but also by findings
from other tests of response inhibition, which generally produce negative
results (Hill, 2004).

However, impaired response inhibition has been shown to occur in people with
ASDs in some tasks and conditions (Raymaekers, van der Meere, & Roeyers, 2004;
Luna, Doll, Hegedus, Minshew, & Sweeney, 2006). The fine cut between tasks in
which people with ASDs can and cannot inhibit responding should be informative

about exactly what makes the latter tasks difficult for people with ASDs. However, the relevant studies have not as yet been carried out.

Disengagement of attention

Although disengaging attention was not found to be a problem for children with ASDs in one of the studies reported in Box 9.1, other more sensitive tests of the ability to disengage attention do indicate a problem. Landry and Bryson (2004) used a well-known experimental test in which the person being tested is asked to look at a stimulus (such as a black dot) in the middle of a screen, and shortly afterwards another stimulus is presented to the left or the right of the central stimulus. On what are termed the 'simultaneous' trials, the central and left or right stimuli are shown together, so that the person being tested has to disengage from focusing on the central stimulus in order to focus on the novel stimulus. On 'successive' trials, the central stimulus disappears as soon as the novel stimulus appears, so there is nothing to disengage from – only a novel stimulus to which to shift attention. Landry and Bryson tested children with ASDs, children with Down syndrome, and younger typically developing children on this task, and found that the children with ASDs were impaired relative to both the other groups in the simultaneous, but not the successive, condition. In other words, they could shift attention to the novel stimulus when the original stimulus was not present, but could not, or were slow to, shift attention when already attending to something else.

Landry and Bryson are not alone in demonstrating problems in the disengagement of attention (see, for example, Rinehart, Bradshaw, Moss, Brereton, & Tonge, 2001b; Van der Geest, Kemner, Camfferman, Verbaten, & van Engeland, 2001). However, their study most neatly demonstrates how defective disengagement might cause the problems of shifting, more technically described as impaired **mental flexibility**, described next.

Problems of Shifting: Mental Inflexibility

Mental flexibility, sometimes referred to as **cognitive flexibility**, is commonly assessed using the Wisconsin Card Sorting Test (WCST) (Heaton, Chelune, Talley, Kay, & Curtiss, 1993). This test uses a set of cards on which are drawn a small number of coloured shapes, for example, two red squares, four blue circles. The cards can be sorted according to colour, shape or the number of shapes represented, and the person being tested is instructed to place each card into the 'correct' pile, as the tester deals them out. They are not told on what basis to sort the cards, but their first sorting strategy is rewarded with approval for a certain number of cards presented. After a run of 'correct' sorting responses, the tester no longer accepts the use of the original sorting strategy, simply saying 'No, that's incorrect'. After a couple of 'No's', most people switch strategy: for example, if they were previously sorting by colour, they switch to sorting by shape or by number. Their responses are then rewarded with approval for a given run of responses. They are then again told 'No, not correct', whereupon they are expected to switch to whichever strategy they have not already used. Both adults and children with ASDs, whether high- or low-functioning, have been shown in numerous studies to have great difficulty in shifting from one sorting strategy to another in this test (Rumsey & Hamburger, 1988; Prior & Hoffman, 1990; Ozonoff et al., 1991). Instead, they continue to sort by the previously rewarded strategy, despite the negative feedback. This behaviour is sometimes described as **perseverative** or **stuck-in-set** in the sense that the individual has developed a mental set (for example, to attend to colour or to attend to number) that they find hard to change.

Stuck-in-set behaviour has also been shown to occur in tests of what is called **intra-dimensional** and **extra-dimensional shift**. In this test, the person being assessed is shown pairs of pictures consisting of shapes and lines, and they learn through a process of trial and error, with feedback from the tester, how to choose the 'right' picture in any pair. At first, the 'right' choice is a particular shape, e.g., the circle, whereas the square is always the 'wrong' choice, and the lines in the pictures are irrelevant. When the person has learnt this rule, some different picture pairs are introduced, also consisting of shapes and lines, and the task is to learn that, for example, the star is the correct choice, the diamond being the incorrect choice, whilst the lines remain irrelevant. At the third stage, these same pairs of pictures are presented again, but now the diamond is 'correct' and the star 'incorrect' (and the lines irrelevant). Up to this point, shape has been the important dimension to attend to, although the person being tested has been required to shift their response to different 'correct' shape stimuli. These shifts are described as being 'intra-dimensional' because they all fall within the dimension of shape. At the critical fourth stage of the test, pairs of stars and diamonds with accompanying lines are presented again, but the task now is to choose a line – for example, the vertical line, not the diagonal line – and to ignore shape. This requires 'extra-dimensional' shift, because *shapes* constitute a different dimension from *lines*. People with ASDs perform relatively well on intra-dimensional shifts, demonstrating that they can shift attention and change their response if this does not involve a shift of the mental set 'respond to shape'. However, they perform poorly in the extra-dimensional shift condition, demonstrating the same sort of stuck-in-set perseveration that occurs on the Wisconsin Card Sorting Test (Hughes, Russell, & Robbins, 1994; Ozonoff et al., 2004).

Problems of Starting

Generativity

Generativity as used in discussions of executive functions means something similar to 'productivity'. It is generally assessed using tests of fluency, where fluency is defined as 'the ability to generate multiple responses spontaneously following a single cue or instruction' (Turner, 1999). So, for example, standard tests of **verbal fluency** involve asking someone to list as many words as they can beginning with a particular letter within a given time or to list names of animals or different sorts of foods. Tests of **design fluency** involve tasks such as drawing as many objects as possible using only four straight lines. Tests of **ideational fluency** may involve asking the person to think up as many uses of a brick or a piece of string as they can.

The results of studies of generativity in people with ASDs are summarised in the paper by Turner, cited above, and in Hill's (2004) review of executive function impairments in autism. The results are not clear-cut. However, they tend to suggest that, when given an informative cue or instruction, fluency is commensurate with overall ability level; but without an informative cue, performance is poor. So, for example, in an early test of verbal fluency, children with ASDs had no problem in generating lists of colour words, animal names or foods, but, when asked to shut their eyes and say 'any words you can think of', they performed significantly worse than controls (Boucher, 1988). In another study, children with autism and ability-matched children without autism were asked over several sessions to draw pictures, each of which should be 'different from what you drew before' (Lewis & Boucher, 1991). Each child's pictures were kept in a folder and shown to them before a new picture, was requested. Children without autism drew quite varied sets of pictures, whereas the children with ASDs tended to draw runs of pictures that were related either by shape or all belonged to a single category, as illustrated in Figure 9.1. In the studies of pretend play described in Chapter 5 a similar problem in generating a succession of dissimilar ideas was demonstrated (Lewis & Boucher, 1995; Jarrold et al., 1996).

Planning

Here again one particular test has been used many times to assess planning abilities. There are different versions of this test, with different names including the 'Tower of Hanoi', 'Tower of London', 'Tower of California' and 'Stockings of Cambridge' tests (test names often reflecting where a particular version was devised). All versions are, however, based on a simple puzzle available from toy shops. In the simplest version of this puzzle, two small wooden bases each support three vertical pegs a few inches high. One of the sets of pegs has a certain arrangement of up to five rings of different sizes and colours stacked on one of the pegs. The other set has the same set of rings stacked in a different order on a different peg. (The number of pegs and rings is increased in more difficult versions of the test). The task is to move the rings on one set to the positions on the other set one at a time in the fewest possible moves, without laying any of the rings aside, and never placing a larger ring on top of a smaller one. Many studies have shown that individuals with ASDs are less able than controls to plan a sequence of moves to achieve an economical solution to this puzzle,

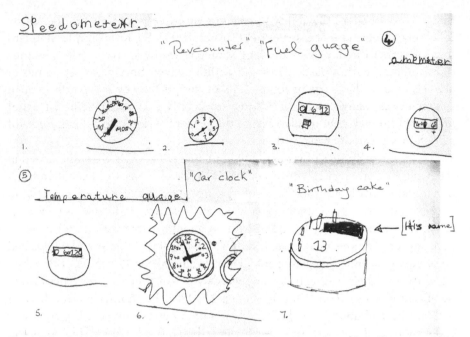

Figure 9.1 A series of drawings by a boy with autism in response to requests to 'Draw something different — something different from what you drew before', showing the tendency to produce a run of related pictures. In this case, the pictures are related by both category and shape.

especially as difficulty level increases and more moves have to be planned ahead (see for example Ozonoff et al., 1991; Hughes et al., 1994).

Action initiation

Action initiation involves more than the generation of a goal for an action and the mental planning of that action. It requires movement preparation, which is a component of motor skills that may be impaired in individuals with ASDs, as mentioned in Chapter 3 (Hughes, 1996; Rinehart, Bradshaw et al., 2001a). However, it also involves **volition** (sometimes referred to as **conation**) defined in terms of wanting or willing to initiate an action, which is closer to an executive function than a motor skill. Again, this is not the same as envisaging the action itself or the goal of the action: we may say 'The spirit is willing...' (I know what I ought to do) '...but the flesh is weak' (I am unable to motivate or bring myself to the point of doing it). Similarly, people suffering from depression may know that they ought to do x, but are unable to summon up the energy or will to carry out the actions required to achieve x.

There is almost nothing in the autism literature on conation or volition so defined. It was suggested in one paper that lack of spontaneous pretend play might result from impaired conation/volition (Lewis & Boucher, 1988), but that suggestion was never followed up. Impaired conation is, however, consistent with behaviour readily observed in people with ASDs. So, for example, people with autism characteristically underuse their skills: they *can* play symbolically but *do not* do so spontaneously; the child in the playground *can* ride a bike, swing, go down the slide, climb on the frame, etc., etc., but they *do not* spontaneously vary their behaviour, despite the fact that all the play equipment is visible and there is no need to generate ideas for more varied play. Instead, they typically do one thing repeatedly or they do almost nothing, demonstrating a kind of behavioural inertia, or what might be more accurately described as impaired **self-activation** or **psychic akinesia**, to use the medical terminology.

Very little has been written about behavioural inertia in people with ASDs, although it is common. Two anecdotes are illustrative (see Box 9.2).

BOX 9.2   Two anecdotes illustrating behavioural inertia contrasting with purposeful activity

Tea-time, and after On arrival at a residential centre for lower-functioning young people with ASDs, I went to the dining room where a dozen or so of the residents were having tea, seated round a table. All were appropriately occupied spreading jam on to bread, stretching out for biscuits, going to the trolley for a second cup of tea. There was little interaction, and the room was oddly silent, but in other respects the level of purposeful and appropriate activity gave no clue to the young people's autism. When the eating and drinking was finished, however, and each individual had cleared away their own plates, mugs etc., no doubt following a well-learned routine, the majority returned to their seats at the table and relapsed into inactivity, not interacting, not looking around, with one or two rocking or engaged in some other self-stimulating activity. The contrast between the normality of the routinised behaviour and the lack of self-initiated purposeful activity at the end of the meal was very striking.

Transformation On another occasion I arrived at a school where I had been working with, amongst others, a teenager with an ASD with whom I had found it difficult to engage because of his pervasive mental and physical apathy, not only towards the activities I had been trying to engage him in, but towards any attempt that I observed to stimulate his interest or to occupy him constructively. On this occasion, however, as I walked from the car park to the entrance of the school I saw a well-built adolescent in running shorts and T-shirt pounding (just a little clumsily) across the playing field a few steps in front of a teacher, reaching the front door of the school and leaning there, panting, looking flushed, alert, and pleased with himself. I thought at the time that the combination of physical activity and a given goal had temporarily transformed this boy, and wondered how and why.

Problems of Organisation and Monitoring

The use of organisational strategies

The use of language-based organisational strategies to facilitate memory has long been known to be impaired in people with ASDs. In their seminal series of psychological tests of young children with autism, Hermelin and O'Connor (1970) showed that, whereas young intellectually disabled children without autism can remember lists of related words (for example, 'Read them your book' or 'Blue, three, red, eight, six, white, green, two') better than lists of unrelated words (for example, 'Book, red, two, car, mouse, fork...'), young children with low-functioning autism were no better at remembering related words than unrelated words. Failure to use language-based strategies in memory tasks has been shown in many subsequent studies of high-functioning as well as lower-functioning individuals (e.g., Tager-Flusberg, 1991; Bowler, Matthews, & Gardiner, 1997; Toichi & Kamio, 2003). The planning, organisation, and control of thought and action is, like memory, facilitated by using language, usually silently in the form of **inner speech**. So, for example, we silently remind ourselves to 'Turn left at the traffic lights' or (in the Wisconsin Card Sorting Test) 'Sort by colour now' or (in the windows test) 'Point to the empty window'. Failure to use strategies of this kind to organise and control actions probably contributes to executive problems in autism (Russell, Jarrold, & Hood, 1999; Biro & Russell, 2001; but see also Williams, Happé, & Jarrold, 2008).

Self-monitoring and action–outcome monitoring

The control of thought and action also involves monitoring what one is doing in the course of carrying out an intended action: where a discrepancy exists between what was intended (the goal in mind) and what one is actually doing, corrections may be made. For example, in serving at tennis, one may intend to throw the ball up high and straight but if, in the course of serving, one realises this has not been achieved, then the positioning and trajectory of the racquet head must be modified to produce an acceptable service, despite the poor throw of the ball. The process of comparing the intended behaviour with the actual, ongoing behaviour, involves self-monitoring. Once one has served, the outcome of the service is also monitored: did it catch the opponent on their weak backhand as intended; or did it go into the net as a result of the poor service action? This involves action–outcome monitoring.

Self-monitoring and action–outcome monitoring both involve the ability to formulate an intention and hold it in mind, also a sense of **agency** (meaning unconscious awareness of oneself as the agent, or doer, of the action). Russell (1996, 1997) hypothesised that people with ASDs might lack a sense of agency and predicted that children with autism would be impaired on tests of self-monitoring and action–outcome monitoring. The prediction was not, however, supported, suggesting that people with ASDs do have the primitive awareness of the self as an agent that is sufficient for self-monitoring and action–outcome monitoring (Russell & Hill, 2001; Hill & Russell, 2002).

Working memory

When researchers began to investigate executive functions in autism, the central executive component of working memory as envisaged in Baddeley and Hitch's model, described above, was thought to be a likely source of problems of organisation and control. Working memory in people with ASDs has, however, proved to be commensurate with mental age (Pennington et al., 1997; Hill, 2004) except for a selective impairment of spatial working memory (Williams, Goldstein, Carpenter, & Minshew, 2005; Luna et al., 2006).

Limitations of Research into Executive Functions in People with ASDs

The research findings reviewed so far greatly enhance *descriptions* of the behavioural inflexibility diagnostic of autism. They do this by characterising these behaviours in terms of the various components of executive function. What emerges is a picture in which the disengagement of attention, mental flexibility, planning, generativity, and the use of organisational strategies all appear to be impaired, whereas response inhibition, self- and action–outcome monitoring, and working memory are mainly spared.

However, the research described so far does little to *explain* behavioural inflexibility in autism. In the first place, the studies described rarely relate their findings 'upwards' to the behavioural inflexibility diagnostic of autism: there is an implicit assumption that the two are related, but little is said about the precise relations. Secondly, few of the studies probe 'downwards' to identify the fundamental cause(s) of the executive function impairments themselves: most of the studies reported have narrowed down the range of possible fundamental abnormalities, but do not attempt to get to the roots of the problem. So, for example, impaired generativity and impaired mental flexibility have been clearly demonstrated, but both these impairments remain to be explained. Studies of attention and attention switching have, however, probed areas in which there may be a fundamental, psychologically irreducible problem (see below).

The small body of research attempting to relate executive problems in autism 'upwards' to specific kinds of behavioural inflexibility, as well as research directed 'downwards' towards identifying the fundamental causes of impaired executive functions in autism, is described next.

LOCATING EXECUTIVE FUNCTION IMPAIRMENTS WITHIN THE CAUSAL CHAIN

'Upwards' Links: Do Impaired Executive Functions Cause Behavioural Inflexibility?

Turner (1997; see also Turner, 1999) tested groups of high- and low-functioning children and adults with ASDs using executive function tests such as those described in the previous section. In addition, parents or primary carers of the individuals taking part were asked to respond to a structured interview designed to assess various different classes of autism-related repetitive behaviours ranging from tics and stereotyped movements through to circumscribed interests. Turner then assessed relations between performance on the executive function tasks and the kinds of inflexible (repetitive, uncreative) behaviours that were reported by parents. She found the following.

- Simple repetition of previous responses on tests of executive function was related to low-level repetitive behaviours such as movement stereotypies.
- Stuck-in-set perseveration was related to higher-level classes of repetitive behaviour such as pursuit of a preferred activity.
- Impaired ideational fluency was related to desire for sameness and circumscribed interests.

Turner suggested that both simple repetition and stuck-in-set perseveration result from defective response inhibition, whereas impaired fluency results from impaired ability to generate novel behaviour. These conclusions were not, however, clearly confirmed in the study reported next.

Lopez, Lincoln, Ozonoff, and Lai (2005) investigated Turner's hypotheses concerning the roles of defective inhibition and/or defective generativity as causes of behavioural inflexibility in autism. The methods they used were similar to those used in Turner's study, except that, instead of identifying different kinds of inflexible behaviours, Lopez et al. measured the overall severity of all types of inflexible behaviours taken together. The results of this study showed that impaired cognitive flexibility (assessed on the Wisconsin Card Sorting Test) is strongly related to repetitive behaviours, as in Turner's study. This finding has been replicated by South, Ozonoff, and McMahon (2007). However, neither impaired planning (assessed on one of the Tower tests) nor impaired generativity (assessed on tests of verbal and design fluency) was related to the undifferentiated measure of behavioural inflexibility in Lopez et al.'s study. From these findings Lopez et al. concluded that no single executive process can fully account for all aspects of behavioural inflexibility in autism. This conclusion provides retrospective support for Turner's method of examining relations between different executive functions and different types of repetitive, restricted and unimaginative behaviours, rather than using a single undifferentiated measure.

The most interesting findings from Lopez et al.'s study were, however, that, although neither response inhibition nor working memory was impaired (consistent with findings from most other studies), both were related to behavioural inflexibility. Lopez et al. concluded that the various forms of inflexible behaviours seen in autism may need to be explained in terms of a combination of intact and impaired executive functions. This conclusion is important in underlining that all the behaviours seen in people with ASDs are shaped at least as much by abilities as by 'deficits' or 'disabilities'.

Jarrold (1997) also considered the possible roles of impaired response inhibition and generativity as causes of repetitive behaviour and lack of imagination, focusing specifically on the impairment of spontaneous pretend play. He used as a basis for his discussion the model of a 'supervisory attention system' that has been identified with the central executive component of working memory (Norman & Shallice, 1986). This model includes an inhibitory component and an excitatory component comparable to the processes of inhibition and generativity identified by Turner as critical to explaining both types of behavioural inflexibility (repetitiveness and lack of imagination) in people with ASDs. However, the supervisory attention system has an additional component that serves the function of representing possible goals of action ('Shall I make coffee now – or tea?'), and goals are selected on the basis of which one wins out in terms of excitation over inhibition. On the basis of evidence available at the time, Jarrold concluded that impaired goal representation, rather than an imbalance between inhibitory and excitatory processes, might be implicated as a cause of impaired pretend play in children with ASDs.

In sum, attempts to relate particular impairments of executive function to the restricted repetitive behaviours and lack of imaginative creativity in autism are few, and have not succeeded in establishing the clear relationships needed to explain these behaviours.

'Downwards' Links: What Causes Executive Function Impairments in Autism?

There are very few suggestions in the literature concerning the fundamental psychological or neuropsychological cause, or causes, of impaired executive functions in people with ASDs. Of the few candidates for a critical cause, two involve one or other facet of executive function as the critical cause of the whole set of executive dysfunctions. Two other theories suggest that impaired executive functions result from some otherwise unrelated cause. These two types of theories are considered separately below.

Theories implicating one facet of executive function as the critical cause of the set of executive dysfunctions in autism

Ozonoff and her co-workers, who have been assiduous in identifying those components of executive function that are most problematic for people with

ASDs, conclude that cognitive flexibility and planning are reliably impaired across the spectrum, and explain these impairments in terms of frontal lobe dysfunctions (Ozonoff et al., 2004). This conclusion would be widely accepted. However, it does not offer an explanation at the psychological or neuropsychological level. The implication might be that impairments of mental flexibility and planning are themselves not reducible psychologically, and map directly on to some facet of frontal lobe function. However, as mentioned above, 'mental flexibility' describes a certain type of behaviour but does not identify the processes involved. Similarly, 'planning' is itself a complex, high-level process.

Impaired ability to disengage attention from one stimulus so as to attend to another is the kind of low-level, developmentally primitive, neuropsychological mechanism that might be capable of explaining mental inflexibility. However, Landry and Bryson (2004), whose work most clearly demonstrates problems with the disengagement of attention, have only studied visual attention. Moreover, problems with disengagement have not been demonstrated in all relevant studies. Nevertheless, deficits in the broad area of attention are a focus of considerable current interest in autism research, as will be discussed in the next chapter, and future studies of attentional abnormalities may shed light on the causes of executive function impairments in autism.

Theories implicating an otherwise unrelated factor as the critical cause of executive dysfunctions in autism

Carruthers (1996) argued that defective mentalising impairs the ability to think about one's own beliefs, desires and thought processes, thereby impairing complex reasoning and executive control. However, given the fact that social impairments and behavioural inflexibility are dissociable characteristics of autism, as shown by studies of the broader autism phenotype, it seems unlikely that impaired mindreading is the critical cause of impaired executive function or vice versa.

Russell's (1996; 1997) defective agency theory proposed that children with autism lack a sense of themselves as an agent, or 'doer', of actions. Russell identified the sense of agency with the first-person self, the 'I', and suggested that this primitive sense of self is required for executive function, and in particular for the ability to exercise self-control and to monitor one's own actions and their outcomes. As has been mentioned above, Russell's exemplary investigations (summarised in Box 9.1) led him to abandon the defective agency hypothesis as originally formulated. However, the nature and development of the self in people with ASDs is increasingly discussed in the autism literature, as was noted in an earlier chapter (see also Chapter 11), and it may be that impaired sense of self contributes to impaired executive function in autism in ways other than those specifically proposed and investigated by Russell.

Critique of Executive Dysfunction Explanations of Behavioural Inflexibility

Pluses There is considerable evidence of specific executive function impairments in people with autism, although some executive functions appear to be intact. It is intuitively likely that those executive function impairments that have been reliably demonstrated (impaired disengagement of attention and cognitive flexibility; impaired generativity and planning), in combination with enhanced reliance on intact abilities (as suggested by Lopez et al.) cause or contribute to the restricted, repetitive and unimaginative behaviours seen in autism. However, the links between patterns of impaired and spared executive function abilities and behavioural inflexibility in autism have not been clearly identified. The strongest conclusion that can be reached, therefore, is that executive function impairments have the potential to explain some aspects of behavioural inflexibility in autism.

Problems Executive functions such as mental flexibility and planning that have been shown to be impaired in autism are relatively high-level and late-developing abilities, and it has proved difficult to demonstrate lower level, early occurring executive function impairments in infants and preschool children (Dawson, Webb et al., 2002; Hill, 2004). Current executive function deficit theories therefore fail to meet the primacy criterion.

Executive function impairments of one kind or another are quite common in other neurodevelopmental disorders and it has not been shown that specific executive functions, or a specific pattern of spared and impaired executive abilities, is unique to people with ASDs. For example, Hill (2004) points out that quite a lot of the evidence of executive function impairments in autism can be explained in terms of intellectual disability rather than autism itself. Thus, explanations of behavioural inflexibility in terms of executive function impairments currently fail to meet the specificity criterion.

OTHER 'CRITICAL CAUSE' THEORIES

Hypersystemising as a Critical Cause of Behavioural Inflexibility

Hypersystemising has recently been proposed by Baron-Cohen (2006) as a cause of behavioural inflexibility in people with ASDs. Systemising has already been mentioned in Chapters 7 and 8 in connection with Baron-Cohen's extreme male brain theory of autism (Baron-Cohen et al., 2005). According to this theory autism is associated with an extreme version of the typical male brain, including an abnormally strong capacity for systemising, or what Baron-Cohen terms hypersystemising. Systemising is defined as the output from a change-predicting mechanism that operates by 'observation... leading to the identification of laws to predict that event x will occur with probability p' (Baron-Cohen, 2006). A mild tendency towards hypersystemising is hypothesised to be present in more able individuals and may be harnessed to achieve academic and professional success. Excessively dominant hypersystemising tendencies, however, are hypothesised to cause non-adaptive behavioural rigidity in LFA. The link between hypersystemising and behavioural inflexibility in LFA is described by Baron-Cohen in terms of resistance to, and inability to cope with, any but the most systematic and predictable forms of change.

Critique of the hypersystemisation theory   There is some evidence of stronger systemising tendencies in typical males than in typical females; and some evidence that systemising tendencies are more dominant in people with an ASD (both males and females) than in the general population (Lawson, Baron-Cohen, & Wheelwright, 2004). However, it has yet to be shown that hypersystemising is specific to people with ASDs (if not, then some other factor must also be involved in causing behavioural inflexibility). Nor has it yet been shown that hypersystemising is universal in people with those forms of ASD that include behavioural inflexibility of the kinds hypersystemising is said to explain.

In addition, the notion of a 'systemising mechanism' is novel and not (as yet) identified with any known neuropsychological function or specific brain system. Baron-Cohen is aware of this, and makes the point explicitly in his accounts of the theory.

Overuse of Spared Abilities as a Critical Cause of Behavioural Inflexibility

Sensory-perceptual anomalies as a contributory cause of behavioural inflexibility

Frith's weak central coherence (WCC) theory (described in detail in Chapter 10) is associated with anomalously good ability to perceive details or parts, but impaired ability to perceive wholes. Frith (2003) has speculated on ways in which WCC might produce certain types of repetitive behaviour seen in individuals with autism. She suggests, for example, that it might underlie the fascination many children with autism have for parts of objects whilst ignoring the whole object, for example, spinning the wheels of a toy vehicle, rather than running it along the ground as if on a road. Similarly, superior attention to, and processing of, detail combined with a weakness in integrating fragments of experience into wholes, may lead the child with autism to repeat small bits of behaviour rather than extended behavioural acts. Thus, whereas the typically developing child repeatedly fills a bucket with sand to make a ring of sand-castles (and is seen as behaving normally), the child with autism repeatedly digs a spade into the sand and watches the sand spill out (and is perceived as behaving abnormally).

Mottron and Burack's (2001) enhanced perceptual function theory (also discussed more fully in the next chapter) suggests that superior low-level per-ceptual functioning might lead to a restriction of interests in favour of preoc-cupation with perceptual processing within a selected domain (Mottron et al., 2006). In his 2006 paper, Mottron and his colleagues also broach the issue of spared creativity in a minority of autistic savants, as described in Chapter 3. They suggest that savants lie at the extreme end of a continuum of preoccu-pation with perceptual inputs within a single domain such as music, drawing or verbal material. Repeated exposure to these inputs leads to unconscious learning of the structural rules embodied in the material (see Pring, 2008). These are utilised in savant performances such as calendrical calculation or for-eign language learning ability. In what Mottron et al. (2006) refer to as 'the ultimate state of savant ability', **implicit** (unconscious) knowledge is comple-mented by **explicit** (conscious, verbalisable) knowledge of the rules and regu-larities within a specialist field, leading to exceptional – but narrowly restricted – achievements in creativity such as musical improvisation, poetry writing or mathematical inventiveness.

The enhanced perceptual function theory is therefore unusual in that it attempts to explain not only the restricted interests diagnostic of autism, but also the rare examples of outstanding creativity that at first sight appear incompatible with the diagnostic descriptions, but which do have to be explained.

Uneven memory abilities as a critical cause of behavioural inflexibility

Occasionally, researchers who argue that hippocampal dysfunction may be important for understanding autism have noted in passing that, whereas hippocampal dysfunction would impair certain kinds of memory and learning, it would leave the acquisition of habits and procedures, and learning of condi-tioned responses, intact. The imbalance in favour of the latter kinds of mem-ory could, it is suggested, lead to some of the kinds of repetitive and restricted behaviours in autism (Bachevalier, 1994; Kemper & Bauman, 1998). Neither Bachevalier nor Kemper and Bauman has developed this theory, however, which has been explicitly argued for only in my own publications with colleagues. This theory will therefore be described more fully in the Personal View chapter at the close of Part II, rather than here.

SUMMARY

Behaviours falling under the descriptions 'restricted and repetitive' and 'lacking in creativity and imagination' are extremely various, both within and across individuals and at different ages and stages of development. There are multiple contributory causes of these behaviours, with different sets of causes operating in different individuals or in the same individual at different times and in different circumstances. Many of these contributory causes are not specific to autism, and include anxiety and stress, maladaptive learning, sensory deprivation, and the presence of co-morbid conditions associated with repetitive behaviour, such as obsessive-compulsive disorder or Tourette's syndrome.

Attempts to identify a critical cause, or set of causes, of behavioural inflexibility specific to and universally present in people with ASDs have not been successful. Attention has focused largely on executive functions, and there is clear evidence that certain aspects of executive control are impaired in autism. Specifically, disengagement of attention, mental flexibility, generativity and planning, and the formulation and use of organisational strategies have generally been shown to be impaired, whereas response inhibition, self-monitoring, action–outcome monitoring, and working memory are largely spared. However, there are some exceptions to these generalisations, which suggests that further clarification of the findings is needed. Moreover, at least one facet of executive function that may have relevance for autism, namely volition and its role in action initiation, has not been investigated.

Research into executive functions in people with ASDs has contributed substantially to descriptions of restricted, repetitive and unimaginative behaviours in autism, but as yet done little to explain these behaviours. In particular, clear links between specific executive function impairments and specific forms of inflexible behaviour have not been established. In addition, the impairments that have been demonstrated have not themselves been explained in terms of fundamental psychological mechanisms. Explanations that have been proposed, but which are unproven, include problems of attentional control, defective mentalising, and impaired sense of self.

A few theories have attempted to identify the critical cause of behavioural inflexibility in autism without reference to executive functions. In particular it has been suggested that hypersystemising would lead to the kinds of restricted and repetitive behaviours typical of people with ASDs. It has also been suggested that overreliance on certain spared abilities to compensate for impaired abilities could be implicated. For example, spared ability to process sensory-perceptual detail in combination with weak central coherence could, it is argued, cause certain repetitive behaviours; as might overreliance on certain intact forms of memory and learning.

In sum, many aspects of the restricted and repetitive behaviours and lack of imaginative creativity seen in people with ASDs are easily explained, or partially explained, in terms of non-specific factors. At the same time the critical, autism-specific causes of behavioural inflexibility remain elusive. It seems likely that executive function impairments are implicated somewhere along the causal chain, but less certain that these impairments are fundamental. There are currently several unproven hypotheses concerning autism-specific causes of behavioural inflexibility, but no convergence of opinion.

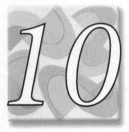

EXPLAINING OTHER UNIVERSAL OR COMMON BEHAVIOURAL CHARACTERISTICS

AIMS
••••
EXPLAINING THE SENSORY-PERCEPTUAL ANOMALIES
What Has to be Explained
Early Theories
Current Theories
Comment
••••
EXPLAINING UNEVEN MOTOR SKILLS
What Has to be Explained
Explaining the Impairments
Comment
••••
EXPLAINING PATTERNS OF LANGUAGE ABILITY AND DISABILITY
What Has to be Explained
Explaining the Autism-specific Language Impairment
Comment
••••
EXPLAINING UNEVEN PATTERNS OF INTELLECTUAL ABILITY
What Has to be Explained
Explaining Intelligence Test Profiles in People with Autism
••••
SUMMARY

EXPLAINING THE SENSORY-PERCEPTUAL ANOMALIES

What Has to be Explained

Sensory-perceptual anomalies that are very common and possibly universal in people with ASDs include the following.

- Both over- and under-responsiveness to stimuli in all the main sensory channels, often co-existing in an individual.
- Superior identification and discrimination of **unimodal** detail, associated with a tendency to attend to individual features of complex stimuli in preference to attending to wholes, sometimes referred to as a preference for local as opposed to **global processing**.
- Impaired detection of visual motion.
- Vulnerability to sensory overload.
- Vulnerability to sensory confusion, or synaesthesia, including idiosyncratic associations between sensory inputs and emotion.
- Possible abnormalities of attentional capacity (monotropic attention).

Abnormalities of sensory-perceptual processing may, like some emotion processing impairments, be among the set of psychologically irreducible abnormalities contributing to autism. However, the precise sensory-perceptual anomalies that might be fundamental have not been identified. Some major hypotheses and findings concerning fundamental sensory-perceptual impairments are reviewed here, beginning with early theories, as in previous chapters.

Early Theories

Ornitz (1974) argued that impaired **sensory modulation** causes not only the over- and under-responsiveness to sensory stimuli seen in people with ASDs, but also self-stimulatory behaviours. He suggested that impaired ability to filter out trivial or background stimuli, and impaired ability to **habituate** to novel stimuli, were related to sensory overload, and to the enhanced autonomic responses that occur in children with autism in response to novelty or increased environmental complexity, or when engaging in motor stereotypies (MacCulloch & Williams, 1971). In company with other researchers, notably Rimland (1964) also Hutt et al. (1964), Ornitz attributed the impairment of sensory modulation to malfunction of the brain stem **reticular activating system**, a structure that modulates arousal levels, amongst other functions. In his later papers Ornitz argued that problems of sensory modulation would have secondary effects on selective and directed attention (e.g., Ornitz, 1989). This linkage of sensory abnormalities of subcortical origin to perceptual and cognitive anomalies involving cortical structures is consistent with current thinking (see Chapters 7 and 11).

Current Theories

The weak central coherence theory

Shah and Frith (1983) showed that children with ASDs have superior ability to pick out a particular detail of a picture representing a whole object or scene. The test they used resembled the kind of puzzle sometimes found in books bought for children to pass the time on a journey, as illustrated in Figure 10.1.

In the same year, Frith and Snowling (1983) reported that children with autism were less able than children with dyslexia to utilise verbal meaning to determine their pronunciation of an ambiguous word. So, for example, children were asked to read aloud the sentence 'In her eye there was a tear', and a little later to read aloud the sentence 'In her dress there was a tear'. Whereas the pronunciation of the word 'tear' by the children with dyslexia was generally consistent with the meaningful context provided at the beginning of either sentence, the pronunciation of the children with ASDs was less likely to be consistent.

In the first edition of her book *Autism: Explaining the Enigma*, Frith (1989) proposed that findings such as the above could be interpreted as reflecting a 'weak drive for central coherence'. The notion of coherence came from work in psychology showing that most individuals have a strong tendency to look for meaning in sensory experience. Frith argued that weak drive for meaning, or what she termed weak central coherence (WCC), could explain not only the results of her studies with Shah and with Snowling, but also some earlier findings: for example, that children with autism solve jigsaw puzzles by attending to the shape of the pieces rather than to the pictures; and that they recall sentences or lists of related words no better than they recall lists of unrelated words (Hermelin & O'Connor, 1970).

Frith (1989) further suggested that superior ability to process detail resulted from impaired ability to integrate parts into wholes. In psychological terminology,

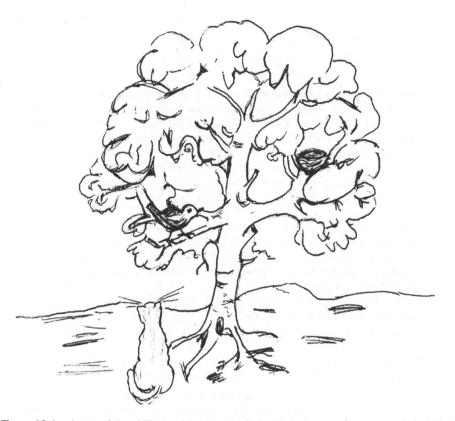

Figure 10.1 A test of the ability to pick out a detail, in this instance a face, concealed within a larger picture

superior **local processing** was hypothesised to result from defective global processing. An explanation in terms of impaired integration fits well with first-hand accounts such as that of John van Dalen, quoted in Box 3.2, who describes the effortful route he must take to assemble in his mind the parts of an object (such as a hammer), the name of the object, and his knowledge of the properties and functions of the object. The suggestion that superior local processing results from impaired global processing is also intuitively plausible: if we are poor at doing one thing, we may compensate by becoming unusually good at doing the next best thing. 'The next best thing', or fall-back option, is often referred to as the **default mechanism**, in this case local processing.

The WCC hypothesis was eclipsed for a time by the impaired ToM/mentalising deficit theory with which Frith was also involved, which figures alongside presentation of the WCC theory in her 1989 book. From the mid 1990s onwards, however, there has been a spate of investigations of phenomena relating to central coherence in people with ASDs. Many of these studies produced findings consistent with the notion of WCC (see Box 10.1 for examples).

Superior recognition of inverted faces Participants are shown several
passport-type photographs of unknown faces. A short while later each face is
shown to the participant again, paired with a face the participant has not seen
before, both faces being presented upside down. The participant is asked:
which of these did you see just now? People with ASDs perform better than
people without ASDs. Conclusion: because it is known that it is the ability to
process upright faces as wholes that makes processing inverted faces difficult
for most people, it may be concluded that people with ASDs do not process
faces as wholes.

Superior (faster than average) performance on the Block Design test People
with ASDs are faster than people without ASDs on this test (described in
Box 3.7). Conclusion: people with ASDs, unlike others, are not slowed down by
seeing the goal pattern as an unsegmented whole: the 'bits' of the pattern are
immediately obvious to them.

Detail-focused and fragmented drawings Participants are shown line drawings and
asked to copy them. People with ASDs are unusually likely to start by drawing
a detail, and to draw fragments of the original picture rather than indicating the
whole.

Inferior ability to assemble a given set of sentences to tell a coherent story
This suggests impaired ability to integrate parts into meaningful wholes.

(Examples are taken from the review by Happé
and Frith, 2006, where relevant references can be found.)

In addition to new evidence consistent with the WCC/impaired global processing theory there was, however, other evidence inconsistent with the theory. Specifically, several studies showed that people with ASDs are able to
perceive wholes rather than parts, and to attend to meaning rather than to
surface appearances or sounds, if directed towards doing so. For example, if
shown a large capital letter 'A' made up of many smaller-sized letter 'H's' and
specifically directed to name the large letter, individuals with ASDs are as fast
and as accurate as comparison groups (Plaisted, Swettenham, & Rees, 1999).
However, if asked simply what letter they see, they show a bias towards
naming the smaller letter in the design (e.g., Ozonoff, Strayer, McMahon, &
Filloux, 1994).

Evidence against impaired global processing led Frith, now working in collaboration with Happé, to modify the WCC theory. They relinquished the suggestion of a deficit in global processing, and suggested instead that the findings
on sensory-perceptual processing in autism could be interpreted in terms of
a preference, or bias, towards processing parts rather than wholes (Happé,
1999). Happé based this suggestion on the assumption that biases towards
global as opposed to local processing are distributed as a continuum within the

general population. Thus 'while the person with weak coherence may be poor at seeing the bigger picture, the person with strong coherence may be a terrible proof reader' (Happé & Frith, 2006: 15). The new suggestion was that people with ASDs have a cognitive style that places them amongst those who are particularly poor at seeing the bigger picture. Happé, Frith, and Briskman (2001) demonstrated that this cognitive style is characteristic of fathers of children with ASDs, suggesting that it is at least partly genetically determined.

In their update of the WCC theory, Happé and Frith (2006) argue that the findings on intact global processing are not particularly robust, whilst findings on a bias towards local processing are consistently strong. They concede, however, that the underlying causes of this bias have yet to be identified, whether at the psychological or neurobiological level of explanation. They discuss various possible causes, including problems of attention switching, whether from one object to another or between a **zoom-in** and a **zoom-out** attentional focus (Mann & Walker, 2003). They also discuss possible causal explanations derived from computer modelling of sensory-perceptual processes, and from theories concerning brain development, organisation and function, some of which are discussed in Chapter 11.

The explanation Happé and Frith now favour involves difficulty in integrating higher-order with lower-order sensory-perceptual information, including the possibility of an impairment of the kind of top-down control normally exerted by executive functions (Frith, 2003; Happé & Frith, 2006). A detailed account of what may be involved in sensory integration at the interface of psychological and neurological processes can be found in Iarocci and MacDonald (2006).

The enhanced perceptual function theory

The enhanced perceptual function theory was articulated by Mottron and Burack (2001) as an alternative to the WCC explanation of anomalous sensory-perceptual processing in people with ASDs. Mottron and Burack use the term 'perceptual' quite broadly to include the detection of what they term 'surface properties' of stimuli, such as the pitch and loudness of auditory stimuli, and the contours and proportions of visual stimuli.

Mottron and Burack were particularly influenced by their investigations of savant abilities in two individuals, one with outstanding musical abilities (Mottron, Peretz, Belleville, & Rouleau, 1999), the other with outstanding drawing ability (Mottron & Belleville, 1993). The young woman with savant musical abilities has **absolute pitch** (sometimes referred to as perfect pitch) and superior ability to identify single notes played within a chord, indicating exceptional perception of auditory detail. These exceptional auditory abilities are not confined to savants, as they are shared by many individuals on the spectrum (Heaton, 2003). The savant draftsman studied by Mottron and

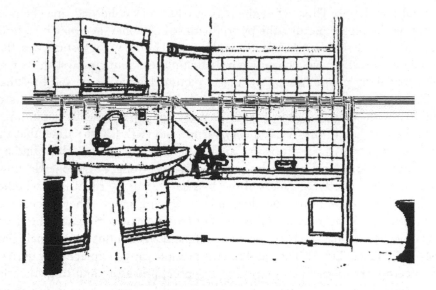

Figure 10.2   A spontaneous drawing by the savant artist E.C. (reproduced from Mottron and Belleville, *Brain and Cognition*, 23: 286, with permission)

Belleville can draw perfect circles and ellipses, and his spontaneous drawings demonstrate exceptionally accurate reproduction of contours, proportions, and perspective, as illustrated in Figure 10.2, demonstrating superior perception of visual detail.

The exceptional local processing abilities of these savants led Mottron and Burack to hypothesise that enhanced processing of the surface properties of visual or auditory stimuli could explain anomalous sensory-perceptual processing in people with ASDs without invoking a deficit in global processing.

In a later account of the enhanced perceptual function theory, Mottron et al. (2006) review evidence that people with ASDs have anomalously good local processing abilities that, nevertheless, do not preclude a capacity for global processing. For example, the savant musician who has absolute pitch also has superior memory for melodies, a capacity that requires global processing. Mottron et al. accordingly suggested that superior low-level processing is associated with overusage of primary sensory areas of the brain with no loss of global processing ability.

The enhanced discrimination–reduced generalisation theory

Plaisted, O'Riordan, and Baron-Cohen (1998a, b) reported a study in which children with ASDs and age- and ability-matched typically developing children were given two visual search tests. In one test children were shown a display of letters and instructed to find, for example, a green 'S' from amongst some red or green 'Ts' or 'Xs'. In this 'single feature' task, children had only to look for

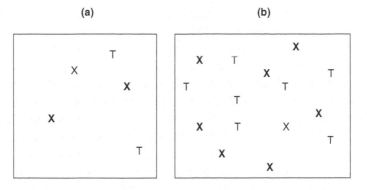

Figure 10.3 Examples of materials used in a conjunctive search task (one easy and one hard version of the task are illustrated). In these examples the target letter is a green 'X' and the distractors are green 'Ts' and red 'Xs' (green is represented by plain font and red by bold font in the Figures) (from Plaisted, O'Riordan, and Baron-Cohen, *Journal of Child Psychology and Psychiatry*, 39: 778, with permission)

the 'S' shape, ignoring colour. In the second test children were instructed to find, for example, a green 'X' from amongst some green 'Ts' and red 'Xs'. In this **'conjunctive search'** task, children had to look for the unique combination of colour and shape distinguishing the target letter from surrounding distractors (see Figure 10.3). Children with ASDs performed as well as the typically developing children on the 'single-feature' task, and outperformed them on the 'conjunctive search' task.

From this experiment (and other related experiments that followed) Plaisted et al. (1998) concluded that superior conjunctive search is inconsistent with the WCC theorists' claim that people with ASDs have difficulty in integrating features, or parts, into wholes. They suggested instead that people with ASDs have superior ability to process the unique features, or feature combinations, of objects such as are utilised in *discriminating* between objects, that is to say, telling them apart. Conversely, people with ASDs are less likely to process the similarities between individual items such as are utilised in *generalising* across objects, that is to say, responding to a novel object on the basis that it resembles previously seen objects. So, for example, a child with an ASD might be exceptionally sensitive to the differences between one make of cornflakes and another, but insensitive to the similarities and therefore reluctant to eat cornflakes of an unfamiliar brand. Plaisted et al.'s interpretation of their findings on conjunctive search led to their **enhanced discrimination–reduced generalisation** theory. This theory differs from the WCC theory in emphasising superior low-level processing as the most likely cause of a bias towards local as opposed to global processing. It differs from the enhanced perceptual function theory in that it emphasises superior discrimination ability, whereas the enhanced perceptual function theory maintains that all aspects of the perception of detail are superior in people with ASDs, including detection, matching, reproduction, and memory, as well as discrimination (Mottron et al., 2006).

Plaisted and her colleagues have continued to investigate the phenomenon of superior discrimination identified in the 1998 paper, using a series of sophisticated tests of auditory as well as visual ability (Plaisted, Saksida, Alcantara, & Weisblatt, 2003; Plaisted, Dobler, Bell, & Davis, 2006). This work is notable because it relates to some of the sensory anomalies that people with ASDs report and that are well documented in the literature, such as hyperacusia and difficulty in detecting speech against background noise. However, Plaisted and her colleagues, like others working in the field, admit some bafflement in their attempts to identify the fundamental problems that may be involved, not least because many of their tests show no differences between people with ASDs and people without ASDs. As they point out, this helps to rule out possible explanations, whilst failing to identify critical causal factors.

Comment

Pluses   The study of sensory-perceptual processes is of undoubted importance for understanding how people with ASDs experience the world around them: what they see, hear, smell, taste and feel, and the sense they make of it or fail to make. In addition, abnormalities in this area, whether in the form of exceptionally good or significantly poor ability, may help to explain some of the interaction impairments in autism, as noted in Chapter 8. Sensory anomalies may also contribute to explanation of some forms of repetitive behaviours, as noted in Chapter 9. This is an example of one causal factor having many possible and varied effects (see the section 'One-to-many' in Chapter 6).

In addition to having broad explanatory potential, the processes that may give rise to anomalies of sensory-perceptual processing in autism, although not finally identified, are of the right kind to qualify as fundamental psychological deficits contributing to autism-related behaviours. This is because they tend to be low-level processes (for example, to do with attentional focus, sensory integration or sensory processes in vision and hearing) that would have consequences for higher-order processing (for example, to do with perceiving the meaning of speech or making sense of facial expressions). Low-level processes are likely to be genetically determined, hardwired processes available to infants from an early age. Impaired or unusual functioning of such processes would have a cascade of effects on brain development as well as on behaviour from the first year of life onwards. Thus the kinds of underlying mechanisms that have been proposed all meet the primacy criterion.

Furthermore, many of the processes identified are pitched at the level of neuropsychology, and thus can be grounded in known brain processes and structures (see Chapters 7 and 11).

Finally, the convergence of several major theoreticians and research groups past and present on to this quite limited area of investigation, and the consistency of this line of research with what people with ASDs tell us about what it is like to be autistic, encourages one to think that part of the answer to the question 'What causes autism?' will be found in the domain of sensory-perceptual processing.

Problems   The precise mechanisms underlying the sensory-perceptual anomalies associated with autism have not been identified, and whether or not any of the currently proposed mechanisms meet the specificity or universality criteria remains to be shown. The bias towards local processing may constitute a common pathway universal and specific to autism. However, the causes of this bias remain controversial. In addition, a local processing bias does not by itself explain phenomena such as synaesthesia or sensory overload that also fall within the set of sensory-perceptual anomalies reported by high-functioning people with ASDs.

EXPLAINING UNEVEN MOTOR SKILLS

What Has to be Explained

In Chapter 3 it was suggested that impairments of motor skills are almost certainly a universal feature of autism, but that some skills are conspicuously spared in at least some individuals, for example, in skilled pianists or agile climbers. Moreover, the patterns of strengths and weaknesses are quite various, and may be different in higher-functioning as opposed to lower-functioning individuals.

Whilst bearing in mind the spared abilities in this domain, the following three forms of motor impairments were identified in Chapter 3:

- motor stereotypies;
- clumsiness and abnormalities of gait and posture;
- selective imitation impairments.

Possible causes of each of these impairments, or sets of impairments, are considered in turn.

Explaining the Impairments

Motor stereotypies

Possible causes of motor stereotypies were mentioned in Chapter 9, where stereotypies were grouped with other forms of repetitive behaviours. Causes that were mentioned include lack of sensory stimulation and a need to self-stimulate; anxiety; hypersystemising tendencies, and impaired response inhibition. However, stereotyped behaviours are not specific to autism (although some forms of motor stereotypies such as toe-walking or hand flapping are highly characteristic), nor are they universal in people with ASDs. The causes of motor stereotypies will not, therefore, be further considered here (see Goldman, Salgado, Florance, Wang, Kim, & Greene, 2006, for further information).

Clumsiness and abnormalities of gait and posture

The clumsiness so frequently noted, especially in people with Asperger syndrome, and the abnormalities of gait and posture more frequently observed in lower-functioning individuals, can be partly explained in terms of abnormal muscle tone or limb dyspraxia. These neuromuscular impairments are unusually common in people with ASDs, as noted in Chapter 3. However, they are not invariably present, and some other factor or factors must also be involved.

In the section on motor skills in Chapter 3 it was noted that several studies have demonstrated problems of motor planning and control such as could be manifested in clumsy and ill-directed movements. Hughes (1996), for example, gave children with LFA a task she called 'the bar game'. In this game, the child sat at a table with a black and white rod-like bar on a stand in front of them, with two discs, one red and one blue, placed just beyond the stand, as illustrated in Figure 10.4 (the apparatus is shown as if the reader was sitting opposite the child being tested). The child's task was to lift the bar using one hand, and place it end-up in one of the discs, following an instruction. The instructions were varied according to whether the bar should be picked up at the black or the white end, and whether it should be placed in the blue or the red disc. Some of the placements are awkward to carry out unless the grip used is varied from 'overhand' (as in the Figure) to 'underhand'. Use of the underhand grip requires the ability to plan and to control a goal-directed movement, and the children with ASDs in Hughes' experiment were less able to do this than either typically developing preschool children or intellectually disabled children without autism.

Problems of motor planning and control might in theory result from executive dysfunctions, rather than from impairments of motor functioning per se. However, a study by Rinehart, Bellgrove et al. (2006) ruled this out, and provided further evidence of difficulties in movement preparation and planning such as were shown in Hughes' study. The study by Rinehart et al. produced two further interesting findings. First, individuals with Asperger syndrome are not as impaired as individuals with autistic disorder (using strict DSM-IV criteria), which may explain differences in the kinds of motor impairments associated with AS as opposed to those observed in other forms of autism. Secondly, a less demanding motor task was worse performed than more demanding tasks, even by the AS participants. Rinehart and her colleagues note that this is consistent with Leary

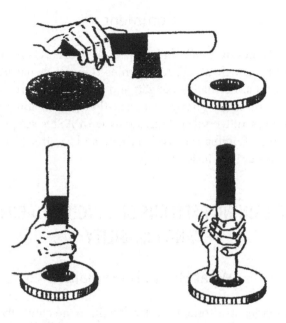

Figure 10.4 Starting off with an overhand grip (top picture) results in a comfortable positioning of the hand when placing the black end of the bar into a ring (lower picture, left). However, it results in an awkward positioning when placing the white end of the bar into the ring (lower picture, right) (from Hughes, *Journal of Autism and Developmental Disorders*, 26: 103)

and Hill's (1996) observation that 'the [autistic] individual who typically experiences severe difficulties with the most simple of movements may suddenly perform complex, skilled movements'. It may be that people with ASDs have problems of action preparation and initiation, as suggested in Chapter 9, rather than problems of action execution. However, other explanations are also possible, and these interesting findings need to be replicated before their cause(s) can be meaningfully investigated.

Selective imitation impairments

As noted in Chapter 3, imitation impairment in people with ASDs is generally confined to the imitation of actions that are body-related, such as touching one's nose with a finger or holding a music box to one ear (although those with additional neuromuscular problems may have more pervasive imitation impairments). The fact that people with ASDs are not universally impaired in the imitation of other kinds of action such as those that involve acting on objects, indicates that motor skills are generally adequate for imitation. Impaired imitation of body-related actions is therefore likely to result from problems of **self–other equivalence** (as mentioned in Chapter 8), rather than from impaired motor abilities.

Comment

The paucity of studies of motor skills in people with ASDs means that no firm conclusions can be drawn, at least concerning the precise nature and origins of the clumsiness and abnormalities of gait and posture that are so characteristic. However, the increasingly strong evidence that motor abnormalities of one kind or another are universal in individuals with ASDs supports the conclusion of Teitelbaum, Teitelbaum, Nye, Fryman, and Maurer (1998), that movement disturbances are intrinsic to autism.

EXPLAINING PATTERNS OF LANGUAGE ABILITY AND DISABILITY

What Has to be Explained

People with Asperger syndrome have, by definition, no clinically significant language impairment. People with ASDs who are high-functioning intellectually are occasionally language- or speech-impaired. The likely causes of such occasional impairments in people with HFA will be mentioned in this section. However, most of the section involves attempts to explain language impairments and anomalies in those people who are mildly or moderately intellectually impaired, and who have some useful language, whilst bearing in mind that a proportion of low-functioning individuals have little or no useful language.

DSM-IV describes the language impairment in autistic disorder as characterised by the following.

- Delay in, or total lack of, the development of spoken language, not accompanied by an attempt to compensate through alternative modes of communication such as gesture or mime.
- Stereotyped and repetitive use of language or idiosyncratic language.

In addition to the above, the profile of **structural language** impairments in LFA was described in Chapter 3 as having the following characteristics.

- Primary problems of comprehension and meaning or semantics.
- Less marked or persistent impairments of grammar or phonology (in the case of spoken language output).
- Apparent superiority of expressive language as compared to comprehension, resulting from the tendency to reproduce echoed or rote-learned chunks of language verbatim.
- Problems with deixis.

Where deprivation, hearing loss, dyspraxia or other co-morbid condition (e.g., Down syndrome, Fragile-X syndrome) is present, a more complex and variable set of language impairments will occur than shown under the bullet points above.

In this chapter, only the causes of *autism-specific* language impairment in lower-functioning individuals as profiled under the bullet points will be considered.

Explaining the Autism-specific Language Impairment

Impaired sequencing

At the time when the major challenge for explanations of autism was still seen in terms of explaining the linguistic and cognitive impairments in LFA, several theories converged on the suggestion that autism involves a fundamental impairment in 'sequencing' (Rutter, 1983; Tanguay, 1984; Lincoln, Allen, & Kilman, 1995). This suggestion was largely based on evidence that autistic children with poor language may have relatively good visual–spatial ability, plus the fact that whereas language involves temporal sequencing, visual–spatial tasks do not. These theories never received wide recognition, not least because they do not address the core social problems, nor the behaviours associated with behavioural inflexibility. However, the suggestion that impaired ability to process information with a temporal dimension might help to explain language impairments in LFA was proposed again by Boucher (2000; see Chapter 12).

Impaired symbolising

Language is defined as 'a set of symbols and rules for combining symbols meaningfully', and the linguistic symbols referred to generally have an arbitrary or conventional relation to the things they stand for. For example, the spoken or written word 'dog' has an arbitrary relation with that kind of animal that has four legs, barks, wags its tail, etc. The arbitrariness is apparent from the fact that someone who does not speak any form of English would be unable to guess what the spoken sounds or written letters 'dog' stand for.

Ricks and Wing (1975) suggested that defective symbolising in the linguistic sense might cause or contribute to impaired language acquisition in autism. This is a plausible hypothesis in so far as defective symbolising would impair the ability to acquire language in any **modality**, whether spoken, written, signed or otherwise conveyed. It is also consistent with the fact that a lack of symbolic pretend play is an early diagnostic marker for autism. However, Ricks and Wing did not suggest exactly how defective symbolising might arise: in other words, what might cause the deficit, in psychological terms. Moreover, those individuals with LFA who have some useful language clearly *can* use symbols and, as argued in Chapter 5, lack of spontaneous pretence is probably related to impaired generativity rather than a difficulty with using symbols.

Hobson (1993) also suggested that defective symbolising might cause or contribute to the language impairment in autism, and was more explicit concerning how such a deficit might arise. He argued that triadic relating (sometimes referred to as secondary intersubjectivity) is a prerequisite for the ability to use symbols and acquire language, and that impaired triadic relating results from a lack of genetically determined readiness to relate emotionally to other people (the theory described in Chapter 8). This argument was based on a classic analysis of the stages that infants go through in acquiring symbols (Werner & Kaplan, 1984). The process is complicated, and will not be detailed here. However, a key point is that the infant must have some minimal (unconscious) understanding of her own mind and of others' minds before she can ascribe meaning to her own utterances or gestures and before she can understand that others can use the same utterance or gesture with the same meaning as her own.

Hobson's argument that impaired social relating of the kind that occurs in autism causes impaired symbolising ability (and thereby impaired language) is thus well grounded in accepted theory. However, as an explanation of impaired language acquisition in LFA the hypothesis is flawed in that it fails to explain why only low-functioning individuals have clinically significant language problems. If all individuals across the spectrum have impaired relating of the kind Hobson describes, and if this leads inevitably to an inability to acquire symbols, as he argues, then it is hard to see why high-functioning individuals with autism are not also language-impaired. The same difficulty arises for theories arguing for a direct link between impaired triadic relating and impaired language without reference to defective symbolising ability, as considered next.

Defective mindreading

Baron-Cohen (1995), following Frith and Happé (1994b), suggested that defective mindreading impairs language acquisition in children with ASDs. To test this hypothesis, Baron-Cohen, Baldwin, and Crowson (1997) assessed the ability of young children with ASDs to use mindreading abilities to learn new words. Baron-Cohen et al. found, as predicted, that children with LFA were less able than age- and ability-matched controls to map a novel word correctly on to a novel object by inferring which object the speaker *meant* to name, that is, by understanding the mental state of 'intention'. A similar finding has been reported by Parish-Morris, Hennon, Hirsch-Pasek, Golinkoff, & Tager-Flusberg (2007). So, for example, if shown two unfamiliar objects and asked to point to the 'moff', a typically developing child will generally point to the one the tester is looking at, whereas children with ASDs do not use direction-of-gaze in this way.

Bloom (2000) agreed with Frith and Happé and with Baron-Cohen that mindblindness will impair the ability of children with ASDs to acquire language. He wrote:

> Learning a word is a social act. When children learn that… rabbit refers to rabbits, they are learning an arbitrary convention shared by a community of speakers, an implicitly agreed-upon way of communicating. When children learn the meaning of a word, they are – whether they know it or not – learning something about the thoughts of other people. (Bloom, 2000: 55)

However, Bloom recognised the problem of explaining why not all individuals with ASDs have delayed or clinically abnormal language, although all do have impairments of mindreading. He concluded that some other route into language, one that minimises the social component in learning, must be available to people with AS/HFA, and suggested that superior rote learning and associative ability might constitute that route. Unusual reliance on rote memory fits well with the fact that language used by children with AS tends to include phrases or whole sentences they have heard adults use, producing the 'little professor' impression first noted by Asperger. Bloom's suggestion that good associative ability may also be heavily relied on fits with the common observation that particular phrases or expressions are often uttered in response to a familiar situation or other cue.

Bloom's explanation also fits well with the theory proposed by Boucher, Mayes, & Bigham (2008), that impaired language in LFA results from a combination of impaired mindreading and a specific pattern of spared and impaired memory abilities, as described in Chapter 12.

Co-morbid specific language impairment

There is little doubt that ASDs and specific language impairments (SLI) are in some way meaningfully related. The evidence comes from various sources.

First, it has long been known that quite a high proportion of children with autism (including some who are not intellectually disabled) have the same kind of language impairments as children with SLI (Bartak et al., 1975). Moreover, one subtype of SLI, pragmatic language impairment, is sometimes accompanied by mild autism, as was pointed out in Chapter 2 (see Box 2.1). Thus there is undoubted behavioural overlap between autism and SLI in some individuals.

Secondly, at least some of the brain areas that appear have been shown to be structurally and functionally abnormal in children with SLI show comparable abnormalities in some children with ASDs (see Chapter 7). However, this could be the result, not the cause, of having a language impairment, and provides only weak evidence that SLI and language impairment are related.

Thirdly, studies of families in which there is one or more individual with an autistic spectrum disorder show a raised incidence of speech and language problems in parents, at least by their own report (Piven & Palmer, 1997; Folstein et al., 1999). In addition, siblings of children with SLI are at higher than normal risk of ASDs (Tomblin, Hafeman, & O'Brien, 2003). There is some (unconfirmed) evidence of shared susceptibility genes for SLI and autism (see Chapter 7).

The question at issue in this section is not, therefore, whether ASDs and SLI are related conditions: they clearly are. Rather, the question concerns the extent to which they may be related and whether or not SLI is the critical cause of the language impairment that differentiates LFA from AS/HFA. Tager-Flusberg and colleagues have suggested that this might be the case (Roberts, Rice, & Tager-Flusberg, 2004). These researchers base their claim on studies of language in children with autism showing that children with ASDs that include language impairment have a pattern of linguistic strengths and weakness that to some extent resembles that of children with SLI. Most importantly, children with autism plus language impairments have two very specific language-related impairments widely seen as **diagnostic markers** of SLI. These are poor memory for nonsense words (e.g., 'klum', 'fegorit') (Kjelgaard & Tager-Flusberg, 2001), and certain errors of verb tense-marking (e.g., walk/s/, walk/ed/) (Roberts et al., 2004).

Tager-Flusberg and her colleagues do, however, point out that the resemblance between the language of some children with autism and that of children with SLI may be superficial only, and may have different causes in the two diagnostic groups. There are, in addition, important differences between the commonest profiles of language impairment in SLI and the typical language profile in autism. In particular, impaired phonology ('articulation') is common in SLI, whereas phonology is generally mental-age appropriate in individuals with LFA, as noted in Chapter 3. Moreover, SLI by definition is diagnosed only in individuals without pervasive intellectual disability, whereas language impairment in autism is generally accompanied by intellectual disability, as discussed below. It is possible, however, that, when language impairments occur in individuals with autism and normal intelligence, this might be explained in terms of co-morbid SLI.

For an extended critique of the theory that co-morbid SLI is the critical cause of language impairment in autism, see Williams et al. (in press).

Hypersystemising

Baron-Cohen's (2005, 2006) extreme male brain theory, described in Chapter 7 and further discussed in Chapters 8 and 9, proposes that people who develop an ASD are unusually poor at empathising and unusually good at systemising. Baron-Cohen suggests that hypersystemising tendencies such as are hypothesised to occur across the autistic spectrum, but most markedly in people with LFA, will reduce the ability to extract rules and regularities from highly variable data such as heard speech. This argument is not, however, clearly articulated, nor is it supported by any directly relevant empirical data. However, 'hypersystemising' might conceivably be equated with overuse of certain processes in procedural memory, bringing it close to part of my own theory of the causes of LFA (see Chapter 12).

Defective mirror neurons

Williams (2005) and Oberman and Ramachandran (2007) have suggested that mirror neurons, which were mentioned in Chapter 8 in connection with imitation in infants, could be implicated in impaired language development. Imitative ability is known to relate to normal language development, and there is evidence to suggest that impaired imitation and delayed language are related in children with ASDs (Toth, Munson, Meltzoff, & Dawson, 2006). As mentioned in Chapter 7, there is evidence from imaging studies of abnormalities of the mirror neuron system in autism. There is also an argument in the broader literature that mirror neurons play a critical role in language evolution and that they play a continuing role in language acquisition (Gallese & Stamenov, 2002).

However, links between mirror neurons and language remain speculative, both in the case of typical development and in autism.

Comment

Whilst none of the theories outlined above offer a full or proven explanation of language impairments in LFA, none of them should be completely discounted. The causes of language impairment in ASDs are likely to be complex, involving many contributory factors. Amongst these may be defective symbolising (especially, perhaps, in the most severely affected individuals); impaired mindreading, which can help to explain the idiosyncratic word meanings commonly observed in autistic language, and also the odd misuse of pronouns and other deictic terms; and the co-occurrence of specific language impairments in a proportion of individuals with ASDs, which might help to explain cases of language impairment in individuals with autism and normal intellectual ability. The hypersystemising and mirror neurons hypotheses are, however, particularly in need of expansion and empirical support.

EXPLAINING UNEVEN PATTERNS OF INTELLECTUAL ABILITY

What Has to be Explained

In Chapter 3 it was suggested that the results of intelligence tests such as the Wechsler scales (Wechsler, 1999, 2004) carried out over many years with different groups of people with ASDs generally show the following.

- Uneven performance across the various subtests, even in individuals with overall high intelligence.
- Verbal quotient (VQ) may lag behind performance (or non-verbal) quotient (PQ) in the preschool years in high-functioning individuals but generally catches up and often overtakes PQ in later childhood, with high verbal intelligence common in older children and adults with AS/HFA.
- By contrast, VQ is almost invariably lower than PQ in low-functioning individuals.

Explaining Intelligence Test Profiles in People with Autism

In this section, the uneven IQ profile in high-functioning individuals will be considered first, followed by a more extended section on possible causes of intellectual disability in lower-functiong autism.

Explaining the uneven IQ profile in people with high-functioning autism

Unevenness in the IQ profiles of people with AS/HFA, a typical example of which is illustrated in Figure 3.2, most commonly presents as poor performance (relative to the individual's other scores) on the Comprehension subtest, and superior performance (relative to other scores) on the Block Design subtest. The Comprehension subtest assesses understanding and knowledge of social situations and conventions, and relatively poor performance on this test is plausibly explained in terms of social impairments. The Block Design subtest benefits from the bias towards local processing discussed earlier in this chapter (see Box 10.1), and it is this feature of autism across the spectrum that is usually thought to contribute to relatively superior performance on this test.

The initial lag in verbal intelligence in high-functioning individuals has not been formally investigated. A plausible explanation might be that lacking the normal social route into language (see Bloom's theory, above) causes some difference, if not delay, in early language development. Some of the verbal subtests of the Wechsler scales depend on verbally acquired knowledge, and limited social interaction in the early years may, in addition, reduce opportunities to acquire such knowledge.

Explaining intellectual disability in people with low-functioning autism

There has been remarkably little research directed towards characterising or explaining intellectual disability in autism, despite the fact that it is extremely common and – in combination with autism and language impairment – extremely handicapping. There appears to be a widespread assumption that intellectul disability is simply another co-morbid condition, probably associated with the extent of brain abnormality, and of no great theoretical interest. This assumption is fatally undermined, however, by the fact that language impairment and intellectual disability almost always occur together when associated with autism. Moreover, autism-specific language impairment is probably genetically related to autism, implying that autism-specific intellectual disability is also related to autism (Bailey, Phillips, & Rutter, 1996). In this section, the close linkage of language impairment and intellectual disability and its relevance for explanations of intellectual disability in autism is considered, and the few theories that attempt to explain this linkage are acknowledged.

As noted in Chapter 3, it is verbal ability rather than non-verbal ability that swings the full scale IQ from the normal to the subaverage range in people with LFA. Non-verbal intelligence, and especially 'general' or 'fluid' intelligence, may be within normal limits in mild to moderately intellectually disabled individuals (Dawson et al., 2007), and facets of visual–spatial reasoning and constructional ability are relatively spared even in severely intellectually disabled individuals (DeMyer et al., 1974). Can intellectual disability in people with low-functioning autism therefore be understood as resulting from impaired language? Clearly the answer is yes, at least in part. However, verbal intelligence is not synonymous with language: more than language is involved in passing these tests, as is clear from the descriptions of a typical set of verbal subtests in Box 3.7.

It is therefore likely that low verbal intelligence in LFA results from a combination of impaired language and some other factor. This additional factor might be unrelated to language. It seems more likely, however, given the tight linkage between language impairment and intellectul disability, that low verbal intelligence in LFA results from a combination of impaired language and some other factor that is related to both the language impairments and the intellectual disability. Three hypotheses are consistent with this suggestion.

1 Ricks and Wing (1975) hypothesised that impaired ability to use symbols would impair the capacity for 'inner speech' and hence the ability to think and reason, as well as impairing language acquisition. As noted in the section on causes of language impairment in LFA, this theory may be relevant to individuals with profound intellectual disability and no language, but is unlikely to be relevant to those individuals who have some language and who are capable of symbolic pretend play. Such evidence as there is concerning the ability to use inner speech, or **verbal mediation**, as it is sometimes called, is mixed, as was noted in Chapter 9 (see e.g., Williams et al., 2008).
2 Baron-Cohen (2005) has argued that extreme forms of hypersystemising, such as are hypothesised to occur in people with LFA, would cause impaired generalisation sufficient to impact on intelligence and breadth of knowledge, as well as impairing language. This hypothesis is not well specified, however, nor has it been empirically tested.
3 Boucher et al. (2008) have argued that a specific type of memory impairment would directly impair crystallised intelligence, as well as impairing language (see Chapter 12).

SUMMARY

Early attempts to characterise and explain anomalous sensory-perceptual processing in autism included some early theories that are consistent with certain strands of current thinking. For example, Ornitz's theory identified impaired ability to filter out background stimuli and impaired ability to habituate to novel stimuli as fundamental deficits, with secondary effects on selective and directed attention. Three current attempts to characterise and explain sensory-perceptual processing anomalies are Frith's/Frith and Happé's weak central coherence (WCC) theory, Mottron et al.'s enhanced perceptual function theory, and Plaisted et al.'s enhanced discrimination–reduced generalisation theory. The WCC theory originally hypothesised that sensory-perceptual processing anomalies result from impaired global processing. This claim was later modified to the suggestion that people with ASDs have an unusually strong bias towards local as opposed to global processing. However, most recently the emphasis in WCC theory has returned to problems of higher-order, or top-down, control such as would involve global integrative processes. The enhanced perceptual function theory, by contrast, has consistently maintained that enhanced ability to process sensory-perceptual input at the level of its surface qualities biases against the usage of more global processing strategies. Plaisted and colleagues' original theory, on the other hand, was that people with autism have unusually good ability to integrate low-level features that serve to discriminate between related stimuli. However, enhanced discrimination comes at the cost of registering stimulus similarities such as are needed for generalisation to occur, with adverse effects on learning about the world. Plaisted et al. have recently been investigating attentional mechanisms in vision and hearing, but have found these to be largely intact. In sum, the precise nature and cause of the wide range of abnormalities of sensation and perception reported by people with ASDs and confirmed by research remain unclear.

Uneven motor skills in some individuals with ASDs may be partly explained in terms of co-morbid problems of muscle tone or neuromuscular control. However, the commonly observed mixture of clumsy movements and gait with dexterity in certain well-practised fine movements cannot be explained in this way. There is some as yet slight evidence to suggest that people with ASDs have a specific difficulty in motor planning and possibly in initiating, as opposed to executing, actions. However this evidence needs replication and extension before conclusions can be drawn from it. The selective impairment in imitating others' body-related movement almost certainly derives from impaired appreciation of self–other equivalence.

Language impairment in people with ASDs across the spectrum may sometimes result from co-morbid conditions such as hearing impairment, Down syndrome or from poor home background. Language output systems, including speech, signing and writing, may also be affected by neuromuscular problems. What has been termed 'the LFA-specific language profile' (see Chapter 3) cannot, however, be explained by co-morbid problems such as the above. Suggested causes include impaired sequencing, in the sense of the capacity to process information that has temporal structure, inability to use symbols, impaired mindreading, specific language impairment, hypersystemisation, and a defective mirror neuron system. None of these theories offers a full or proven explanation of the LFA-specific language profile. However, mindblindness is certain to be a factor; impaired ability to use symbols might help to explain complete lack of language in the least able individuals; and SLI probably occurs co-morbidly in a proportion of language-impaired individuals. Further investigation of the more recent theories is needed.

There has been remarkably little investigation of the intellectual impairment associated with low-functioning autism. However it is clear that the impairment derives at least in part from impaired language, and there are suggestions that impaired language and intellectual impairment may, in addition, have some common cause. Impaired use of symbols and hypersystemisation have been proposed as possible common causes, but the argument for impaired symbolisation is weak and the argument for hypersystemisation is untested.

EXPLAINING AUTISM AS A WHOLE: ATTEMPTS AT A SYNTHESIS

AIM
••••
INTRODUCTION
••••
PSYCHOLOGICAL EXPLANATIONS OF AUTISM: AN EMERGING
SYNTHESIS
Past: The 'Three Theories' Explanation
Present: Advances on the Three Theories
Future: New Directions
Comment
••••
LINKING LEVELS: BRAIN–BEHAVIOUR EXPLANATIONS
OF AUTISM AS A WHOLE
Brain–behaviour Theories Consistent with a Dedicated Systems Model
Brain–behaviour Theories Consistent with an Emergence Model
Possible Objections to Disconnectivity Theories, and a Defence
Comment
••••
FROM FIRST CAUSES TO AUTISTIC BEHAVIOUR: LINKING THE
EXPLANATIONS TOGETHER
••••
SUMMARY

AIM

The aim of this chapter is to consider ways in which the material presented in preceding chapters in Part II may begin to fit together into a multi-level, coherent explanation of autism as a whole, indicating the kinds of explanation that are emerging, although the details of a full explanation are not known.

INTRODUCTION

In Chapter 6 it was suggested that attempts to explain autism should focus on a limited agenda consisting of the interaction impairments (social, emotional, and communicative), behavioural inflexibility (restricted, repetitive and unimaginative behaviours), sensory-perceptual and motor anomalies, spared abilities, and the language impairment and intellectual disability that distinguish lower-functioning autism from Asperger syndrome and most forms of HFA. This agenda provided the topics covered in previous chapters in Part II, and will remain the focus of the present chapter.

It was also noted in Chapter 6 that there are three major levels at which autism may be explained: etiological, neurobiological, and psychological; and that another simplifying strategy is to examine explanations at each of these levels separately in the first instance, before considering how explanations at the different levels may fit together. Consistent with this strategy, Chapter 7 examined explanations at the etiological and then at the neurobiological levels, and in the next three chapters psychological explanations of each of the agenda topics were considered separately. However, ways in which the psychological theories described in Chapters 8–10 might fit together to explain autism as a whole were not examined. The present chapter therefore starts by attempting a synthesis of the psychological theories covered in the preceding three chapters. Following this, attempts to link together explanations at the psychological level with theories of the brain bases of autism will be considered. In the final main section of the chapter, attempts to link explanations across all three levels will be considered.

The third simplifying strategy argued for in Chapter 6 will also be utilised here. This is to focus on the search for the critical causes of the various facets of autism-related behaviours, ignoring for the time being the multiplicity of additional contributory factors that are certainly involved.

PSYCHOLOGICAL EXPLANATIONS OF AUTISM: AN EMERGING SYNTHESIS

Past: The 'Three Theories' Explanation

Three groups of psychological theories concerning the causes of autism dominated the literature in the last decade of the twentieth century: defective theory of mind/mentalising deficit/mindblindness theories, executive dysfunction theories, and the weak central coherence/enhanced perceptual function/enhanced discrimination–reduced generalisation group of theories (see Rajendran & Mitchell, 2007 for a review). For brevity, these three groups of theories will be referred to in this section as 'defective ToM theories', 'executive dysfunction theories' and 'WCC theories'.

The ToM and WCC theories were each originally presented as 'single deficit theories', or 'single common pathway' theories, and were the last of a string of theories of this kind. Once studies of relatives of people with ASDs had established that behaviours associated with autism can occur independently of each other, single deficit theories became untenable, and attempts to identify a single psychological cause of ASDs were abandoned. This opened up the possibility that each of the three types of psychological deficit identified in the theories is the critical cause of one particular set of autism-related behaviours, as illustrated in Figure 11.1(a).

For various reasons, however, it is certain that the three theories are only stepping-stones towards a full and coherent explanation of autism at the psychological level. Most of the reasons for this conclusion can be found in the critiques included within Chapters 8, 9 and 10. However, they are summarised here.

1 All three psychological impairments, or kinds of psychological impairment, identified in the theories are in need of further expansion and explanation themselves. The ToM theories and executive dysfunction theories in particular fare poorly when assessed in terms of the specificity and primacy criteria.
2 If impaired ToM is the critical cause of the social and communicative impairments in autism, and executive dysfunction is the critical cause of behavioural inflexibility, then defective ToM and executive dysfunction should be independent, or dissociable, causal factors. This follows from evidence from the broader autism phenotype that socio-communicative impairments and behavioural inflexibility are dissociable. However, there is a great deal of evidence indicating that performance on ToM tests (notably false belief tasks) is related to executive abilities in typically developing children as well as in individuals with ASDs, although the nature of the relationship is controversial (Russell, 1997; Perner & Lang, 1999; Leslie et al., 2004).

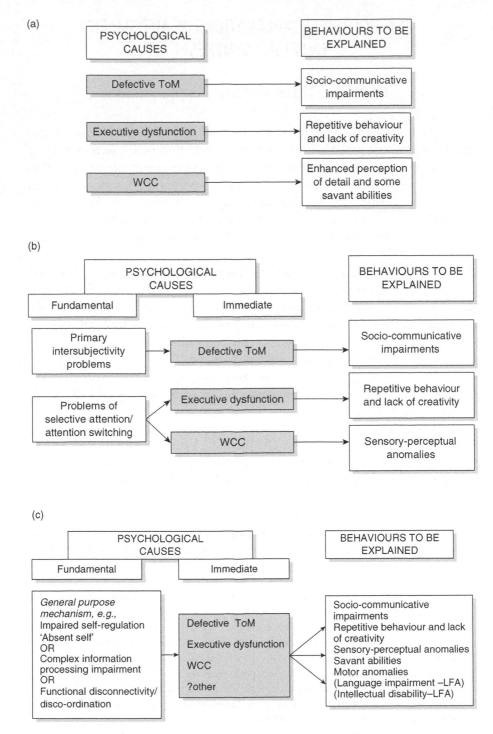

Figure 11.1 Theoretical formulations of the psychological causes of behaviours associated with ASDs: (a) recent; (b) current; and (c) possible future formulations

3   The three theories say nothing about uneven patterns of motor skill, almost nothing about anomalous emotion processing, and little about spared abilities with the exception of enhanced perceptual processing. Nothing is said, for example, about superior rote memory, a characteristic noted from Kanner onwards. Nor do the theories provide an adequate explanation of the language and intellectual impairments in LFA. Although this latter point is not a major criticism, because the three theories aim only to explain 'pure' autism, at some point the links between autism, language impairment and intellectual disability will have to be elucidated.

4   An additional problem for the set of ToM theories is that they were proposed at a time when the analogy between computers and the human mind and brain was dominant in psychology. However, by the end of the twentieth century the limitations of this model were increasingly recognised, and some of the assumptions underlying this group of theories are now widely rejected. This point was touched on in Chapter 7, in connection with the degree to which brain development is tightly genetically controlled as opposed to relatively flexible or 'plastic'. In addition to the argument that brain development shows more plasticity than is assumed within the computer-inspired 'modularist', or **dedicated systems,** model, two other criticisms may be mentioned. The first is that computers are quite unlike human brains and minds in that they are disembodied machines that *react* to a limited set of highly specified environmental inputs, but do not *interact* with their environment. The second is related to the first in that computational modelling methods associated with the computer-inspired model do not adequately reflect the overall course or character of human learning and behaviour.

Present: Advances on the Three Theories

Attempts to explain autism at the level of psychology have developed since the three theories model held sway, as noted in previous chapters. Newer developments are illustrated in Figure 11.1(b). Some advantages of these developments are considered next, enumerated so as to correspond with the problems listed in the previous section.

1   The focus on primary intersubjectivity in place of the higher-level ToM theories, and on attentional processes in place of less well-specified executive function theories, offers psychological explanations of major features of autistic behaviour that have improved potential to satisfy the specificity and primacy criteria.

2   Low-level causal factors of the kinds invoked in primary intersubjectivity theories are more likely to be dissociable from executive functions than are the kinds of high-level complex cognitive abilities involved in theory of mind.

3   Most of the primary intersubjectivity theories, unlike the ToM group of theories, are designed to be able to explain the emotional as well as the socio-communicative impairments.

4   Only one of the primary intersubjectivity theories (Baron-Cohen's empathising deficit theory) is based on the dedicated systems model that has been widely criticised; and two of the theories (Klin et al.'s and Loveland's) are explicitly based on the **constructivist or emergence** model that is taking its place (see below). An additional gain from the reformulation represented in Figure 11.1(b) is outlined next.

5 Three major features of autistic behaviour, namely socio-emotional-communicative impairments, behavioural inflexibility, and sensory-perceptual anomalies, can be explained in terms of two, rather than three, underlying psychological deficits, or kinds of deficit. The suggestion that attentional abnormalities underlie, or contribute to, both the behavioural inflexibility and the sensory-perceptual anomalies also helps to explain why central coherence and executive functions are at least partially related, not only in individuals with ASDs (Pellicano, Maybery, Durkin, & Maley, 2006) but also in typically developing individuals (Pellicano, Maybery, & Durkin, 2005).

Future: New Directions

From dedicated systems and connectionist modelling to constructivism, emergence, embodiment, and dynamic systems modelling

Through the 1990s, several neuroscientists began to argue for what was variously called an emergence (Elman et al., 1996), constructivist (Quartz, 1999), or neo-constructivist (Karmiloff-Smith, 1998) model of brain–mind development to replace the dedicated systems model. What will be referred to here as the constructivist emergence model, or sometimes just the emergence model, allows for considerable plasticity in brain development, which is seen as largely dependent on experience, guided by innate but low-level attentional biases and basic learning mechanisms (see Figure 11.1(c)). The **domain-specific** information-processing systems that are found in the adult brain are thus seen as the products of construction over time, and as being genetically guided rather than genetically determined.

Over the same period, the disembodied nature of the dedicated systems model, noted above, was criticised by philosophers (e.g., Clark, 1997) as well as psychologists (e.g., Varela, Thompson, & Rosch, 1991). Clark, for example, subtitled his book *Putting brain, body, and world together again*, and argued that the mind 'emerges' from each individual's bodily experiences resulting from their interactions with the environment. He used the term **embodied mind** to summarise his argument. Thus the concepts of emergence and embodiment are closely related.

As noted above, the computational modelling methods associated with the dedicated systems model do not adequately reflect the overall course or character of most of human learning and behaviour. Connectionist or neural network models, for example, although useful for exploring how small facets of learning progress, take no account of the continuous processes of interaction occurring between the environment, bodily experience, and the brain emphasised by Clark and others.

Dynamic systems modelling is now widely seen as providing a more appropriate method of simulating embodied learning than connectionist, or 'neural network', modelling can provide. The body-environment-brain/mind system is 'dynamic' because a change in any part of the system affects the operation of the whole, causing continuous reorganisation and change, rather as a flock of birds will form, reform, and reform again in constant motion but acting as a whole. Correspondingly, in dynamic systems modelling, the acquisition of skills and knowledge as well as ongoing behaviour are viewed as emerging from the cumulative effects of small changes in a multiplicity of components of the overall system, mathematically represented.

The shift from a modularist, or dedicated systems, model to a constructivist emergence model is reflected in some psychological theories of autism. For example, the concept of the embodied mind underpins Klin, Jones, Schultz, and Volkmar's (2003) **enactive mind** theory. According to this theory, infants who will develop autism lack the normal preferential attention to social stimuli that is so conspicuous in typically developing infants. As a result, these infants never experience those interactions with others that become embodied in real-life social skills. Loveland's (2001) 'impaired affordances' theory, also outlined in Chapter 8, is based on an older but not dissimilar **ecological** model of the development and function of the human brain and mind (Gibson, 1979). According to Gibson's ecological model each organism and its environment constitute an interactive whole, as is assumed also by the concepts of embodiment, constructivism and emergence.

Fuller accounts of emergence and dynamic systems modelling, and how these novel approaches apply to typical development and potentially to an understanding of autism, can be found in Bowler (2001, 2007).

Increased recognition of the possible role of the self

As briefly noted in Chapter 5, there is increasing interest in the role of the self, and possible abnormalities relating to the self, as causally implicated in autism. This is not a new focus of interest, as is evident from the summary presented in Box 11.1. However, Frith (2003) and Hobson, Chidambi, Lee, and Meyer (2006) are notable autism researchers who have re-emphasised the possible centrality of an impaired sense of self.

BOX 11.1   Do people with ASDs have a sense of self that is different from that of people without ASDs?

This question has intrigued researchers for decades. Creak (1961) noted an apparent lack of personal identity. However, in the 1980s it was shown that children with ASDs recognise themselves in a mirror at about the same age as children without autism, if overall ability is taken into account (Dawson & McKissick, 1984; Spiker & Ricks, 1984). Moreover, a study by Lee and Hobson (1998) also showed that children and adolescents with mid- to lower-functioning autism are as good as non-autistic youngsters of comparable ability at answering questions about their own physical attributes, their activities, abilities, and psychological processes.

(Cont'd)

However, the young people in Lee and Hobson's study were less able to answer questions about themselves as social beings, a finding interpreted in terms of an impaired 'interpersonal self' (see also Hobson, 1990, 1993; Hobson et al., 2006). They also performed poorly on probes about self-understanding, such as 'Do you change at all from year to year?', 'What makes you different from other people you know?' or 'What do you like best about yourself – what are you most proud of?' This impairment suggests that, despite straightforward knowledge of themselves as physical and psychological beings, people with ASDs nevertheless have a more limited sense of themselves than do other people.

This conclusion is consistent with Powell and Jordan's (1993) suggestion that people with ASDs lack an 'experiencing self' that provides a personal dimension for ongoing events – the feeling that '*I* am doing this' or '*I* was there at the time'. Millward, Powell, Messer, and Jordan (2000) suggested that people with ASDs remember real-life episodes less well than other people because they have no 'experiencing self', a suggestion further explored by Lind and Bowler (2008). Frith (2003) also notes the loss or impairment of an experiencing self in her 'absent self' theory. She points out that all three major theories of the psychological roots of autism entail an absence of the 'I' that reflects on mental states, that exerts executive control, and that has access to integrated coherent experience (see also Frith and Happé, 1999).

Possible brain correlates of impaired sense of self in people with ASDs have been proposed by Ben Shalom (2000b).

From domain-specific to general-purpose mechanisms

As noted above, Loveland sets her view of autism within a Gibsonian ecological model of an organism–environment system. According to this model, processes of **self-regulation** play a key role in the organisation and control of the overall system, and Bachevalier and Loveland (2006) interpret evidence of impaired function within the social brain in terms of an impairment of self-regulation.

Notably, 'self-regulation' identifies a **general-purpose mechanism** operating across many facets of behaviour. Some other theories of the psychological causes of autism also identify general-purpose mechanisms as important for understanding the causes of autistic behaviour. One example is Minshew and colleagues' hypothesis that autism is caused by a generalised impairment of complex information processing (Minshew, Goldstein, & Siegel, 1997). The re-description of WCC in terms of a lack of top-down control such as could affect many domains of behaviour is another example. Executive functions, whether identifying response inhibition, attention switching, self-monitoring or indeed self-regulation, are also general-purpose mechanisms. It might even be said that Baron-Cohen's (2006) concept of a systemising mechanism ranks as a general-purpose rather than a domain-specific processing mechanism, in that systemising is hypothesised to affect many different aspects of learning and behaviour.

All these theories represent a move away from explaining autism in terms of multiple independent deficits, and towards the effects that a single *kind* of problem might have on this or that facet of learning and behaviour, either separately or together (Frith, 2003; Happé & Frith, 2006). The route to autism that is being proposed by general-purpose mechanism theories is illustrated schematically in Figure 11.1(c).

Theories invoking general-purpose mechanisms have the potential to explain why certain behaviour anomalies in different domains co-occur in people with ASDs. For example, hypersystemising is hypothesised to affect behavioural flexibility, language acquisition, and intelligence. A lack of top-down control could affect the planning and control of non-routinised movements and the flexible use of strategies in problem solving just as much as the ability to bind parts into wholes in perceptual experience. Impaired ability to process complex information would affect both memory function and the acquisition of conceptual knowledge (Minshew, Meyer, & Goldstein, 2002).

Nevertheless, theories such as the above that identify a single *kind* of deficit or anomaly that has effects on many domains of behaviour face certain challenges. In particular, they must be able to explain why many facets of development and psychological function are completely or relatively intact in people with ASDs. Explaining some fine cuts, where one of a pair of closely related behaviours is impaired and the other spared, may prove particularly difficult for the broad brush of general-purpose mechanism theories. These theories must also defend themselves from the possible charge of constituting single-factor explanations of autism, of the kind argued against in Chapter 6. These challenges are easier to respond to in terms of the brain bases of autism than in terms of psychology alone, and are considered again later in the chapter.

Comment

The 'three theories' have justifiably dominated psychological thinking about the causes of autism for over two decades, generating between them an immense increase in our understanding of the things people with ASDs do well, the things they find difficult, and the things they do differently. None of the three theories is going to go away. However, the ToM and executive function theories in particular have proved insufficient by themselves, at least in their present form, to explain either the interaction impairments or the behavioural inflexibility diagnostic of autism, let alone other universal or common autism-related characteristics.

The major problem with the ToM theories is that, although they identify what is almost certainly a *necessary* common pathway to autism, they do not offer a *sufficient*, nor a sufficiently *early occurring*, explanation of social and communication impairments (nor of emotional impairments). The newer primary intersubjectivity theories seem likely to supply the missing link(s). The major problem with various versions of the executive function theories is similar, in that those executive dysfunctions that have been most reliably demonstrated (e.g., mental inflexibility, impaired planning) may constitute common pathways to autism, but are in need of explanation themselves. Here, unfortunately, less progress has been made. However, the investigation of possible links with WCC and lack of top-down processing may prove fruitful.

The WCC group of theories has proved more resilient than the other two theories, and is greatly strengthened by the fact that it is consistent with, and has contributed to, the kinds of neurobiological explanations of autism that are the topic of the next main section of the chapter. Impaired integrative functions and impaired top-down control are, in addition, general-purpose mechanisms of the kind that are consistent with a constructivist emergence model of brain development and function, now seen to offer a more appropriate approach than a dedicated systems model to understanding the causes of autism.

Gaps remain in psychological explanations of autism, notably relating to some facets of behavioural inflexibility, uneven motor skills, spared abilities, and impaired language and intellectual disability in lower-functioning individuals. Some suggestions as to how to fill these gaps are offered in Chapter 12.

LINKING LEVELS: BRAIN–BEHAVIOUR EXPLANATIONS OF AUTISM AS A WHOLE

The same tension exists at the level of brain bases of autism as exists at the level of psychological explanation, namely that between a dedicated systems model as opposed to a constructivist emergence model that gives more emphasis to developmental processes and the brain as an integrated whole. In what follows, attempts to establish relationships between specific brain abnormalities and specific psychological deficits will be described first. Attempts to identify the origin(s) and course of abnormal brain development in autism using a constructivist model, and to relate this to the *kind* of consequences there would be for psychological functions and behaviour across a number of domains will then be described.

Brain–behaviour Theories Consistent with a Dedicated Systems Model

Brain correlates of impaired mindreading, executive dysfunction, and weak central coherence

In Chapter 7 it was stated that there is reliable evidence of abnormalities in people with ASDs of brain structures and functions within 'the social brain', or what is sometimes called 'the social cognition system', supporting theories of impaired triadic relating and theory of mind. Reviews of this evidence can be found in Pelphrey et al. (2004) and Schultz (2005). Mundy (2003) has reviewed evidence of impaired mediation of social reward by structures within the social brain, supporting some primary intersubjectivity deficit theories. Dapretto et al. (2006) and Hadjikhani et al. (2006) have demonstrated abnormal mirror neuron function in people with ASDs, supporting another group of primary intersubjectivity deficit theories.

Reliable evidence of abnormalities related to executive function impairments has proved more elusive, especially as concerns structural abnormalities in the frontal lobes. However, as noted in Chapter 7, studies using technically sophisticated methods of examining brain structure have begun to show some of the expected frontal lobe abnormalities (Courchesne & Pierce, 2005; Casanova et al., 2006). Moreover, the fact that the cerebellum contributes to executive functions, together with the fact that cerebellar abnormalities have been reliably demonstrated in the brains of people with ASDs, suggests that executive function impairments in autism may originate at this level of the brain circuit subserving executive control (see Hill, 2004, for a review of the evidence).

The WCC theory differs from the other two theories in that it was not predicated on any system-specific brain abnormalities. Instead, when Frith (1989) introduced the theory she speculated that there might be a problem in 'binding' brain activity in one area of the brain with activity in another, causing a fragmentation of neural activity resulting in the psychological phenomena associated with weak central coherence. Brock, Brown, Boucher, and Rippon (2002) elaborated this suggestion. Utilising evidence and theories from mainstream neuropsychology they suggested that impaired **neural binding** could result from impaired synchronisation of activity across several local networks, such as would normally summate into a global network. The concept of impaired binding, and the related suggestion that a lack of connectivity in the brain can explain many of the behavioural impairments in autism (Just et al., 2004; Geschwind & Levitt, 2007), are discussed at greater length below.

In sum, each of the three theories that dominated the psychological literature in the last decade of the twentieth century can be linked to what is known about the brain bases of autism, even if the evidence is not strong (in the case of executive function impairments) or if it is unproven (in the case of WCC and related theories). In the section on psychological explanations of autism it was, however, pointed out that the three theories leave much of autism unexplained. Two attempts to formulate a more comprehensive explanation of autism in terms of brain–behaviour correlates are described next.

Brain correlates of autism as a whole: (1) Dawson et al.'s theory

Dawson, Webb et al. (2002) identify six areas of psychological functioning that are generally impaired in people with ASDs, which they refer to as phenotypic traits. Figure 11.2 shows the brain–regions hypothesised to contribute to each of the six traits.

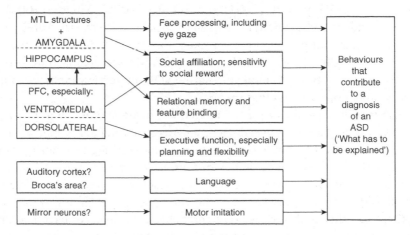

Figure 11.2 Diagram showing the brain structures and systems hypothesised to underlie the six phenotypical traits identified in Dawson et al.'s model (extracted from the text of Dawson et al., *Development and Psychopathology*, 14: 581–611) MTL = medial temporal lobe. PFC = prefrontal cortex.

The six phenotypic traits between them cover all the behaviours identified in the present book as in most immediate need of explanation. Thus impaired face processing and impaired processing of social reward/affiliative behaviour and impaired imitation together are seen as causing the socio-emotional-communicative interaction impairments; impaired executive function relates to behavioural inflexibility; impaired **feature binding** relates to sensory-perceptual anomalies; and impaired motor imitation relates in part to the uneven motor skills noted in the present book. Impaired language ability, the fifth of Dawson et al.'s phenotypic traits, has also been identified in the present book as in need of explanation.

Dawson et al.'s proposed brain–behaviour explanations of the interaction impairment, behavioural inflexibility and sensory-perceptual abnormalities are consistent with findings on brain anatomy and function in autism reviewed in Chapter 7, and with the most recent psychological theories detailed in Chapters 8, 9, and 10. Their theory does not, however, address the issue of motor abnormalities in full. Nor is their proposed brain–behaviour explanation of language impairments in low-functioning autism fully consistent with such evidence as is available (see Chapter 10).

Brain correlates of autism as a whole: (2) Waterhouse, Fein, and Modahl's theory

Waterhouse and colleagues (1996) also hypothesised that several different abnormalities of brain function might be needed to explain the whole set of autism-related behaviours. Each of four brain abnormalities identified in their model was hypothesised to cause a particular impairment at the level of psychological description, and each of these psychological impairments was hypothesised in turn to cause or contribute to facets of autism-related behaviour. An outline of Waterhouse et al.'s complex hypothesis is represented in Figure 11.3.

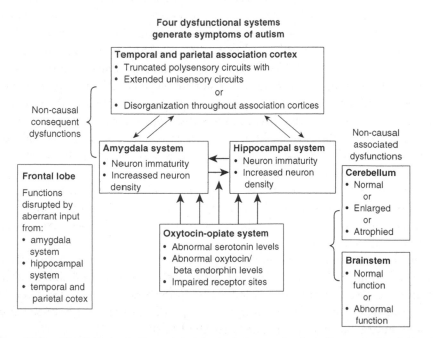

Figure 11.3 Waterhouse et al's model of the brain bases of autism. The centre block identifies four dysfunctional systems hypothesised to cause behaviours diagnostic of ASDs, indicating the kinds of abnormality that may be present. Blocks to the left and right of the centre identify systems that would be secondarily affected (from Waterhouse, Fein, and Modahl, *Psychological Review*, 103: 460, with permission)

The full paper should be read by anyone with particular interest in brain–psychology–behaviour relationships in autism: it is a good example of the kind of account that is needed to explain autism in all its complexity and variety, and much in the paper prefigures current theories. It is, in fact, transitional between dedicated systems explanations and emergence-based theories such as are outlined in the next section, which is why I describe it after Dawson et al.'s theory, although it is an older theory. Ways in which Waterhouse et al.'s theory prefigures current views include the following.

First, there is specific rejection of a narrowly modular account of typical development, and of the development of autism. However, some degree of brain specialisation is assumed. Thus the hippocampus has the specialised role of integrating information from various sources during the registration of ongoing experience of all kinds; the amygdala assigns significance to social stimuli (but also to non-social stimuli); the oxytocin opiate system subserves the kinds of social bonding mechanisms contributing to primary intersubjectivity (but may also subserve some non-social functions); and polysensory association areas in the temporal and parietal lobes form part of the global networks needed for the perception of complex wholes.

Secondly, just as structures such as the amygdala and neurochemical systems such as the oxytocin opiate system subserve both social and non-social functions ('one-to-many'), so each facet of autism-related behaviours is seen as having multiple causes ('many-to-one'), not only at the level of psychological explanation but also at the level of brain function. Thus all four brain abnormalities are seen as contributing to all of the behaviours diagnostic of autism. However, the contribution of each to the various facets of autism-related behaviour varies; the degree of dysfunction in the four systems is also seen as varying in different individuals, allowing for variation within the autism phenotype.

Thirdly, the brain abnormalities are seen as resulting from abnormal neuronal growth and organisation during brain development, the effects of some initial abnormality being cumulative.

Fourthly, abnormal neuronal growth and organisation is seen as associated with excess neural tissue resulting from excessive neuron proliferation prenatally or abnormal increase in white matter or abnormally decreased neural pruning and cell death.

Fifthly, abnormalities within the frontal lobes are seen as secondary consequences of the initial abnormalities. (The existence of structural abnormalities within the cerebellum is acknowledged by Waterhouse et al., but not seen as of causal significance. This is an important point of difference between their model and two important theories described next.)

Brain–behaviour Theories Consistent with an Emergence Model

Impaired connectivity theories

By the turn of the century most neuroscientists engaged in the study of autism were assuming a (neo)constructivist or emergence model of brain development in which, as prefigured in Waterhouse et al.'s theory, brain abnormalities are seen as resulting from an initial abnormality or abnormalities with cumulative effects. Terms such as 'disconnection' and 'impaired connectivity' were also increasingly used to characterise brain structure and function in people with ASDs, with decreasing emphasis on any single structure or brain area as *the* location of a particular functional impairment.

Carpenter, Just, Keller, Cherkassky, Roth, and Minshew (2001), for example, described autism as having differential amounts of co-ordination within, as opposed to between, system components, and explained this in terms of abnormal connectivity. This group of researchers has continued to interpret its detailed investigations of brain–behaviour relations in people with ASDs in terms of abnormal connectivity (Just et al., 2004; Koshino et al., 2005). Minshew, who is a member of this group, sees impaired connectivity as the brain basis of the impairment of complex information processing that she and her colleagues hypothesise to be the cause of autism at the psychological level of description (see the section on 'general-purpose mechanisms' above).

Brock et al. (2002), as also mentioned above, proposed that the brain basis of weak central coherence is impaired binding of neural activity across diverse local networks to achieve global network activity. Rippon, Brock, Brown, and Boucher (2007) subsequently equated impaired binding with a reduction in long-distance connectivity combined with overconnectivity within isolated neural assemblies. This hypothesis echoes Carpenter et al.'s description of the brain in people with ASDs as having more within-system co-ordination than between-system co-ordination, as a result of lack of connectivity.

The most fully articulated theories of brain–behaviour relations in autism consistent with emergence models are, however, those of Courchesne and Belmonte and their colleagues. Courchesne's and Belmonte's theories are very similar, and these two researchers sometimes collaborate. There are some differences in emphasis, however, and in what follows Courchesne's and Belmonte's theories are presented separately, but commented on as a single theory.

Courchesne's theory

Courchesne and his colleagues have studied the cerebellum in individuals with ASDs over many years, reporting various abnormalities within this complex structure (Courchesne, 2004, provides a summary). As noted in Chapter 7, reduced numbers of Purkinje cells in the cerebellum has been a consistent finding in postmortem studies (Bailey et al., 1998). These cells constitute the main route for transmission of information from the cerebellum to other brain regions, having a mainly GABA-mediated inhibitory function.

Courchesne and his colleagues have also been at the forefront of investigations of brain size in people with ASDs. As noted in Chapter 7, brain size is normal at birth in children who are later diagnosed with an ASD, but increases abnormally rapidly during the first two years of life. Following early overgrowth there is what Courchesne refers to as 'premature arrest of brain growth', the net result being that maximum brain size in autism is reached by five years of age or earlier, up to ten years sooner than is normal.

Building on these two strands of his research, Courchesne (2004) proposed that the cerebellum is a site of initial abnormality in people with ASDs, reduced numbers of Purkinje cells being critical. He argued that reduced numbers of these cells results in a lack of inhibitory control of neural activity. Excessive excitatory output from the cerebellum is argued to overstimulate brain growth in regions with which the cerebellum is connected from birth, namely those regions of the limbic system and the temporal and frontal lobes that are critically involved in mediating early social and emotional learning and behaviour, language, and higher-order cognitive functions. By contrast, the premature arrest of brain growth that follows is argued to result in a lack of structural connectivity between the frontal lobes and non-frontal brain regions. This would impair the ability to integrate information from many parts of the brain and to exert top-down influence from the frontal lobes to lower-level systems. This in turn, Courchesne suggests, may trigger overconnectivity amongst local networks subserving lower-level functional systems. He concludes:

> In this sense, autism may be an unusual disconnection disorder with sparing (or perhaps even enhancement) of lower-level basic processing, but also with an impaired capacity to fully integrate lower-level detailed information into high-order meaningful contexts. (Courchesne, 2004: 109)

Belmonte's theory

Belmonte et al., (2004a; Belmonte et al. 2004b) are in agreement with Courchesne's (2004) hypothesis that a reduction in Purkinje cells in the cerebellum would release cerebellar outputs from inhibition, and that the resulting excessive excitation would cause activity-dependent overgrowth in regions to which the cerebellum projects. They also agree with Courchesne that this overgrowth underlies the rapid increase in brain size in infants subsequently diagnosed with an ASD, and that following a period of overgrowth there is a relative lack of brain growth in the later childhood years affecting in particular the long-range connectivity necessary for higher-order control of lower-level functions.

The differences between Courchesne's and Belmonte et al.'s statements of their theory concern the greater emphasis that Belmonte et al. place on impaired connectivity and how it should be understood; and in the more ambitious scope of the latter theory, especially as articulated in Belmonte et al. (2004a).

Regarding clarification of what may be understood by 'abnormal brain connectivity', Belmonte et al. make the following points.

- Physical connectivity (actual nerve tracts and synapses) can be differentiated from functional connectivity (the transmission of information between neurons and within circuits).
- There can be too much or too little physical connectivity (and these can co-exist), and both have adverse effects on functional connectivity.
- Abnormal functional connectivity will affect both brain development and brain function and behaviour.

The net result of abnormal physical connectivity is, according to Belmonte et al., an abnormal **signal-to-noise ratio** in the neural transmission of information, with the signal being reduced relative to noise: an overconnected network passes so much noise that it swamps the signal; an underconnected network passes so little signal that it becomes lost in the noise. In either case, there is a loss of information-processing capacity.

Belmonte et al. place their theory explicitly within a constructivist emergence model of brain development, and suggest the following sequence of likely causes and effects. They suggest that physical overconnectivity in the primary sensory processing regions of the brain (which develop early) causes hyperarousal in the infant, who is unable to direct attention selectively to competing sensory inputs. The resulting flood of input to those brain regions that would normally subserve higher-order functions, such as control of attention (executive functions), social cognition and language, causes overgrowth and reduced information transmission in these regions, also within the first two years of life. To compensate for what Belmonte et al. refer to as a bottleneck in higher-order cognition, the brain develops a mode of functioning that avoids reliance on higher-level integrative processing and instead emphasises low-level features. This mode of functioning underlies what Frith described as weak central coherence and what Mottron and his colleagues have termed enhanced perceptual function. This detail-focused bias leads in turn to a further set of behavioural abnormalities that have in common failure to integrate the components of complex experience, including social experience. Poverty of social experience, it is suggested, may then contribute to failure to develop domain-specific brain systems for face processing, language, and mindreading.

As is clear from this description, one abnormality is seen as leading to another, usually with consequences for both brain and behaviour; different in detail for different individuals but always leading to the same set of autism-related behaviours. Belmonte et al. use the expression 'fan out' to describe how the effects of an initial lack of inhibitory activity in the cerebellum could spread and ramify, leading to autism. They use the term 'fan in' to describe how a variety of risk factors, both genetic and environmental, might converge to produce the initial cerebellar abnormalities from which, according to their theory, autistic behaviour grows. It is this attempt to articulate a theory embracing not only the fan out effects of an initial brain abnormality but also how fanning in from first causes might occur that makes Belmonte et al.'s theory ambitious in scope. Their attempt to explain the 'fan in' process is considered in the final main section of the chapter.

Possible Objections to Disconnectivity Theories, and a Defence

Certain objections to, or concerns about, impaired connectivity theories are foreseeable. In particular, why do disconnection theories not constitute single deficit theories of the kind argued against in Chapter 6 and how can this kind of theory explain the various full forms of ASD (AS, HFA and LFA) as well as the partial or atypical forms (as in PDD-NOS and the broader autism phenotype)? And if the answer to the latter question is that the critical causes of the universal or very common characteristics of autism are dissociable, then why are some quite diverse facets of autistic behaviour apparently related? Each of these questions will be considered in turn.

Why are disconnection theories not single deficit theories?

A response to this question falls out of points made in the preceding paragraphs: impaired connectivity probably takes various forms resulting from different sets of etiological factors, with different effects on different neural circuits. It does not, therefore, constitute a single discrete causal factor, but rather a *kind* of brain pathology that can affect one or more circuits in the brain. This explanation may be clarified by a comparison with tuberous sclerosis, a condition described in Chapter 3. Tuberous sclerosis is characterised by a particular *kind* of brain pathology, namely tuberous growths, that can occur in various parts of the brain that are not always the same in all affected individuals. No single cause of behavioural impairments is therefore implied.

How can this kind of theory explain all the various forms of ASD?

Because 'disconnectivity' does not constitute a single discrete causal factor, but rather a kind of brain pathology that can affect one or more circuits in the brain, it is not in principle incompatible with the numerous different patterns of spared and impaired abilities that fall within the autistic spectrum. So, for example, disconnectivity within the amygdala prefrontal circuitry that subserves emotion processing and social behaviours may be different in kind and differently caused from disconnectivity affecting top-down control from frontal lobes to sensory or motor regions. Equally, disconnectivity affecting the hippocampal region prefrontal circuitry subserving declarative memory and learning may be different in kind, and differently caused, from disconnectivity within the social brain or between the frontal lobes and 'lower' brain regions. It follows that socio-emotional-communicative impairments can occur independently of behavioural inflexibility, and both can occur independently of memory and learning impairments: the various strands of autism-related behaviours are thus dissociable.

If dissociable, why do some of these behaviours appear to be related?

The argument that key strands of autism-related behaviours are dissociable because they result from different sites and kinds of disconnectivity, associated with different combinations of etiological risk factors, might seem to raise a problem of explaining why, when they co-occur in individuals, some of the major behavioural characteristics of ASDs appear to be related. Thus, impaired performance on ToM tests (notably false belief tasks) is related to executive abilities in typically developing children as well as in individuals with ASDs, as noted earlier in the chapter. There is also ample evidence to show that performance on ToM tasks is related to language ability in neurotypical individuals as well as in individuals with autism, although here again the nature of the relationship is controversial (Tager-Flusberg, 2000; Slade & Ruffman, 2005). Weak central coherence and some facets of executive function may also be related (Rinehart, Bradshaw, Moss, Brereton, & Tonge, 2000; Pellicano et al., 2005).

Any problems are, however, more apparent than real so long as one focuses on the kinds of fundamental (neuro)psychological deficits identified in Chapters 8, 9, and 10 (see also Figure 11.1(b)). So, for example, it has not been shown that impaired primary intersubjectivity in infants who will become autistic is related to any kind of executive dysfunction, or infant language. On the contrary, it has been shown that impaired joint attention occurs independently of executive dysfunction in young children with ASDs (Dawson, Munson et al., 2002). The fact that performance on tests of theory of mind is associated with executive ability and with language is irrelevant and unsurprising, given the cognitive and linguistic demands of most of the tests that have been devised.

Similarly, an association between certain facets of executive function and WCC is unsurprising given that executive functions include processes of top-down control that may be reliant on some of the same circuits that subserve the integration of perceptual features. Other types of executive function, for example, generativity and planning, might not relate to WCC because they are not reliant on shared circuitry.

Comment

This short review of brain–behaviour theories is representative, although necessarily selective, of current attempts to explain autism at this combined level. The increasing convergence of views, from Waterhouse et al.'s comprehensive theory published in 1996 to the theory presented by Courchesne, Belmonte and their many collaborators ten years later, is striking, and suggests that there is now enough known about brain–behaviour development in general, and about brain development and function in autism in particular, to begin to understand rather than to guess at the processes involved.

Despite these broad areas of agreement, however, much of the story remains hypothetical and more research is needed. There is also some disagreement even within the small group of theories described. In particular, neither Waterhouse et al., nor Dawson, Webb et al. consider cerebellar abnormalities to be the origin of subsequent brain **dysgenesis**, both these research groups placing more emphasis on primary abnormalities within the limbic system (see also Bachevalier & Loveland, 2006; Loveland, Bachevalier, Pearson, & Lane, 2008). Other current theories propose quite different initial abnormalities, for example within the brain stem (Rodier & Arndt, 2005) or vagus nerve (Porges, 2005). Moreover, although some degree of consensus is emerging concerning how autism might be the end point of a fan out process, there is no consensus concerning how first causes might fan in to a single initial brain abnormality – if, indeed, this is what happens, as discussed next.

FROM FIRST CAUSES TO AUTISTIC BEHAVIOUR: LINKING THE EXPLANATIONS TOGETHER

The process of understanding how genotypes emerge as phenotypes is rather like building a tunnel starting at both ends and hoping to meet in the middle. At one end, psychologists work back from manifest behaviour to the hidden psychological determinants of the behaviour. At the other end, geneticists explore how genes and environments interact to construct and maintain human bodies and brains from conception to maturity and thereafter. In the middle is the embodied brain, studied by neuroscientists.

A good deal of the work at the psychology end has been done, for typically developing individuals and for individuals with ASDs. The advent of magnetic imaging techniques is enabling rapid progress to be made in understanding the neuropsychology of autistic behaviour, in other words in linking behaviour back to its brain bases in terms of brain regions and circuits. However, less is known about the brain in terms of abnormalities of neurochemistry and cellular structure. This is where brain bases and first causes must link together, which is why space was given in Chapter 7 to summarising what is known about the neurochemistry of autism, despite the fact that the evidence here is extremely incomplete.

In addition, research into the processes by which genes and environments build brains in typically developing individuals is in its infancy, and the even more difficult task of unravelling connections between genes and psychological processes in typical development has hardly begun (see Fisher, 2006, for a warning against the 'gene for x and gene for y' oversimplications that abound). Tracking the effects of even a single abnormal gene on brain development and function, and thereon to psychological functions and behaviour, is therefore exceedingly difficult (Karmiloff-Smith, Scerif, & Thomas, 2002; Bishop, 2006). As noted in Chapter 7, autistic behaviour is almost certainly the end point of several genetic and environmental susceptibility factors in various combinations, and these are not yet certainly identified. Constructing a full explanation of autism from first causes up to what is known about brain bases, and thereon to psychological deficits or anomalies, is therefore not yet possible. However, there are many hypotheses concerning what the links from first causes upwards might be. Some indication of the state of knowledge is included below.

Hypotheses concerning links from first causes to brain bases

Regarding hypotheses that have been proposed concerning links from first causes to brain bases, some of the areas of research interest were indicated in Chapter 7. Genes known to be involved in the production and **metabolism** of neurochemicals influencing brain development as well as brain function, and for which there is some evidence of abnormality in autism, have attracted particular interest. Thus genes whose products include serotonin, dopamine, GABA, oxytocin and vasopressin, or whose products include regulators of serotoninergic, dopaminergic, GABAergic, etc., metabolism figure in a number of hypotheses (Bauman & Kemper, 2005b, provides a representative sample). Similarly, gene variants or teratogens known to cause cerebellar abnormalities including reduced Purkinje cells in animals are central to other hypotheses (see for example, DiCiccio-Bloom et al., 2006).

Hypotheses concerning links from first causes to behaviour

Hypotheses concerning possible links from genes to behaviour or from environmental factors to behaviour (with or without speculation concerning the intervening processes) are also numerous. For example, it is hypothesised that abnormalities of certain gene loci on chromosome 15 may contribute to the behavioural characteristics of 'insistence on sameness' and superior visual–spatial constructional abilities; abnormalities of the vasopressin receptor gene may contribute to the lack of normal social behaviours; abnormalities affecting genes sited on chromosomes 2 and 7 may contribute to language impairments in LFA; and exposure to chemicals engendered by high levels of maternal stress during pregancy may contribute to increased vulnerability to anxiety.

There are also many hypotheses based on possible links from behaviour back to genes. Quantitative trait loci (QTL) studies (see Box 7.1) are predicated on the assumption that a particular behavioural trait that occurs in people with ASDs, such as impaired face recognition or impaired set shifting, has a genetic origin, and that the genes in question may show abnormalities in a significant proportion of close relatives. A good example of hypotheses derived in this way can be found in the paper by Dawson, Webb et al. (2002). These authors suggest that the six phenotypic traits identified in their paper, namely face processing, sensitivity to social reward, motor imitation, declarative memory/feature binding, executive function, and language ability, should be targeted in a programme of QTL studies in an attempt to identify the genes that may contribute to each of these autism-related behaviours.

A hypothesis linking first causes to brain bases to psychology and behaviour

Not surprisingly, given the current sketchy understanding of the etiological factors in autism and how they link to what is known about the brain bases of autism, there are not many attempts to construct theories explaining autism as a whole, from root causes through brain bases to behaviour. One such attempt can be found in the paper by Belmonte et al. (2004a) referred to at some length in the section on brain–behaviour relations in autism. The gist of Belmonte et al.'s theory is reported here to give an idea of the kind of links that need to be made.

These authors suggest that many subtle genetic, biochemical, immunological, and other factors at the neural level may be involved in the etiology of autism, and their paper includes an extended discussion of genes governing neural growth, the substances that govern gene expression, and the substances involved in neural transmission of information. They suggest that combinations of these factors distort brain development in ways that cause abnormal connectivity of various kinds, all with the net result that there is reduced signal-to-noise ratio in neural transmission. Thus, a multiplicity of causal factors are all seen as capable of causing a single *kind* of functional abnormality: they 'fan in' to produce the abnormality. From this convergence point, or common pathway, the effects on brain development and behaviour ramify and fan out as described earlier in this chapter (noting the scope for heterogeneity in outcomes). The paper by Belmante et al. closes with a section on 'Research imperatives', emphasising the research that needs to be done to confirm or disconfirm the hypothetical links proposed. There are also some interesting comments on possible implications for physical treatments, should certain of their hypothesised causal factors prove to be implicated.

SUMMARY

Attempts to explain autism at a psychological level focused for many years on impaired ToM, executive dysfunction, and WCC/enhanced perceptual processing. Each of these three theories was argued to be able to explain at least one major facet of autism-related behaviour. The three theories are all important for understanding the causes of autism. However, the ToM and executive function theories proved incomplete as fundamental explanations of autism-related behaviours, and attention has shifted to primary intersubjectivity impairments as the likely critical cause, or set of causes, of interaction impairments, and to problems of attention (possibly related to WCC) as implicated in behavioural inflexibility. This tentative two-factor model of the psychological causes of ASDs has several advantages. However, as a full explanation of autism it remains underspecified and incomplete.

A shift in the prevailing psychological model of how the mind develops and operates, from a computer inspired model to a constructivist emergence model, is reflected in some newer theories. Most importantly, it seems likely that future explanatory theories will identify general-purpose psychological mechanisms as critically impaired, rather than domain-specific mechanisms. The WCC group of theories survives this shift well, not least because it maps on to current theories of behaviour–brain relationships, as below.

At the combined brain and psychology levels of explanation, the computer-inspired model led to attempts to pair psychological deficits with pathology affecting specific brain structures or circuits. So, for example, impaired primary and secondary intersubjectivity and theory of mind are generally agreed to involve structures within the social brain, including the amygdala and specific regions of the prefrontal cortex. Impaired executive function is generally described as resulting from frontal lobe pathology. Notable attempts to explain the whole of autism by identifying psychological deficits and their brain correlates can be found in the models proposed by Waterhouse et al. in 1996 and by Dawson, Webb et al. in 2002. Waterhouse et al.'s model in particular prefigures current views, based on a constructivist emergence model of brain–mind development. Current theories emphasise ways in which brain development in autism increasingly deviates from the norm as a result of some initial pathology. For example, both Courchesne and Belmonte hypothesise that abnormal brain growth in autism stems from disinhibited neural output from the cerebellum, which overstimulates growth in limbic and some frontal regions, resulting in too much structural connectivity. Premature arrest of brain growth in later childhood causes too little connectivity, especially between the frontal lobes and more distant brain regions. Impaired connectivity, however caused, fits well with psychological theories focusing on impaired integration, including the WCC group of theories and also several primary intersubjectivity deficit theories. It is also compatible with the suggestion that problems of higher-level executive functions may reflect a lack of frontally mediated top-down control.

Too little is known for certain about the etiology of autism for clear links to be made across all three levels of explanation. However, there are numerous hypotheses concerning links from first causes to brain bases, and quantitative trait loci studies are increasingly being used to investigate links backwards from specific psychological deficits to susceptibility genes. Belmonte et al. review the kinds of evidence that will contribute to an eventual three-level explanation, and suggest strategies for future research.

12

WHAT CAUSES AUTISM: PERSONAL VIEW

AIMS

••••

INTRODUCTION

••••

THE MEMORY HYPOTHESIS AND WHAT IT MIGHT EXPLAIN
Background
The Updated Memory Hypothesis
Uneven Memory Abilities as a Critical Cause of
Language Impairment in LFA
Uneven Memory Abilities as a Critical Cause of
Intellectual Disability in LFA
Uneven Memory Abilities as a Critical Cause of Certain Forms of
Behavioural Inflexibility Across the Spectrum
Uneven Memory Abilities as an Explanation of Some Spared and Savant
Abilities in LFA
Uneven Memory Abilities and Paradoxical Motor Skills
Conclusion

••••

THE TIME PROCESSING HYPOTHESIS
The Hypothesis
Evidence
How the Time-processing Impairment Hypothesis Fits Into
the Broader Picture

••••

A MODEL OF THE CRITICAL NEUROPSYCHOLOGICAL
CAUSES OF AUTISM

••••

CONCLUSION

AIMS

The aim of this chapter is to outline my own model of the causes of autism. As a psychologist rather than a geneticist or a neuroscientist, the emphasis is on psychological explanations of ASDs. However, these are linked to what is known about the brain bases of autism, and are thus neuropsychological rather than purely psychological. Most elements of the model are adopted from others' theories and research, as described in earlier chapters. Some elements are, however, original, and these are the main focus of this chapter.

INTRODUCTION

It will be clear from the critique sections of Chapter 8 that I am optimistic that the underlying psychological cause(s) of the social, emotional, and communicative impairments associated with autism are close to being understood. Almost all the primary intersubjectivity theories outlined in that chapter either explicitly or implicitly invoke a lack of integration of the perceptual, emotional, and cognitive contents of infants' social experience. I assume, with many others, that this lack of integration reflects disconnection or discoordination of function amongst key structures of the social brain, as described in Chapter 11.

It will also be evident from material in Chapter 10 that I am optimistic concerning the potential power of the WCC, enhanced perceptual function, enhanced discrimination–reduced generalisation group of theories to explain anomalous sensory-perceptual processing and some kinds of savant ability. In the past I have been impatient with the WCC theory because it seemed simply to redescribe the phenomena to be explained (as, indeed, do the names of the other two theories in this group). But when these theories were linked to the notion of impaired neural binding, which Jon Brock introduced me to (Brock et al., 2002), and as the evidence and arguments for conceptualising ASDs as a group of disconnection disorders becomes increasingly persuasive, the 'redescriptions' map neatly onto their probable brain correlates and secure their place in any causal model of autism.

It will be equally evident from the discussion sections of Chapter 9 that I consider the critical causes of behavioural inflexibility are poorly understood at the psychological (and neuropsychological) level. Similarly, in Chapter 10 I argued for the importance of gaining a better understanding of the causes of language impairment and intellectual disability in lower-functioning autism. I also pointed out that the uneven patterns of motor skills observed across the spectrum are not well understood, nor are many facets of spared ability explicable in terms of current psychological theories. In this chapter I will outline my own view of how these unexplained characteristics might be explained.

The major hypothesis to be presented concerns different profiles of spared and impaired memory functions across the spectrum. The different profiles of uneven memory abilities are hypothesised to have different effects in high-functioning as compared to lower-functioning forms of ASDs, especially on language and learning ability, but also to some extent on the kinds of restricted and repetitive behaviours that occur, and on patterns of spared ability. This hypothesis constitutes a return to something I was interested in when I started to research into the causes of autism many years ago, and I will point out how the hypothesis has changed and developed since it was first proposed.

A second hypothesis, presented more briefly, concerns impaired 'time processing'. This hypothesis has a long history in the study of autism without ever having achieved wide recognition. I will suggest how impaired time processing may be compatible not only with the memory hypothesis that I propose, but also with the overall model of autism presented in the final section of the chapter.

THE MEMORY HYPOTHESIS AND WHAT IT MIGHT EXPLAIN

Background

Early studies

My first studies of autism carried out in the 1970s were motivated by a hunch that the hippocampus might be an important structure for an understanding of at least some facets of autism. I was influenced by two quite different strands of work: studies of adults with acquired global amnesia who were known to have hippocampal-region pathology; and studies of animals with experimental lesions of the hippocampus and adjacent structures.

From the first set of studies I learned that adults with acquired global amnesia 'stood still' in terms of new learning of most kinds; that their sense of an ongoing changing self, their sense of the passing of time, their ability to live in anything but the immediate present, were grossly impaired. It seemed to me that a congenital or very early acquired form of global amnesia might go a long way towards explaining impaired language and intellectual disability in the children I was working with (all of whom were low-functioning, because high-functioning forms of ASD were not recognised in those days). Their apparent lack of a sense of personal identity and their disorientation, including temporal disorientation, also seemed to me to be compatible with their having at least some degree of hippocampal-type amnesia.

From the second set of studies I learned that rats and monkeys with hippocampal lesions produce repetitive behaviour associated with reduced habituation and reduced response to novelty. These findings also appeared to have potential relevance for understanding the repetitive behaviour and desire for sameness in the children I was working with.

I was further encouraged by the fact that Rimland (1964), whose book I revered, noted that hippocampal pathology might be important for an understanding of autism. Elizabeth Warrington, an authority on acquired brain disorders, was also encouraging in that she had privately conjectured that there might be a parallel between autism and global amnesia. My early studies of children with lower-functioning autism were therefore studies of memory and of habituation and response to novelty, all motivated by a hippocampal hypothesis. These studies all produced positive findings (Boucher & Warrington, 1976; Boucher, 1977, 1981a). (Unknown to me at the time, DeLong (1978) was investigating a similar hypothesis.)

From the early 1980s onwards, however, it was clear that the socio-emotional-communicative impairments and behavioural inflexibility characteristic of autism can occur in the absence of language and learning impairments. A global amnesia hypothesis has little relevance to the first set of characteristics, and is positively contraindicated by the high intelligence and superior language of many individuals with HFA or Asperger syndrome. Moreover, various researchers tested memory abilities in people with AS/HFA and found them to be largely intact (e.g., Minshew & Goldstein, 1993, 2001; Renner, Klinger, & Klinger, 2000). The memory hypothesis therefore has nothing very obvious to contribute concerning the causes of 'pure' autism (but see below).

Some authors, however, notably DeLong (1992) and Bachevalier (1991, 1994), continued to argue for the possible importance of hippocampal-related memory and learning impairments for an understanding of the broader group of ASDs. I also continued to believe that memory impairments might help to explain language impairment and intellectual disability in lower-functioning autism, but could not see the links clearly enough to develop a detailed hypothesis. I also suspected that impaired memory and impaired generativity are closely related (for reasons described below), and I switched to investigating this facet of the hypothesis in a series of studies, again with generally positive results (see Chapters 5 and 9; also below).

Subsequent developments

A great deal more is now known about normal memory and about memory impairments in conditions other than autism than was known when I carried out my early studies of memory in people with LFA. These developments offer a greatly strengthened argument for the role of uneven patterns of memory as a contributory cause of language and learning impairments in LFA, and of other facets of autistic behaviour across the spectrum.

Human memory is now widely considered to consist of five partially independent systems: **episodic** (memory for personally experienced events);

semantic (memory for impersonal factual information); **procedural** (memory for skills, associations, habits, sequences, and the unconscious extraction of regularities from experience); **perceptual** memory for single items (e.g., a flower, a scene); and working memory, including **immediate** memory (Tulving, 1995).

Semantic and episodic memory involve the retrieval of consciously accessible representations about which there is a feeling of memory ('I can recall', 'I know I know...'). These representations can be reflected on and reported, and such memories can be described as **declarative** or **explicit**. Declarative memory is dependent on two underlying processes: **recollection**, which is a form of recall that makes the major contribution to episodic memory; and **familiarity**, the feeling of knowing or recognition in the absence of contextual detail, that makes the major contribution to semantic memory.

Procedural memory, however, includes memory for acquired skills, habits and associations that are generally inaccessible to conscious retrieval, and about which there is no conscious feeling of memory, but which are nevertheless evident in behaviour. Procedural memory can thus be described as non-declarative or **implicit**. Perceptual memory is also implicit, or non-declarative, and is defined as memory for the 'raw' perceptual information from which declarative memories are derived.

Immediate memory holds recently perceived information in unmodified form for a limited time. However, the contents of immediate memory can be rehearsed, maintained and manipulated within working memory, as described in Chapter 9.

With regard to developments in what is known about different forms of organic memory impairment, studies of rare cases of **developmental amnesia** show that congenital or early acquired lesions restricted to the hippocampus cause a selective impairment of episodic memory (Vargha-Khadem, Gadian, Watkins, Connelly, van Paesschen, & Mishkin, 1997). Studies of adults with acquired lesions confirm that if only the hippocampus is affected, a selective impairment of episodic memory results, associated with impaired recollection. Only when hippocampal lesions are combined with lesions of the adjacent **medial temporal lobe** cortex, involving in particular the **perirhinal cortex**, does an additional impairment of semantic memory result, associated with impaired familiarity (relevant studies are reviewed in Mayes & Boucher, 2008). Global amnesia, or what is sometimes referred to as 'the amnesic syndrome', results when a combination of hippocampal and perirhinal lesions impairs both recollection and familiarity, with a combined loss of episodic and semantic memory.

The Updated Memory Hypothesis

In Boucher et al. (2008) the following are hypothesised.

- High-functioning individuals with autism have a selective impairment of recollection, hence episodic memory.

- Lower-functioning individuals have a more pervasive impairment of declarative memory affecting both recollection and familiarity, hence both episodic and semantic memory.
- Most non-declarative, implicit forms of memory are intact across the spectrum (except possibly in individuals with profound intellectual disability).
- Immediate and working memory are also mainly intact.
- The selective impairment of recollection in individuals with AS/HFA is associated with damage or dysfunction affecting the neural circuit of which the hippocampus is an integral part; whereas the combination of impaired recollection and familiarity is associated with damage or dysfunction extending beyond the hippocampal circuitry to include perirhinal and possibly other medial temporal lobe cortices.

The hypothesised profiles of memory strengths and weaknesses in higher- and lower-functioning autism are summarised in Table 12.1.

Table 12.1   *Hypothesised memory profiles in higher- and lower-functioning autism*

	AS/HFA	LFA
Long-term Memory Systems		
Episodic memory retains memory for personally experienced events, including a conscious awareness of remembering and of having experienced these events in the past. Mainly dependent on recollection.	Impaired	Impaired
Semantic memory retains impersonal, factual information, including the feeling of knowing this information. Mainly dependent on familiarity.	Spared	Impaired
Procedural memory retains habits, skills, simple associations (A with B) and also strings, or sequences, of invariant associations (A to B to C to D – as in rote learning) below the level of conscious awareness.	Spared	Spared
Perceptual memory holds single-item percepts below the level of conscious awareness.	Spared	Spared
Short-term Memory Systems		
Immediate memory holds very recently experienced information in the form in which it was experienced, and for a matter of seconds.	Spared	Relatively spared
Working memory holds and manipulates verbal-linguistic information and visual-spatial information short term. It may also hold and manipulate episodic information in the short term (Baddeley, 2000).	Mainly spared	Mainly spared

Evidence for the hypothesis

Ben Shalom (2003) preceded us in proposing that 'pure' autism is characterised by a selective impairment of episodic memory, associated with structural or functional disconnection or discoordination within hippocampal-prefrontal circuitry. She suggested that impaired episodic memory would be evident in impaired source memory, temporal order memory, and memory for personally experienced events, and reviewed evidence in support of these predictions. Some of the studies reviewed (e.g., Bennetto, Pennington & Rogers, 1996; Klein, Chan, & Loftus, 1999; see also Bowler, Gardiner, & Berthollier, 2004) demonstrated intact semantic memory co-existing with impaired episodic memory in AS/HFA.

A study of adults with Asperger syndrome using a test that discriminates between the contributions of recollection and familiarity to declarative memory provides further evidence in support of this part of the hypothesis (Bowler, Gardiner, & Grice, 2000). The test used by Bowler et al. is verbally demanding. We developed a less verbally demanding test that measures recollection and familiarity separately, and showed that young children with AS/HFA have, as predicted, impaired recollection in combination with intact familiarity (Anns, Bigham, Mayes, & Boucher, 2008).

That part of the hypothesis that concerns a more pervasive impairment of declarative memory, including a combined impairment of recollection and familiarity in lower-functioning individuals with ASDs, is supported by most but not all currently available evidence, as below.

Tests of recall are mainly dependent on recollection, and most studies requiring explicit recall by lower-functioning individuals show impairment. Specifically, recall of words and pictures, and especially of meaningful word groups or sentences, is impaired (Hermelin & O'Connor, 1967; Boucher & Warrington, 1976; Fyffe & Prior, 1978; Tager-Flusberg, 1991). Impaired recall of personally experienced events has been shown in studies by Boucher (1981b), Boucher and Lewis (1989), and Millward et al. (2000).

Tests of recognition are mainly dependent on familiarity, and studies of explicit recognition by individuals with LFA tend to show impairment. However, clear and consistent evidence is lacking. Thus, Ameli, Courchesne, Lincoln, Kaufman, and Grillon (1988) reported impaired visual recognition for non-meaningful, but not for meaningful, visual stimuli in a mixed ability group; however, their control group was not matched for verbal ability. Summers and Craik (1994) reported impaired word recognition. Barth, Fein, and Waterhouse (1995) reported visual recognition impairment, although the impairment was not evident when non-verbal ability was controlled for. Dawson, Meltzoff, Osterling, Rinaldi, and Brown (1998b) showed impaired performance on a test of delayed non-matching to sample (a recognition memory test), but subsequently concluded that this resulted from impaired reward-association mechanisms rather than recognition impairment per se (Dawson, Osterling, Rinaldi, Carver, & Partland, 2001). Boucher, Bigham et al. (2008) demonstrated impaired recognition in teenagers with LFA relative to language ability-matched typically developing children, but not relative to age- and language ability-matched teenagers without autism. (Face recognition is impaired, but is a specific ability normally mediated by dedicated brain structures not relevant to the declarative memory hypothesis).

In a forthcoming study we plan to clarify findings on familiarity in lower-functioning individuals, using the test referred to above that provides separate measures of recollection and familiarity. Meantime, our prediction of a combined impairment of recollection and familiarity is unproven. However, it should be noted that individuals with milder forms of LFA, such as are able to co-operate with formal tests, would not be expected to have severely impaired familiarity.

That part of the hypothesis that concerns mainly intact perceptual and procedural memory is supported by studies of **priming**, where some prior experience exerts an unconscious influence on current experience and judgement (e.g., Renner et al., 2000; Hala, Paxman, & Glenwright, 2007). The successful use of behaviourist intervention techniques with individuals with ASDs confirms that associative learning and conditioning is also generally intact, with the exception of amygdala-related fear conditioning (Gaigg & Bowler, 2007). Habit formation, which is related to associative learning, has not been directly investigated. However, the diagnostic criteria for ASDs imply intact habit formation, as evident in adherence to routines and resistance to change.

There is, on the other hand, some evidence suggesting that sequencing is impaired (Mostofsky et al., 2000; note also that several early theories suggested impaired sequencing as a cause of language impairment and intellectual disability in autism). 'Sequencing', however, covers many different kinds of learning, sometimes involving simple succession (A followed by B followed by C...), sometimes involving hierarchical organisation, as in the acquisition of complex movement or grammatical language. Moreover, the acquisition of complex sequences may initially involve declarative memory (learning to play a new piece on the piano), only later being stored in procedural memory (playing a familiar piano piece without the music).

The claim that immediate memory and working memory are mainly intact across the spectrum is supported by phenomena such as echolalia, by the relative sparing of performance on the Digit Span subtest of the Wechsler tests even in lower-functioning individuals, and by numerous experimental demonstrations of relatively intact immediate recall of word strings and intact working memory apart from certain types of spatial working memory (see Chapter 9). Findings on immediate and working memory in autism are reviewed in Poirier and Martin (2008).

Finally, the memory hypothesis presented here is consistent with data indicating hippocampal abnormalities extending into the perirhinal and parahippocampal cortex in mixed ability groups of individuals with autistic spectrum disorders (ASDs) (Bauman & Kemper, 2003; Boucher et al., 2005). It is also consistent with reports of individuals with extensive medial temporal lobe damage, autism, and severe language and intellectual impairment (DeLong & Heinz, 1997). On the basis of such evidence, others before us have suggested that lower-functioning autism results when medial temporal lobe abnormalities extend beyond the amygdala into the hippocampus and adjacent regions (e.g., Kemper & Bauman, 1998; Bachevalier, 1991, 1994, 2008). There is, however, some negative evidence relating to structural hippocampal abnormalities (e.g., Bailey et al., 1998; Piven, Bailey, Ranson, &

Arndt, 1998), and conflicting evidence concerning the kinds of abnormalities that may be present (e.g., increased or decreased volume; generalised or selective pathology).

Uneven Memory Abilities as a Critical Cause of Language Impairment in LFA

The hypothesis

In Chapter 10 several theories concerning possible causes of language impairment in ASDs were described. These were: impaired sequencing theories (e.g., Rutter, 1983; Tanguay, 1984); Ricks and Wing's (1975) impaired symbolisation theory; Hobson's (1993) and Bloom's (2000) impaired mindreading theory; Baron-Cohen's (2006) hypersystemisation theory; the mirror neurons theory; and the suggestion made by various authors over several years that language impairment in autism is caused by co-morbid specific language impairment (SLI).

It was concluded that sequencing theories received some empirical support but were never widely accepted; the impaired symbolisation theory might be relevant to individuals with severe or profound inability to acquire language but could not explain milder forms of language impairment; impaired mindreading is certain to contribute to language anomalies (even if subtle) across the spectrum; the hypersystemisation and mirror neurons theories are in need of further specification and empirical support; and the co-morbid SLI theory may well explain language impairment when it occurs in individuals who are not globally intellectually impaired, and may also exacerbate and complicate language impairment in a proportion of individuals with LFA, but cannot explain the LFA-specific language profile.

The theory proposed in Boucher, Mayes et al., (2008) was also mentioned in Chapter 10. However it was not fully described there, because it is novel and has not as yet been widely peer-reviewed. In that paper (see also Boucher, Bigham et al., 2008) we propose that the critical cause of language impairment in LFA is a combination of impaired mindreading plus an impairment of declarative memory that affects both recollection and familiarity.

The importance of declarative memory for language acquisition was initially inferred by us on the basis of studies of adults with global amnesia showing that, although implicit category formation is unimpaired, explicit recall or recognition of items encoded during category formation is impaired (Knowlton & Squire, 1993). We reasoned that this observation is consistent with the fact that individuals with LFA (except those with profound intellectual disability) are generally well oriented in familiar surroundings: they know that spoons are for eating with, chairs for sitting on, shoes for wearing, even if they do not understand or use words such as 'spoon', 'eat', etc. In this they resemble prelinguistic infants whose procedural learning abilities enable them to learn a great

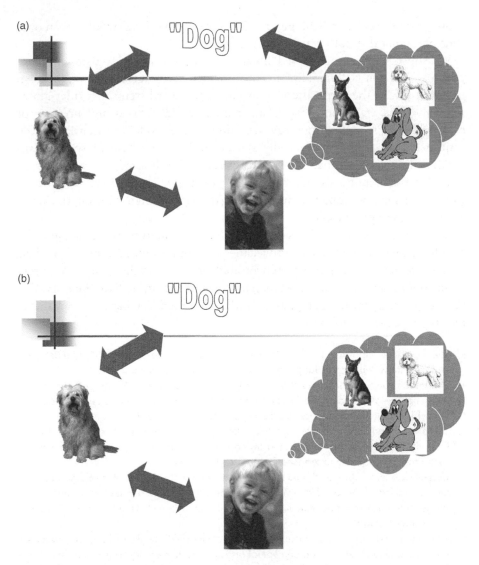

Figure 12.1 (a) The boy learns that the word 'dog' refers both to a particular dog currently present and to the class of dogs in general. (b) The boy learns only that 'dog' refers to the particular dog currently present (from Boucher, Mayes & Bigham, (2008) *Memory in Autism*, Cambridge University Press, with permission)

deal about their surroundings and the routines in which they participate, although they do not yet have access to explicit, declarative forms of memory.

The disconnection that we envisaged as occurring between categorical knowledge of the world *implicitly* acquired by a young child with an ASD, and the words that should be *explicitly* linked to that knowledge (rather than to items 'out there') is illustrated in Figures 12.1a and b. The net result of such a disconnection would be that words would tend to be learned as if they were proper names. For the boy in Figure 12.1, for example, 'dog' would mean only 'this particular dog' rather than 'dogs in general'.

We subsequently learned of Ullman's model of the prerequisites for language acquisition (Ullman, 2001, 2004), which gives declarative memory an essential role in the acquisition of lexical items (word stems, irregular grammatical forms, e.g., /ran/, /feet/, and regular word suffixes and prefixes or **morphemes**). Procedural memory, according to the model, is essential for the acquisition of grammar, especially syntax, and (in the case of spoken language) phonology. Ullman's model provides an additional, strongly argued basis for our hypothesis that declarative memory impairment is a critical cause of language impairment in LFA (though Ullman himself does not ascribe to the hypothesis).

If, as we propose, individuals with LFA have impaired mindreading and the profile of memory strengths and weaknesses summarised in Table 12.1, their routes into language will be severely limited. Specifically, they will have to rely to an abnormal degree on perceptual, procedural and immediate memory. The autism-specific profile of language abilities identified in Chapter 3 can therefore be explained as follows.

- The language impairment is amodal because a declarative memory impairment (also mindblindness) will impair language acquisition regardless of modality.
- The impairment is characterised first and foremost by problems of comprehension and meaning (semantics) because impaired declarative memory mainly affects the acquisition of lexical items, and these are the major bearers of linguistic meaning.
- There is 'limited ability to integrate linguistic input with real-world knowledge' (Lord & Paul, 1997: 212) because implicit knowledge of the world will not be fully reflected in such language as is acquired (see Figure 12.1(b)).
- Grammar is less impaired than semantics because intact procedural memory subserves the acquisition of syntax. However, morphemic errors occur because morphemes and irregular word forms are lexical items, acquisition of which is affected by impaired declarative memory.
- There is a tendency to reproduce echoed or rote-learned chunks of language verbatim because of default reliance on perceptual and immediate memory. This contributes to the impression that expressive language is superior to comprehension.
- Knowledge of the sound system of spoken language (phonology) is also largely unimpaired because it is acquired implicitly, via intact perceptual and procedural memory.
- Idiosyncratic words or phrases and problems with deictic terms are common because mindblindness interferes with the acquisition of shared meaning and especially person-centred meaning.

Evidence for the hypothesis

Support for the impaired memory component of this explanation of language impairment in LFA would involve showing that individuals with LFA have the predicted memory impairment and, in addition, that performance on tests of memory correlates with performance on tests of lexical and semantic knowledge. In Boucher, Bigham et al. (2008) we showed precisely this: that impaired recognition in teenagers with LFA correlates with lexical and semantic knowledge, which is not the case in matched groups of those without autism.

Support for that part of the hypothesis that concerns abnormal word learning as illustrated in Figure 12.1 comes from two studies. In the first of these (Perkins, Dobbinson, Boucher, Bol, & Bloom, 2006), a detailed linguistic analysis of spontaneous language in young adults with moderate to low-functioning autism led to the conclusion that 'lexical knowledge in autism may not be reflected in lexical use'. Results of the second study (Preissler, 2008) demonstrate why this may be the case. In her study, Preissler showed pictures of unfamiliar objects to typically developing young children and older children with LFA, and taught the children to name the pictures. When a child had learned to name a picture, for example 'whisk' as illustrated in Figure 12.2(a), they were shown the picture and a real object, as illustrated in Figure 12.2(b) and

(a) Line drawing of a whisk used during training

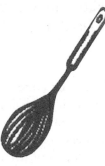

(b) Line drawing and real whisk presented together at test

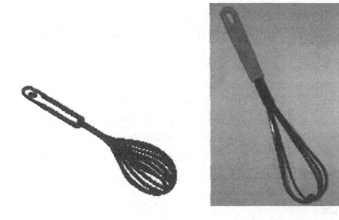

Figure 12.2 Examples of materials used in Preissler's word-learning experiment (adapted from *Autism*, 2008, Sage, with permission)

asked 'Which is the whisk?' Whereas most of the typically developing young children now pointed to the real object, most of the children with autism pointed to the picture. This is consistent with our suggestion that children with LFA tend to associate a word to a single exemplar 'out there'; in other words, they treat words as if they were proper names. Young typically developing children, on the other hand, know that words stand for implicitly-acquired categories of real objects of variable appearance, rather than to individual exemplars.

Also consistent with our overall hypothesis is evidence from a test of category formation and recognition in high-functioning children with ASDs (Molesworth, Bowler, & Hampton, 2005). These high-functioning children, unlike the amnesic adults in Knowlton and Squire's (1993) study, had normal memory for exemplars used in a category formation task (although their category formation was qualitatively different from that of typically developing children, see also Bott, Brock, Brockdorff, Boucher, & Lamberts, 2006).

Uneven Memory Abilities as a Critical Cause of Intellectual Disability in LFA

The hypothesis

In Chapter 10 it was noted that there are very few attempts in the literature to explain why intellectual disability and language impairment occur together in people with LFA. Only Ricks and Wing's (1975) impaired symbolisation theory, and Baron-Cohen's hypersystemisation theory attempt an explanation, and neither theory is well developed or defended.

We suggest (Boucher, Mayes et al., 2008) that intellectual disability in LFA results both directly and indirectly from a broad impairment of declarative memory, as argued above. A direct effect occurs because memory for factual information (semantic memory) is necessary for acquiring the kinds of general knowledge about the world that contribute to crystallised intelligence. An indirect effect occurs because, according to our hypothesis, declarative memory impairment limits the acquisition of lexical knowledge of the kind explicitly assessed in some verbal subtests. Delayed and limited language acquisition will, in addition, reduce the ability to use verbal mediation ('inner speech') in reasoning and problem solving. Fluid intelligence, or 'g', however, is intact or relatively spared because it is not dependent on processes associated with declarative memory.

The evidence

The evidence from intelligence tests described at length in previous chapters is consistent with the hypothesis, because it gave rise to the hypothesis.

Empirical studies that have reported relatively spared fluid intelligence (Dawson et al., 2007) or 'g' interpreted as speed of processing (Scheuffgen et al., 2000) provide further evidence consistent with the hypothesis.

Uneven Memory Abilities as a Critical Cause of Certain Forms of Behavioural Inflexibility Across the Spectrum

At various points in previous chapters I have stressed that many of the repetitive and restricted behaviours characteristic of autism can be explained by non-specific factors such as anxiety or maladaptive learning. In Chapter 9 I also discussed the large body of research into executive functions in people with ASDs, concluding that either a low-level problem in disengaging attention or a problem of top-down control might help to explain lack of mental flexibility and some types of repetitive behaviour in autism.

These explanations, however, leave the problems of generativity and planning, including some forms of imaginative creativity, unexplained. There may, in addition, be factors fuelling the restricted and repetitive behaviours other than anxiety, maladaptive learning or executive dysfunctions, as highlighted in previous chapters. In this section I suggest ways in which uneven patterns of memory and learning ability might contribute first to impaired generativity and planning and, secondly, to restricted interests and repetitive behaviour.

An impaired memory – impaired generativity and planning hypothesis

Impaired declarative memory would impair generativity and planning in each of three ways outlined below.

Problems with accessing stored information   I investigated generativity in some of my early research (see Chapters 5 and 9 for references) because my prior research on memory suggested that children with lower-functioning autism have memory problems of a kind that make it difficult for them to access information from their store of knowledge, unless given an informative prompt or cue of some kind. So, for example, answering the question 'What did you do on the weekend?' is difficult for them, whereas answering the question 'What did you do at Granny's house on the weekend?' is easier. I reasoned that if the children I had been working with had difficulty in retrieving uncued information in memory tests, they would have difficulty in retrieving uncued information in tests of generativity. A selective impairment of spontaneous, or uncued, generativity was shown in my own studies with colleagues, and also in tests reported by Turner (1999). This does not prove a link between impaired declarative memory and impaired generativity: to prove this link it would have to be shown that memory and generativity impairments are closely correlated, and this has not been done. However, my view remains that the link is plausible, if not inevitable.

Limited material from which to extract 'event grammar'   Impaired memory for personally experienced episodes would make it difficult to acquire knowledge of event structure from the usual sources – one's own episodic memories. Creative pretend play, story writing, and event planning (all of which are dependent on knowledge of event structure) would be affected as a consequence, as I have suggested elsewhere (Boucher, 2001, 2007).

Impaired mental time travel   With regard to impaired planning, there are at least four single case reports of adults with selective episodic memory loss who were impaired in 'future thinking', in the sense of being able to plan for their personal future (Atance & O'Neill, 2001). Future thinking is related to what has been called **mental time travel,** defined as the ability to project oneself mentally into the past to re-experience an event or into the future to 'pre-experience' future events (Suddendorf & Corballis, 1997). There is considerable discussion in the broader psychological and philosophical literature concerning relationships between episodic memory, mental time travel, and the kind of self-awareness (referred to as **autonoetic awareness**) that may be required to project an experiencing self into thoughts about the past or the future (Wheeler, Stuss, & Tulving, 1997; Hoerl & McCormack, 2001; Moore & Lemmon, 2001; Atance and O'Neill, 2005).

In the case of autism it is tempting to suggest that episodic memory and future thinking are impaired as a result of impaired development of a sense of self (see the various theories concerning self-concept outlined in Box 11.1). However, the fact that adults with episodic memory impairment lack future thinking, even though they have presumably had a normal self-concept up until the time of their memory loss, argues against this interpretation. It seems more probable that what is lost is the ability to integrate representations of 'an experiencing self' (Powell & Jordan, 1993) with other constituents of past episodes or future plans (see Lind & Bowler, 2008, for discussion of the issues as they relate to autism).

The suggestion of links from impaired episodic memory to impaired generativity and to impaired planning receives some informal support from Vargha-Khadem's report (personal communication) that individuals with developmental amnesia (who, like individuals with AS/HFA, have a selective impairment of episodic memory of developmental origin) have 'reduced drive to generate new plans and ideas'. Vargha-Khadem attributes this to 'a memory impairment, in that for an idea to be pursued and actively developed, one has to keep the goal in mind and work towards its accomplishment'.

Finally, Atance and O'Neill (2001) reported that one individual described in their paper was able to apply 'structured routines' to compensate to some degree for impaired planning. This anticipates a point to be made in the next section, concerning ways in which loss of one memory capacity forces increased reliance on intact memory capacities, a point made strongly by Ullman (2001).

An intact memory system – repetitive behaviour hypothesis

The more pervasive an individual's declarative memory impairment, the more that individual will be reliant on their intact memory systems. The fact that high-functioning individuals have intact memory for impersonal factual information (but impaired episodic memory) might thus help to explain why many able individuals with ASDs excel in accumulating factual knowledge concerning their particular subject area or topic of interest.

Lower-functioning individuals do not, according to the main hypothesis, have intact semantic memory, and are not able to amass factual information. Their learning is therefore heavily reliant on intact perceptual, procedural, and immediate memory systems. This may help to explain the preference for invariant environments and routines in lower-functioning individuals, as has been suggested by Kemper and Bauman (1998) and by Bachevalier (1994, 2008) as well as in my own publications (for example, Boucher et al., 2005; Boucher, Mayes et al., 2008).

Uneven Memory Abilities as an Explanation of Some Spared and Savant Abilities in LFA

An unusual degree of dependence on intact perceptual, procedural, and immediate memory systems can also help to explain some peak abilities, including some savant abilities, in low-functioning individuals. In particular, intact or relatively spared perceptual and immediate memory is consistent with the frequently noted peak of ability in rote learning. Optimisation of intact procedural memory in the absence of declarative memory abilities is also consistent with the explanation of some savant abilities proposed by Mottron et al. (2006), Pring (2008) and others.

Uneven Memory Abilities and Paradoxical Motor Skills

In Chapter 10 an intriguing observation made first by Leary and Hill (1996) was noted. This was that less demanding motor tasks tend to be performed less well than more demanding tasks by individuals with ASDs. It was also noted in Chapter 10 that this observation is consistent with the apparently paradoxical skilled fine movement observed in at least some individuals with ASDs, including some who are low-functioning (Wing, 1996).

Skilled fine movements, such as are required for playing the piano, using a keyboard or tying shoelaces, are initially acquired utilising explicit learning systems, involving the kinds of explicit movement preparation and planning shown to be impaired by Rinehart, Bradshaw et al. (2006), and others. With practice, dependence on explicit learning systems decreases and the role of implicit, procedural processes increases to the point where highly practised skilled movements are carried out automatically, with no conscious control. This observation might help to explain the apparently paradoxical fine movements that have been observed in some individuals. Where some neuromuscular impairment such as hypotonia or dyspraxia is present, as is commonly the case, skilled fine movement will not of course be observed, which could explain why good fine movement is not observed in all individuals with ASDs. **Automatisation** of motor skills in people with ASDs has been very little investigated, although one study supports the suggestion that it may be intact, at least in high-functioning individuals (Mostofsky et al., 2004).

Conclusion

The suggestion that different patterns of spared and impaired memory abilities are characteristic of individuals with higher-functioning as compared to lower-functioning forms of autism, as summarised in Table 12.1, has the potential to explain most of the important characteristics of ASDs that are currently unexplained. However, more behavioural research is needed, as has been indicated at various points in the foregoing sections. The brain correlates of the hypothesised memory impairments in AS/HFA as opposed to LFA also remain to be tested. Some of these further investigations are currently under way.

THE TIME PROCESSING HYPOTHESIS

The Hypothesis

First-hand accounts of autism and reports of parents, teachers and other 'insiders' suggest that people with ASDs have a very poor sense of time. A selection of the types of reports that are common, if not universal, is reproduced in Box 12.1.

Crucially, these problems are not to do with being able to keep track of time using clocks, watches, calendars or diaries: more able people with ASDs are competent at using external measures and markers of time and are, indeed, heavily reliant on them. The problems have more to do with sensing the passage of time, with bodily timing, and with thinking about the past and the future. For brevity, the term 'time processing' will be used here to cover all these forms of time-related processing, whether sensory-perceptual, cognitive or motor.

Anomalous time processing in people with ASDs has been noted for decades, as is evident from an extract from Hermelin and O'Connor's *Psychological Experiments with Autistic Children*, published in 1970:

> Anthony (1958) sees autism as... a derangement of sensory input. The (autistic) child has no time sense and his sensory input structure lacks hierarchical organisation. He deals with the world in an ad hoc fashion without reference to history, temporal series, or spatial organisation. (Hermelin and O'Connor, 1970: 9)

One early theory concerning the origins of (low-functioning) autism was that cognitive and linguistic impairments in particular are caused by impaired 'sequencing', as noted in Chapter 10. Taking a rather different approach, some clinician theorists have stressed the possible importance of lack of timing in social exchanges as a cause, or contributory cause, of impaired social interaction, communication, and emotional reciprocity in autism, as outlined in Chapter 8. Evidence in support of impaired sequencing and impaired social timing was cited in Chapters 10 and 8, respectively. There is also biochemical evidence suggestive of abnormalities of **circadian rhythms** in people with ASDs (Nir, 1995; Tordjmann, Anderson, Pichard, Charbury, & Touitou, 2005) and reports of the kinds of sleep disorders that can be associated with disruption or malfunction of the internal 24-hour clock (as commonly experienced in jet-lag) (Richdale & Prior, 1995; Limoges, Mottron, Bolduc, Berthiaume, & Godbout, 2005; Hare, Jones, & Evershed, 2006).

In Boucher (2001; see also Boucher, 2000) I attempted to pull these strands of evidence together and understand aspects of autism-related behaviours in terms of a disturbance within a set of hierarchically organised and integrated cyclic timing mechanisms. These mechanisms were identified with cyclic neural and physiological processes with frequencies ranging from very high-frequency electrical oscillations within the brain to the c. 24-hour 'body clock'. I hypothesised that the ability to utilise very high-frequency oscillators such as are involved in speech perception and articulation, and in the execution of fine movements, is generally intact across the spectrum, but that lower-frequency 'brain waves', and especially the integration of neural and physiological timing mechanisms operating at very different frequencies, is increasingly impaired as the severity of autism and associated language and learning impairments increases. The theory differs from the earlier 'sequencing' theories in that it emphasises impaired integration of hierarchically organised timing mechanisms (see the quote about Anthony, above) explicitly excluding problems of temporal sequencing in the sense of A then B then C. I used the phrase 'time parsing' to emphasise the kinds of integrative problems envisaged.

Evidence

As argued in Boucher (2001), it is hard to overestimate the effects that congenital problems in time processing would have on a range of behaviours relevant to autism. At the least, time-processing problems of the kinds envisaged would inevitably impair primary intersubjectivity (Trevarthen & Aitken, 2001; Feldman, 2007), motor skills (Gowen & Miall, 2005), and the sleep–wake cycle.

Direct positive evidence of impaired time processing at the behavioural level is, however, sparse and sometimes contradictory. A study by Boucher, Pons, Lind, and Williams (2007) demonstrated a significant bias towards present-focused thinking as opposed to thinking across time from past to present to future. A study by Szelag, Kowalska, Galkowski, & Pöppel (2004) showed impaired ability to estimate temporal duration. However, two other studies of temporal duration judgement found no impairment (Mostofsky et al., 2000; Wallace & Happé, 2007), which is suprising in view of the concensus in first-hand reports of problems in experiencing the passage of time. Impaired processing of very high-frequency (extremely rapid) temporal information was shown to be intact in individuals with AS but not in individuals with LFA (Cardy, Flagg, Roberts, Brian, & Roberts, 2005).

Biochemical evidence of impaired circadian rhythm is more copious and stronger, although findings from different studies do not always agree (see Tordjmann et al., 2005, for a review). The suggestion of impaired oscillatory brain activity, and especially the suggestion that the integration of cyclic brain activity is impaired, has not been explicitly tested. However, it is consistent with the now common agreement that neural activity in different brain regions is poorly synchronised (Brock et al., 2002) and disco-ordinated (Courchesne, 2004; Geschwind & Levitt, 2007) in individuals with ASDs (see Chapter 11).

At the etiological level, Nicholas et al.'s (2007) study of 'clock genes', cited in Chapter 8, provides potentially important support for the impaired time processing hypothesis, although their findings are in need of replication and extension. Clock genes are defined as those several genes that contribute to the formation and function of timing mechanisms ranging from circadian rhythms to the very high-frequency neural mechanisms required for rapid movement, amongst other things. These genes are present in all animal species, and have been extensively studied in fruit flies, some studies with mice, and a few studies in humans that have focused on sleep disorders (see Nicholas et al., 2007, for references).

Most interestingly from my own personal view of the causes of ASDs, certain clock genes are thought to contribute to the normal development of limbic and prefrontal connections in the mammalian brain (Reick, Garcia, Dudley, & McKnight, 2004). Consistent with this claim, the elimination of particular clock genes in animal models has been shown to be associated with impaired memory for past experience (Sakai, Tamura, Kitamato, & Kidokoro, 2004) and with impaired fear conditioning (Garcia et al., 2000).

How the Time-processing Impairment Hypothesis Fits Into the Broader Picture

The fit with an uneven memory abilities hypothesis

The time-processing impairment hypothesis as I have proposed is consistent with the memory hypothesis proposed earlier in the chapter. Specifically, impaired integration of oscillatory neural activity at different frequencies, however caused, would impair both timing and the ability to co-ordinate and relate the multimodal constituents of episodic memory.

The time-processing impairment hypothesis as argued for by Wimpory et al. (2002), the findings on clock genes in people with ASDs (Nicholas et al., 2007), and Reick et al.'s (2004) finding concerning the contribution of clock genes to the formation of limbic prefrontal circuitry involved in declarative memory are also consistent with, and could strengthen the suggestion of, a link between time processing and memory in autism.

The fit with explanations of autism as a whole

The combined 'memory and time' hypothesis is entirely consistent with the concept of ASDs as a group of disorders involving disconnectivity and disco-ordination of activity between neural circuits. As I have stated it, the combined hypothesis simply adds forms of declarative memory and the ability to process temporal information to the widely accepted list of capacities that would be affected by impaired connectivity. In fact, the link between impaired declarative memory and disconnectivity is anticipated in Dawson, Webb et al.'s (2002) model in which impaired declarative memory and impaired feature binding are ascribed to the same underlying deficit (see Figure 11.2).

There is a possible conflict, however, between the emerging consensus outlined in Chapter 11 concerning the origins of impaired connectivity and the suggestion of a critical role for clock genes as a cause of abnormal brain development and function, as argued for by Wimpory and her colleagues. I have no view here. Although the clock genes hypothesis strengthens my argument that impaired time processing is important in understanding autism, it is not essential to it. Disruption and disco-ordination of neural activity in the brain however caused would impair at least some forms of time processing. The neuropsychological model of the causes of autism presented next is, in fact, more closely based on the theories described in Chapter 11 than on a clock genes hypothesis.

A MODEL OF THE CRITICAL NEUROPSYCHOLOGICAL CAUSES OF AUTISM

A model of the critical neuropsychological causes of autism is summarised in Figure 12.3.

Figure 12.3 indicates a lack of co-ordinated function within two neural circuits in particular:

- the amygdala–orbitofrontal circuit that includes other structures (superior temporal gyrus, ventromedial prefrontal cortex, and fusiform gyrus) that constitute the social brain;
- the hippocampal (perirhinal)–dorsolateral prefrontal cortex circuit.

In addition, Figure 12.3 indicates:

- a lack of fully functioning pathways from the frontal cortex to other relatively distant brain regions, including the occipital, parietal and temporal lobes.

The cerebellar vermis (in the cerebellum) containing Purkinje cells is shown in Figure 12.3 because, following the evidence and theories concerning brain dysgenesis in autism described in Chapter 11, I assume that malformation and malfunction within the circuits identified under the first two bullet points derive from abnormal outputs from Purkinje cells in the cerebellum.

The brain stem is shown for two reasons. First, because there is some evidence to suggest that the initial cause of brain dysgenesis may involve abnormalities within the brain stem (Rodier & Arndt, 2005) and, secondly, because nuclei within the brain stem have a role in generating and modulating oscillatory neural activity involved in hippocampal-mediated **relational memory** (Jackson & Bland, 2005).

At least as important as the dysfunctional circuitry indicated in Figure 12.3 is the assumption that many brain areas and their associated functions are

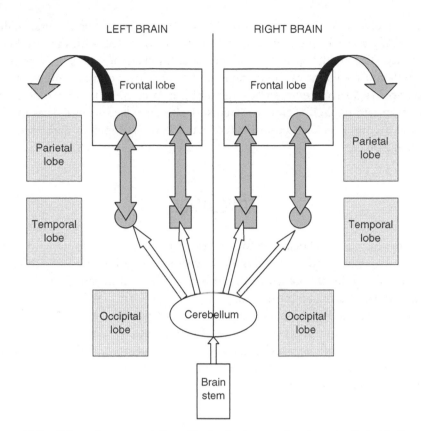

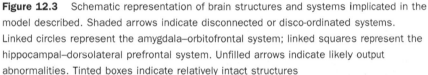

Figure 12.3 Schematic representation of brain structures and systems implicated in the model described. Shaded arrows indicate disconnected or disco-ordinated systems. Linked circles represent the amygdala–orbitofrontal system; linked squares represent the hippocampal–dorsolateral prefrontal system. Unfilled arrows indicate likely output abnormalities. Tinted boxes indicate relatively intact structures

intact, or relatively intact, at least in higher-functioning individuals. Brain regions assumed to be mainly intact include the primary sensory processing regions in the occipital and parietal lobes, some regions of the frontal and temporal lobes (that would be available to take over some higher-order functions), and most of those subcortical structures that subserve more basic functions, including the various forms of non-declarative memory and learning that are grouped together as perceptual and procedural memory.

The model draws in particular from Bachevalier's research over the years (for an example and a review, see Loveland, Bachevalier et al., 2007; Bachevalier, 2008) and more recently from Ben Shalom's work (Ben Shalom, 2003; Faran & Ben Shalom, 2008). The model overlaps with those proposed by Waterhouse et al. (1996) and by Dawson, Webb et al. (2002), described in Chapter 11 (see Figures 11.2 and 11.3). The model is also consistent with theories such as Belmonte et al.'s (2004a), highlighted in the previous chapter, that conceive of ASDs as 'fanning out' from a single *kind* of brain abnormality, specifically a lack of integrated neural function associated with impaired connectivity. The model goes beyond previous models, however, in offering a more detailed account of the possible effects of selective impairments of hippocampal region-related memory impairments in combination with predominantly spared implicit memory systems. It also goes beyond previous models in identifying a lack of co-ordinated activity with impaired neural timing mechanisms.

CONCLUSION

The autism puzzle is beginning to yield its secrets and able people with ASDs, as well as parents and those who work with and care for people with ASDs, should feel cautiously optimistic about being able to understand the causes of autism in the reasonably near future.

For researchers it is an exciting time to be working in this field, especially given the opportunities afforded by new technologies. Whether or not my own particular model of the psychological causes of autism and their brain bases proves to be correct is neither here nor there; the important thing is that progress continues to be made.

PART III

Practical Issues

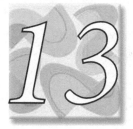

ASSESSMENT, DIAGNOSIS AND SCREENING

AIMS
••••
ASSESSMENT: INTRODUCTORY REMARKS
••••
DIAGNOSIS
Why Diagnose?
When Should a Diagnosis be Made?
Diagnosis by Whom, and Where?
Methods for Diagnosing Autistic Spectrum Disorders
Methods for Diagnosing Subtypes of Autism-related Disorders
Supplementary Assessments Contributing to Differential Diagnosis
••••
SCREENING
Introduction
Methods of Screening for Autistic Spectrum Disorders
Methods of Screening for Subtypes
••••
SUMMARY

ASSESSMENT: INTRODUCTORY REMARKS

Assessments in the field of autism are carried out for a variety of different purposes. The most obvious of these is to make a diagnosis. There are, in addition, many assessment procedures designed to estimate the probability that an individual has an ASD, or a particular subtype of ASD, but which fall short of yielding a reliable diagnosis. These are generally referred to as screening tests (but see below for a different usage of the term 'screening').

In addition to diagnosis and screening, however, assessment may be carried out for numerous other purposes: for example to help determine educational placement or progress, monitor response to an exclusion diet or make a case for awarding disability allowance. Apart from these narrow and specific uses of assessment, a full investigation of an individual's particular pattern of strengths, weaknesses and interests helps those who work with or care for the individual to understand and cater for that individual's unique set of needs.

Assessments for diagnosis or screening are designed to determine whether or not an individual may belong to a particular diagnostic group, whereas assessments relating to intervention education and care are designed to evaluate the achievements, problems, needs, etc. of individuals. The contrasting aims of assigning individuals to groups as opposed to focusing on individuals echo the contrast made earlier in the book between the generalised descriptions of autism-related behaviours that are given in the diagnostic manuals, and the particular or manifest behaviour of individuals at different life stages and in different contexts. Assessments for diagnosis or screening gather information that is relevant to generalised descriptions of autistic behaviour, whereas assessments for intervention, etc. gather detailed and particular information about individuals. There should be no conflict or sense of competition between the two types of assessment: they serve different functions, both of which are important.

This chapter focuses exclusively on diagnosis and diagnostic assessment methods, and on preliminary screening methods. Assessments used in specialist fields of intervention, education and care are too numerous and varied for even summary coverage to be attempted here. However, information can be found in the various specialist literatures (for example, concerning neurological assessment, speech and language assessment, self-help skills assessment, financial assessment). For a discussion of the assessment of individuals for the purposes of developing programmes of intervention and care, see Jordan (2005a).

DIAGNOSIS

Why Diagnose?

Diagnosis is a tool, not an end in itself. It has a number of uses, the most important of which are indicated below.

Uses of diagnosis

To help people with ASDs themselves and their families   The main purpose of diagnosis is to achieve useful ends for people with ASDs themselves, their families and other carers. So, for example, in the case of a young child, a diagnosis of an ASD can do all of the following.

- Give parents a lever with which to obtain appropriate education or other intervention for their child.
- Help parents to make sense of their child's problems ('so that's why she never looks at me', 'that's why he has a tantrum if I try to get him to wear new shoes').
- Guide parents' hopes and expectations for their child.
- Help parents and others to share their problems and learn from others (by joining a parents' group, reading, attending conferences, workshops or discussion groups).
- Protect parents from negative reactions from others ('Some people with autism have a very sensitive sense of smell – I'm afraid she doesn't like your perfume', 'He doesn't mean to be rude – he's autistic and doesn't like being touched').

Similarly, a diagnosis of an older child or an adult can help to explain why an individual is different from most others in certain ways, alleviating the frustration and distress resulting from misunderstanding or misinterpreting the individual's behaviour. For example, it may be frustrating and upsetting to parents that their teenage son does not want to go out with friends in the evenings and is bullied and labelled a swot by his peers, until they know why their son prefers to be alone and to study his special interest subjects. A husband's undemonstrative behaviour and lack of emotional warmth may be misinterpreted as lack of love and commitment, until the reason for it is understood. Diagnosis of an older child or adult may also enable them or their carers to access practical things such as respite care, free transport to and from school or college or assistance in obtaining sheltered accommodation. For more able individuals it may enable them to obtain social skills training, counselling or psychotherapy if these or other similar interventions are likely to be beneficial.

To facilitate communication between practitioners   Diagnosis is also useful as an aid to communication amongst practitioners and professionals. For example, a family doctor writing a referral for a child for a hearing test may write 'Joe has mild autism' in place of a more detailed description of Joe's autism-related behaviours that may be relevant to the audiologist's administration and interpretation of the hearing test. Similarly, mention of a diagnosis of 'autism', 'autistic features' or 'Asperger syndrome' on documents preceding a child's enrollment at a new school instantly conveys important preliminary information to teaching staff. Use of a diagnostic label for communication between practitioners is, of course, only as good as their shared understanding of the terms used. It also conveys a limited amount of information, not specific to the individual, which may be enough for some purposes but not for others (e.g., Preece & Jordan, 2007).

To provide information needed for the provision and financing of services   Statisticians, policy makers and administrators concerned with the provision and financing of health, educational and social services need information concerning the incidence and prevalence of ASDs based on authoritative diagnoses. If diagnoses are not made, then provision will not be made. Of course, even when good diagnostic services are available and operating well, it may not ensure that the best possible provision will be made because there are always limiting factors. At least, however, the information is there on which to base claims. The anecdotes recounted in Box 13.1 illustrate how critical a diagnosis is for the allocation of scarce resources at local level.

BOX 13.1   Tales of two cities: The use and abuse of diagnostic labels for obtaining appropriate educational provision

In *City A* there was for a time a strong lobby amongst educationalists against diagnosing children, on the grounds that 'labelling' was stigmatising, and that it would lower teachers' expectations of children or create prejudice against them. These are reasoned arguments based on legitimate fears. However, the net effect of not using an autism diagnosis was that children with ASDs were described instead as having 'communication difficulties' (and sent to special units for language-impaired children) or as having emotional or social difficulties (and sent to schools for children with emotional and behaviour problems) or as simply learning-impaired (and sent to schools for 'slow learners'). No special educational provision for children with ASDs was made until, eventually, parent pressure and government legislation forced the city's Local Education Authority to recognise that there is a group of children for

---

whom a diagnosis of an ASD is appropriate and useful, and that for these children the diagnosis signals a very particular set of educational needs that should be provided for.

City B, by contrast, has long recognised that an autism-related diagnosis provides an indicator of a child's special needs, and excellent educational provision is made for children on the autistic spectrum from infancy to post-16. In this city, however, somewhat less good provision is made for children with certain other kinds of special educational needs. As a result there is pressure from some parents of children who are not autistic but who have some social, emotional, communicative or learning difficulty, for the child to be diagnosed as autistic or as having autistic features of behaviour. These parents hope that this may qualify their child for the special teaching and support available to children with autism (even if not entirely appropriate for their child).

To ensure comparability between participants assessed in different research studies Suppose that two studies of a particular method of preparing high-functioning young adults for job interviews produced radically different results, one showing the methods to be very useful, the other suggesting that they made no difference to interviewees' success. One possible explanation of the discrepant results is that the participants in the two studies were not comparable. Perhaps one group was made up of individuals with Asperger syndrome strictly defined as in the diagnostic manuals (see Chapter 1), whereas the group in the second study was made up of individuals whose personal records used the description 'Asperger syndrome' without specifying the criteria used. The likely difference between the two groups taking part means that results of the two studies are not comparable. Given that one of the aims of scientific research is to build up a body of findings replicating an effect across many comparable studies, failure to ensure that groups taking part in autism research have been diagnosed according to agreed categories and criteria undermines the usefulness of research.

Arguments against diagnosis

Despite the many uses of diagnosis, there are some counter arguments and occasional misuses or abuses.

Adverse effects for individuals and families In Box 13.1 it was mentioned that a diagnosis can have stigmatising effects that might include lowering teachers' expectations of particular children or creating prejudice against them. Stigmatising effects are in fact more likely to be experienced in the wider world where knowledge and understanding are more limited than in most schools. The words 'autism' or 'autistic' conjure up for many people ideas of incomprehensible difference that they find personally threatening, and they may react accordingly. So a child known to have an ASD may be omitted from the class-wide invitation to a birthday party; a family that is open about their child's autism may be refused a booking for an activities holiday; an adult with 'autism' on their CV may not be considered for a job interview, however strongly recommended as suitable.

The extent and severity of the stigmatising effects of what is sometimes pejoratively called 'labelling' are related to the degree of ignorance that exists and the scope for stereotyping that ignorance provides. One of the arguments for educational **inclusion** is to help to reduce ignorance within the general population (see Chapter 15). National and local autistic societies also work hard to dispel the ignorance, prejudice and stereotyping that underlie stigma. In this they are sometimes helped, but sometimes hindered, by the media. Most importantly, individuals themselves and families face down stigma by speaking openly about their experiences, writing about them and, above all, being able to laugh about them. Martin Ives and Nell Munro who are parents of a child with an ASD, write:

> Sooner or later most parents reach a point where they feel less sensitive about what other people might think or say. It is this tougher skin combined with a liberal sense of humour that sees most parents through. (Ives and Munro, 2002: 70)

Ironically, use of diagnostic labels is essential for dispelling ignorance and stigma: it is not possible to demystify autism and take the fright out of it without using the term. In addition, not using diagnostic labels does not make people's perceived differences go away, nor does it prevent other people from reacting negatively. Claire Sainsbury, who has Asperger syndrome, writes:

> When I didn't have an official diagnostic label my teachers unofficially labelled me as 'emotionally disturbed', 'rude' and so on, and my classmates unofficially labelled me 'nerd', 'weirdo' and 'freak'; frankly I prefer the official label. It's the stigma attached to being different that's the problem, not the label. (Sainsbury, 2000: 31, quoted in Ives and Munro, 2002)

Fortunately, the truth of Claire Sainsbury's last statement is more widely recognised now than it was a decade or two ago when arguments against diagnostic 'labelling' were being strongly aired. Unfortunately, however, prejudice and stigma remain.

Overuse or misuse of diagnosis   The question of the possible over-diagnosis of ASDs was considered in Chapter 4, in the section dealing with the apparent rise in the prevalence of ASDs. The large-scale study by Baird et al. (2006) referred to in that chapter, found no evidence of overuse in the sense of diagnosis of an autism-related condition having been given to individuals who did not qualify for this diagnosis using current diagnostic criteria and current interpretation of these criteria. However, these authors note that diagnostic criteria may be looser, or interpreted more loosely, than in the past. If this is of benefit to individuals who now receive a diagnosis, the charge of overuse does not apply.

However, within the set of diagnoses that may be made (Asperger syndrome, autistic disorder, PDD-NOS, atypical autism, ASD, HFA or LFA), two diagnostic descriptions may be preferred over others, for clinically justifiable reasons. The first of these is a diagnosis of 'ASD', with no further qualification or description. This has been recommended by some advisory bodies on the grounds that the next stages of assessment should be directed towards delineating each individual's strengths and needs, rather than towards allocating the individual to a categorical subtype (see below).

The second diagnosis that may be preferred by clinicians, and overused by the standards of DSM-IV, is Asperger syndrome. A diagnosis of AS carries less stigma than a diagnosis of autism, and the long-term outlook for people with AS is usually better than that for people with classic autism, allowing for greater optimism. Giving a child with mild intellectual disability a diagnosis of AS rather than a diagnosis of autism may therefore help some parents to accept their child's differences and to go forward, rather than reacting in more negative ways detrimental to the child and the family. A particular school may accept children with a diagnosis of AS but not children with a diagnosis of autism. A late diagnosis of AS in an intelligent teenager with persistent language impairments is less damaging to self-esteem than a strictly 'correct' diagnosis of autism or autistic disorder. These are only a few of the reasons why the diagnosis of Asperger syndrome is sometimes stretched beyond its strict limits by clinicians. An example of an instance where this was done is described in Box 13.2.

BOX 13.2   An example of the justifiable 'misuse' of the diagnosis of Asperger syndrome

Jane at age 20 had problems in making and sustaining relationships, with limited interests. She had had speech therapy as a child, and was later diagnosed with dyslexia, leaving school with no formal qualifications. However, Jane was an accomplished pianist, pretty, with 'active but odd' social behaviour and a desire for friendships. When she left school she obtained employment playing the piano in the restaurant of a local hotel, but was asked to leave when she was rude to a customer. It was not the first incident of this kind, and Jane's parents, who had long resisted the suggestion that she was not 'just a little slow', finally arranged for

(Cont'd)

her to see a psychiatrist. She was diagnosed with AS, rather than with autism, probably partly to maintain the parents' optimistic attitude; partly to maintain Jane's self-esteem; partly with the thought in mind that an AS diagnosis might not prevent her from finding work again, whereas an autism diagnosis would be a greater bar; and partly, one feels sure, because Jane was talented, pretty and socially engaging.

Less justifiable overuse of the term 'Asperger syndrome' occurs in the everyday speech of certain groups of people who apply it to any relations, acquaintances or work colleagues who may be unusually reserved, not very empathic or a bit rigid. The people referred to might, on investigation, be described as belonging to the broader autism phenotype. However, we are not yet at the stage of broadening diagnostic criteria to include such people. Nor do they need the diagnosis, because most are leading satisfactory, 'normal' lives.

Abuse of diagnosis   An example of the abuse of diagnosis can be found in the story of City B in Box 13.1, where parents may sometimes have persuaded clinicians to describe their language-impaired, emotionally disturbed or intellectually disabled child as being on the autistic spectrum to obtain specialist education for their child within the excellent autism teaching units in that city.

In sum   Some objections to diagnosis can be made, and occasionally diagnosis is misused. However, the legitimate and important uses of diagnosis, correctly used, outweigh any objections.

When Should a Diagnosis be Made?

Young children

In view of the potential usefulness of a diagnosis for the parents of a young child with an ASD, the obvious answer to the question 'When should a diagnosis be made?' might appear to be 'As soon as possible'.

There are dangers, however, in assuming that early diagnosis is always best for the child and the family. Some research suggests that a proportion of children who appear to warrant a diagnosis of an ASD at two years old no longer warrant the diagnosis at age four years (Sutera et al., 2007). This is consistent with large-scale surveys that show the diagnosis of very young children with social and communication delays is not 100 per cent accurate, given the methods currently available. The diagnosis of an ASD in their child, even if it comes as some kind of relief from doubt and frustration, is always painful and sometimes traumatic for parents, requiring many adjustments of relationships and expectations within the family. If the diagnosis is overturned a year or two later, the family's anxieties and attempts at adjustment may have been needless.

A safer answer to the question 'When?' might therefore be 'As early as it can be done with reasonable certainty.' This, however, begs the question of when that might be, given that all children develop differently, and given the problems of **differential diagnosis** (see Chapter 2). A preferable answer might be 'As soon as the benefits of diagnosis for the child and family outweigh any adverse effects of possible misdiagnosis'.

In the event, each clinician or clinical team has to make a judgement on each individual case. A strategy recommended by a government-led working party in the UK is to proceed towards diagnosis in stages, with the initial stage focusing on the child's and the family's immediate needs rather than on giving a name to the child's problems (Le Couteur, Baird, & NIASA, 2003). According to the strategy elaborated on in Le Couteur et al., the assessments needed for making a reliable diagnosis should proceed in stages that could take up to 18 months in complex cases (see Table 13.1).

Older children and adults

With older children and adults with mild autism or with sufficiently high ability to compensate well, the answer to the 'When?' question is again pragmatic: 'When the diagnosis tool helps them to understand themselves or to be better understood by those around them or to receive needed intervention or support' (see Box 4.1 for an example).

With older children and adults whose severe intellectual or physical impairments may have masked their autism or overshadowed the individual's autism in terms of earlier needs, there is again a pragmatic answer to the 'When?' question: 'Never too late if having the autism diagnosis achieves better provision for their needs' (Bennett, Wood, & Hare, 2005).

Diagnosis by Whom and Where?

Infants and young children

Practitioners involved in diagnosis, and places where diagnosis may be carried out, vary from country to country, and from region to region within countries; there are also national and regional variations in the stages that must be gone through to obtain a diagnosis (see Volkmar, 2005, for information about national differences). An ideal progression and timescale as advised by a working party in the UK is summarised in Table 13.1, overleaf. The reality is, however, often less than ideal, as outlined next.

Parents are usually the first to notice that there is something unusual about their infant or young child, although sometimes it may be a grandparent, clinic nurse or experienced nursery school teacher who first voices some concern.

Table 13.1 *Summary of the stages through which diagnostic assessment should ideally proceed, the actions to be taken at each stage, and the approximate timescale of the staged process (based on Le Couteur et al., 2003)*

STAGES	ACTIONS		TIMESCALE
	INVESTIGATIONS	*OTHER*	
Concerns identified		Referral for general developmental assessment	Within six weeks
Stage 1	*General developmental assessment* Developmental history Full examination of the child Appropriate further tests	Feedback to family Plans for provision begin	Within a further seven weeks
		If ASD suspected, named keyworker appointed	Within a further four weeks
Stage 2	*Assessment for differential diagnosis baseline of skills and difficulties* ASD-specific developmental history Observation across more than one setting Cognitive assessment Communication assessment Assessment of mental health and behaviour Full physical examination and investigations Family assessment		Within a further 17 weeks
		Written report and co-ordinated programme of intervention including care plan, discussed with parents	Within a further six weeks
		Professional knowledgeable re. ASDs visits home and preschool/ school placement	
Stage 3 if required in case of diagnostic doubt, case complexity or if additional specific advice needed	(As required)	(Referral for additional assessments) (Second opinion sought)	Within a further 30 weeks

Once concerns have been raised about a young child's development, the first professional to be consulted is generally the family doctor. What happens next is dependent on a range of factors, including the degree of delay and difference in any particular child's development, the knowledge and experience of autism of the doctor first seen, and the availability of specialist facilities in the area in which the family lives. At best, the child will be immediately referred to a multidisciplinary child development clinic for assessment. The professionals who may be involved in this assessment would probably include a paediatrician or paediatric neurologist, a clinical or educational psychologist, a speech and language therapist (pathologist), and a preschool education or family liaison specialist (consistent with the multi-agency assessments indicated in Table 13.1).

Child development clinics offering multidisciplinary assessments are not, however, available in all regions. Children may then be referred for diagnostic assessment by a child psychiatrist or paediatrician, or by a clinical or educational psychologist specialising in autism-related problems. However, it would be unusual for a diagnosis to be made by a single professional without reference to information from others, and reports from other specialists would probably be requested before making a diagnosis. It is particularly important for more than one professional to be involved in the process of making a diagnosis, because it has been shown that collaborative assessment leads to more reliable and earlier diagnosis than diagnosis by a single person, however experienced (Risi et al., 2006).

Prompt referral to a multidisciplinary centre or other diagnostic clinic is, unfortunately, not what reliably happens as a result of an initial visit to the family doctor. Doctors who are in genuine doubt as to whether they are looking at a child who might have a significant developmental problem or a child who is just a little on the slow side developmentally, may refer the child for assessments that might help to clarify the nature and cause of the child's behavioural anomalies but which are not designed to assess the child for possible autism. For example, the child might be referred to an audiologist for hearing assessment, a speech and language therapist for assessment of communicative development, an educational psychologist for assessment of developmental level or intelligence, a neurologist for investigation of motor abnormalities or to the preschool clinical psychology service or family therapy clinic if the GP suspected emotional problems related to difficulties within the family (which could, of course, result from stresses centred on the child). Referrals such as these may be useful in helping to rule in or rule out some possible causes of the child's developmental differences, and thus contribute to differential diagnosis (see below). However, none of these assessments by themselves are sufficient for an authoritative diagnosis of an ASD, and referring the child for a succession of specialist assessments can introduce undesirable delay.

At worst, the family doctor will give unwarranted, if well-meant, reassurance of the kind 'She's fine; you've nothing to worry about' or a temporising response such as 'He's probably just a slow starter' or 'He may have had a virus you didn't notice at the time; let's see how he's doing in six months'. In the case of misguidedly reassuring or temporising responses, further visits to the doctor will be required before the process of obtaining a diagnosis can begin, again causing the delay and frustration that are all too common (Howlin & Asgharian, 1999; Mansell & Morris, 2004).

Older children and adults

Older children and adults who have not previously been diagnosed with an ASD are often at the more extreme ends of the spectrum. In very low-functioning individuals, the predominance of needs relating to physical and intellectual disabilities may lead to signs of autism being overlooked until, as sometimes happens, intractable behaviour problems bring their autism to the attention of psychologists or psychiatrists working in the learning disability services (see also Box 3.9).

In very high-functioning individuals, however, autism-related behaviours may be well compensated for or masked by superior academic achievement. The structure provided by home and primary school may also help high-functioning children to cope without excessive stress. Coping mechanisms may, however, break down in the more demanding and less structured environments of secondary school, college, and independent adulthood, with relationship failure and stress-related depression or anxiety bringing high-functioning older children or adults to the attention of educational or clinical psychologists or psychiatrists (see, for example, Box 4.1). There is a slight risk that high-functioning adults are misdiagnosed with a mental health problem, the chronic problems associated with the individual's autism being overlooked, and inappropriate treatment prescribed. Careful differential diagnosis (for example, from schizoid personality disorder or anxiety disorders) is therefore particularly important for these people.

Methods for Diagnosing Autistic Spectrum Disorders

There are currently no methods for diagnosing ASDs using physical tests. This is because the genetic and neurobiological bases of ASDs are unknown (see Chapter 7). It is likely that physical tests will become available as the physical causes of ASDs become known (Hu-Lince, Craig, Huentelman, & Stephan, 2005). However, because the physical causes that can lead to autism are almost certainly various, a number of different tests may be required. Each of these might identify a subgroup of people with ASDs or the results might support a diagnosis of an ASD whilst not constituting incontrovertible evidence. Nor can ASDs be diagnosed on the basis of physical appearance, such as provides an initial diagnostic indicator of numerous congenital medical conditions; nor on the basis of the kinds of behavioural tests that produce clear-cut evidence of, for example, visual impairment or cerebral palsy; nor on the basis of consistent adverse reactions to certain foods or other environmental influences or a looked-for response to a certain physical treatment; or on the basis of any other kind of physical test or natural indicator.

Instead, diagnosis must be made by assessing an individual's developmental history and current patterns of behaviour, and comparing the results of these assessments with the diagnostic criteria for autism-related conditions set out in DSM-IV and ICD-10 (see Chapter 1) or the criteria for an autistic spectrum disorder (see Chapter 2). In the next subsections, some formal and well-authenticated methods of collecting information about the individual in the past and present are described. By 'well authenticated' is meant that the methods have been shown to be both **reliable** and valid, and can therefore be used with reasonable confidence. (For discussion of the concepts of reliability and validity in relation to diagnostic tests, see Lord and Costello, 2005.)

The Autism Diagnostic Interview-Revised (ADI-R)

The ADI-R (Rutter, Le Couteur, & Lord, 2003) is sometimes described as constituting the 'gold standard' for diagnosis of an autistic spectrum disorder. It consists of a semi-structured interview in which a parent or primary caregiver is questioned by a trained clinician using a set of questions designed to obtain the information summarised in Box 13.3.

Box 13.3   Topics on which information is elicited in the ADI-R

- The family background, education, previous diagnoses (if any) and medications (if any) of the child or adult who is being assessed.
- Their behaviour, in general terms.
- Early development and developmental milestones.
- Language acquisition and any loss of language or other skills.
- Current functioning with regard to language and communication.
- Social development and play.
- Interests and behaviours.
- Other clinically relevant behaviours, such as hearing impairment, self-injury or epilepsy.

The interviewer records and codes responses in a standardised way that provides both an overall score and scores on three key domains of behaviour, namely reciprocal social interaction, language/communication, and restricted repetitive and stereotyped behaviours and interests. If scores in each of these domains reach certain levels, then a diagnosis of autism based on DSM-IV criteria can be made. The severity of an individual's autism, in terms of problematic behaviours within each domain, is also rated, allowing some indication of whether the individual might qualify for a diagnosis of Asperger syndrome as opposed to autistic disorder or PDD-NOS. However, the interview is not designed to yield authoritative subtype diagnoses.

Autism Diagnostic Observation Schedule (ADOS)

In a best practice diagnostic assessment, the ADI-R is supplemented by information from the ADOS (Lord, Rutter, DiLavore, & Risi, 1999). The ADOS consists of four sets, or modules, of specified activities to be initiated by the clinician, who both interacts with and observes the child or adult being assessed. Each module is designed for use with individuals within a particular age and ability range. So, for example, Module 1 activities are designed for observation of preschool children with little or no expressive speech, and include bubble play, having a snack, and having a pretend birthday party. Module 1 is also designed to provide situations that might elicit specific behaviours, including response to name, responsive social smile, and joint attention. Module 3 activities are designed for older children with some fluent spontaneous language, and include describing a picture, talking about friends, and carrying out a construction task. The observer, who must be trained in the procedures and scoring methods to be used, codes the child's behaviour according to items listed on the schedule, either immediately after administration of the session (which lasts approximately 30–45 minutes) or subsequently using video.

Although the ADOS is described as a diagnostic instrument, it is particularly useful in providing practitioners with information concerning an individual's current functioning and needs, and how these might be responded to. It can also be used on repeated occasions to assess behavioural change. The ADI-R and ADOS together, therefore, provide both a method for assigning an individual to a group as in diagnosis, and a method of obtaining information about an individual's current strengths and needs. Because diagnosis is rarely undertaken in a vacuum independent of considering needs and provision, this dual function is advantageous despite the time and effort that may be involved.

The Diagnostic Interview for Social and Communication Disorders (DISCO)

As with the combined ADI-R and ADOS assessment procedures, the DISCO (Wing, Leekam, Libby, Gould, & Larcombe, 2002) involves an extended parental interview supplemented by observation focussing on areas in which information has been elicited in the interview. In addition to the interview and the observations, information from psychological assessment and any past reports can also be used to make the final judgement concerning the items in the DISCO. The information obtained covers the topics summarised in Box 13.4.

BOX 13.4   Topics on which information is elicited in the DISCO

- Infancy history.
- Age of any setback in development.
- Gross motor skills.
- Self-care, e.g., feeding, dressing, domestic skills, independence.
- Communication.
- Social interaction with adults and with age peers, including social play.
- Imitation.
- Imagination.
- Skills, e.g., reading and writing, number, money, dates and time, special abilities.
- Motor and vocal stereotypies.
- Responses to sensory stimuli.
- Repetitive routines and resistance to change.
- Emotions.
- Activity pattern.
- Maladaptive behaviour.
- Sleep pattern.
- Catatonic features.
- Quality of social interaction.
- Any history of psychiatric conditions or sexual problems.

Scores based on information entered into the assessment schedule can be used to make either a diagnosis of ASD according to Wing's criteria or a diagnosis of autism according to ICD-10 and DSM-IV criteria (Leekam, Libby, Wing, Gould, & Taylor, 2002).

The DISCO differs from the ADI-R/ADOS in a number of ways. First, when used as part of a whole day assessment of a child, time is generally set aside for observation of the child's behaviour in an informal, unspecified setting. This provides a less structured and less repeatable observation method than is provided by the ADOS. However, the upside of this is that it allows experienced clinicians to form more intuitive judgements of the child's behaviour than is permitted by the standardised scoring of the ADOS. Risi et al.'s (2006) important study of 'what works' in the field of diagnosis, referred to above, showed that, contrary to what might be expected, informally derived clinical judgement is at least as reliable and valid a method of diagnosis as use of standardised tests, and an important part of any diagnostic assessment.

Secondly, the DISCO was initially developed by clinicians as a method of assessing individual needs, whereas the ADI was originally devised as a method of selecting bona fide cases of autism for the purposes of research. The history of the DISCO as a clinical tool explains why such a broad range of characteristics is assessed, compared to the behaviours assessed by the ADI-R.

Thirdly, the DISCO was based on a dimensional model of developmental disorders and was designed to establish a profile from which a diagnosis of an autistic spectrum disorder might be made or, alternatively, a borderline or overlapping condition might be identified. Only later was it modified to yield a diagnosis using ICD-10 and DSM-IV criteria. When the criteria for an ASD are used rather than the ICD-10 and DSM-IV criteria, the DISCO identifies a broader, more loosely defined group of individuals with autism-related disorders than the ADI-R.

Other diagnostic instruments

Numerous other diagnostic checklists, rating scales and observation schedules have been developed over the years, each designed to identify individuals with autism according to whatever diagnostic criteria were current. Some of these have stood the test of time or been updated as diagnostic criteria have been modified. These include the Autism Behaviour Checklist (ABC) (Krug, Arick, & Almond, 1980), the Childhood Autism Rating Scale (CARS) (Schopler, Reichler, & Renner, 1988), and the Ritvo-Freeman Real-Life Rating Scale (RLRS) (Freeman, Ritvo, Yokota, & Ritvo, 1986). None of these instruments, however, can be relied on as safely as the ADI-R (especially in combination with the ADOS) or the DISCO in making a diagnosis, though they may be very useful as screening tools (see below). This does not imply that the ADI-R/ADOS or DISCO are 100 per cent reliable and will not themselves be modified or superseded. In fact the ADI-R and the ADOS, also the DISCO, are still being elaborated and refined. Furthermore, if the diagnostic criteria for ASDs change in the forthcoming new edition of the *Diagnostic and Statistical Manual*, these current diagnostic assessment procedures will inevitably change.

Methods for Diagnosing Subtypes of Autism-related Disorders

At present, there is no reliable and valid way of diagnosing subtypes of autism, in particular PDD-NOS and Asperger syndrome. Various groups of clinical researchers are currently engaged in trying to develop methods of differentiating these subtypes from 'autism' or 'autistic spectrum disorder' more generally. It has been suggested, for example, that individuals who score within a certain range of points below the threshold for a diagnosis of autism on the ADI-R might warrant a diagnosis of PDD-NOS. However, a cut-off point has not been agreed. Gillberg's group in Sweden have had some success in developing a reliable and valid method of differentiating Asperger syndrome from other forms of autism with their Asperger Syndrome Diagnostic Interview (ASDI)

(Gillberg, Gillberg, Rastam, & Wentz, 2001). However, this diagnostic instrument uses criteria for Asperger syndrome that differ slightly from the criteria in DSM-IV and ICD-10, reducing the likelihood that it will be widely used. The Asperger Syndrome Diagnostic Scale (ASDS) (Myles, Bock, & Simpson, 2005) may prove more useful (Boggs, Gross, & Gohm, 2006; but see also Campbell, 2005). Attempts to diagnose autism subtypes using behavioural data are, however, based on the assumption that there are reliable behavioural differences between the putative subtypes. In view of the fact that reliable behavioural differences have not been demonstrated (see Chapter 2), attempts to achieve differential diagnosis behaviourally may be based on a false assumption.

Supplementary Assessments Contributing to Differential Diagnosis

As highlighted in Chapter 2, ASDs have fuzzy boundaries with various other developmental and mental health disorders. As a result it is sometimes difficult to discriminate between individuals for whom the most appropriate and useful diagnosis may be of an ASD as opposed to, for example, diagnosis of a specific language disorder that includes pragmatic language impairment, an attachment disorder, non-verbal learning disability, schizoid personality disorder, obsessive compulsive disorder or combinations of other difficulties, for example, hearing loss plus learning difficulties. Examples of assessments that include supplementary procedures contributing to differential diagnosis in diagnostic work-ups (see Table 13.1) can be found in Rapin (1996) and Klin, Saulnier, Tsatsanis, & Volkmar (2005).

SCREENING

Introduction

Screening in the field of medicine is used to identify those who may be at significant risk for a particular disease or disorder. It may be carried out across a whole population, for example screening all women within a certain age range for early signs of breast cancer. Alternatively, screening may be carried out with a selected group of individuals thought to be at increased risk of developing a disease, for example women with a family history of breast cancer. Those found to have the disease that is being screened for will be offered treatment. Those thought likely to have the disease, or to be at high risk of developing it at a later date, may be referred for fuller diagnostic assessment, precautionary treatment or advice and future monitoring. Information about some of the concepts and terms used in the literature on screening is summarised in Box 13.5.

Screening tests are used mainly for clinical purposes, as outlined above. However, they may also be used by researchers to check (a) that the participants in the group targeted in a study do, in fact, have the condition under investigation and (b) that the participants in any comparison group do not have the condition, even in very mild form.

Fuller accounts of screening in general can be found in the reviews of autism screening by Coonrod and Stone (2005) and Williams and Brayne (2006).

Methods of Screening for Autistic
Spectrum Disorders

Infants and very young children

In view of the difficulties of diagnosing autism reliably in very young children and the undesirability of diagnosing incorrectly (see above), the development of effective 'at risk' screening instruments for use with young children is highly desirable. If screening suggests that a child is at significant risk for autism, appropriate actions can be instituted; at the same time, a firm diagnosis is withheld until the child can be assessed more reliably when a little older, avoiding possible misdiagnosis.

There are currently no screening tests for very young children that meet all three of the criteria for effective screening listed in Box 13.5. However, those described below are relatively effective, particularly when used with selected groups of children ('Level 2' screening, in US terminology). All the tests described are in the process of modification and improvement.

The Checklist for Autism in Toddlers The Checklist for Autism in Toddlers (CHAT) (Baron-Cohen et al., 1996; Baird et al., 2000) is designed for use by doctors and nurses during routine check-ups of toddlers aged approximately 18 months. The CHAT consists of nine questions to the parent or other primary caregiver, all of which have YES/NO answers, and two of which are critical probes for possible autism-related behaviour. The critical probes are:

> Does your child ever PRETEND, for example, to make a cup of tea using a toy cup and teapot, or pretend other things?
>
> Does your child ever use his/her index finger to point, to indicate INTEREST in something?

In addition, five observations are made, the following three of which are critical and involve attempting to elicit certain behaviours from the child.

- Following a point (looking towards a toy the adult is pointing to).
- Producing a point, using an index finger, when asked to 'Show me (the toy)'.
- Pretending to make or drink tea when given a miniature cup and teapot and asked 'Can you make a cup of tea?'

Children who fail all five critical items are considered to be at high risk for autism. Children who do not produce a point, either according to their parent's report or when the adult tries to elicit a point, but who succeed on all the other items of the checklist, are considered to be at medium risk for autism. Failure on the critical questions and observations has been shown to be quite *specific* to autism: the CHAT does not often identify false positives. However, the CHAT is not highly *sensitive* to autism, and has quite a high rate of false negatives (Baird et al., 2000; but see Scambler, Hepburn, & Rogers, 2006, for a report of modifications leading to improved **sensitivity**).

The Modified Checklist for Autism in Toddlers The Modified Checklist for Autism in Toddlers (M-CHAT) (Robins, Fein, Barton, & Green, 2001) is an extended version of the CHAT designed for use with children of approximately two years of age. The **specificity** and sensitivity of this checklist is satisfactory when used with selected groups of children, as shown in preliminary studies (Williams & Brayne, 2006). Modifications of the M-CHAT to increase its effectiveness as a whole population screening test are discussed in Robins and Dumont-Mathieu (2006).

Other screening tests for use with infants and very young children   Other screening tests showing varying degrees of effectiveness include the Screening Tool for Autism in Two-year-olds (STAT) (Stone, Coonrod, Turner, & Pozdol, 2004); the Pervasive Developmental Disorders Screening Test – Stage II (PDDST-II) (Siegel, 2004); and Early Screening of Autistic Traits Questionnaire (EST) (Dietz, Swinkels, van Daalen, van Engeland, & Buitelaar, 2006), a promising whole population screening test designed for use with children aged 14–15 months.

School-age children and adults

The Autism Spectrum Quotient (AQ) was initially developed as a quick and easy whole population self-screening method for high-functioning adults with AS, HFA or autism-related traits (Baron-Cohen, Wheelwright, Skinner, Martin, & Clubley, 2001; Woodbury-Smith, Robinson, Wheelwright, & Baron-Cohen, 2005). The initial study showed the AQ to have high sensitivity. However, specificity was low because the test was not designed to exclude the identification of individuals with autistic traits, and some of the individuals tested (especially any mathematicians or scientists) were predicted to have such traits. The AQ has subsequently been modified for use with pre-teen children and adolescents. A study in which the children's AQ was adminis-tered to groups of higher- and lower-functioning individuals with ASDs and typically developing controls, showed acceptable levels of both sensitivity and specificity (Baron-Cohen, Hoekstra, Knickmeyer, & Wheelwright, 2006). Further tests of the AQ by independent groups are, however, needed.

The Autism Spectrum Screening Questionnaire (ASSQ) (Ehlers, Gillberg, & Wing, 1999; Posserud, Lundervold, & Gillberg, 2006), like the AQ, is designed to assess autism-related behavioural traits in whole population screening. Also, like the Autism Spectrum Quotient, results from the ASSQ support the con-cept of a spectrum of autism-related disorders, with no clear cut-off points between individuals who might warrant a clinical diagnosis and those who have autism-related traits, short of diagnostic significance.

Other screening methods suitable for use with individuals of various ages include some of the older checklists, rating scales and observation schedules mentioned in a previous section. These are well tried and tested methods, although they have now given way to the ADI-R/ADOS and the DISCO for use in diagnostic assessment.

Methods of Screening for Subtypes

Screening is particularly important for individuals with high-functioning forms of ASD who have not been diagnosed in their early years, but who are having problems in later childhood or adulthood. Various rating scales designed either to diagnose Asperger syndrome or to screen for high-functioning autism are reviewed by Campbell (2005), using a rigorous set of criteria. The procedures reviewed included: the Asperger Syndrome Diagnostic Scale (ASDS) (Myles et al., 2005, already mentioned in the section on diagnosis); Gilliam Asperger's Disorder Scale (GADS) (Gilliam, 2001); the Childhood Asperger's Screening Test (CAST) (Scott, Baron-Cohen, Bolton, & Brayne, 2002); and Krug's Asperger's Disorder Index (KADI) (Krug & Arick, 2003). None of these screening procedures fare well in Campbell's review, although the KADI is the least heavily criticised. However, work continues to refine and evaluate some of the procedures (see, for example, the report on CAST by Allison et al., 2007).

SUMMARY

Assessment in the field of autism is used for a variety of purposes, most notably for diagnosis and screening, but also for assessing individuals' strengths, needs and progress with regard to intervention, education and care. Assessments for diagnosis and screening (the topic of the present chapter) are designed to determine group membership, whereas assessments associated with intervention, education and care focus on individuals.

Diagnosis is a tool with certain functions. The most important of these is to assist individuals with ASDs and their immediate families and carers to understand themselves (or their child), to access services and other forms of support, and to plan for the future. However, diagnosis also facilitates communication between practitioners with knowledge of ASDs, in that diagnostic terms act as shorthand to convey information that would otherwise have to be detailed. Diagnosis is also necessary for estimating prevalence and, thus, for the estimation of provision for the educational, health and social needs. Finally, diagnosis is needed to ensure comparability between participants assessed in different research studies.

It has sometimes been argued that 'labelling' individuals with a diagnosis is stigmatising, creating prejudice and lowering expectations of that individual. In response it has been argued that it is the condition itself, and the fact that individuals with ASDs are perceived as 'different', that creates stigma, not the labelling process.

The appropriate time for a diagnosis to be made is as soon as the gains to be made for the individual and their family outweigh the disadvantages of possible misdiagnosis (which can occur in the case of infants and very young children). The processes of obtaining a diagnosis vary from country to country and regionally within any country. For infants and young children, the process at best starts with the family medical adviser and moves quickly to a specialist diagnostic centre offering multidisciplinary diagnostic assessments. Another reasonably satisfactory route to diagnosis involves referral from the family doctor to a specialist practitioner, who then obtains information from other specialists such as may be needed to arrive at a secure diagnostic decision.

Unfortunately, many families even in developed countries encounter delay and difficulty in having their young child fully and efficiently assessed. Individuals whose overall abilities place them at the extreme ends of the spectrum are often not diagnosed until later in life, for contrasting reasons. Differential diagnosis between an ASD and a mental health condition is particularly important for highly able individuals.

The most authoritative diagnostic instruments are the Autism Diagnostic Interview-Revised (ADI-R) and the Autism Diagnostic Observation Schedule (ADOS) used in combination, and the Diagnostic Interview for Social and Communication Disorders (DISCO) used in combination with informal observation. Clinical judgement, also consensus between more than one experienced professional, have been shown to be important. Supplementary assessments (for example, of communication and language, learning ability, and neurological status) are widely used, especially to assist differential diagnosis. There is currently no valid and reliable diagnostic method for discriminating between putative subtypes of ASD.

Screening in the autism field is used to identify individuals at significant risk of having an ASD, rather than to produce a reliable diagnosis. An effective screening method has high specificity, sensitivity, and **predictive value**. Screening whole populations, or selected populations, of very young children for ASDs is important because of evidence suggesting that early intervention is more effective than later intervention. The Modified Checklist for Autism in Toddlers (M-CHAT), developed from the earlier CHAT procedure, rates reasonably well on the three criteria. Several other procedures for screening very young children have been published and evaluated, with varying degrees of success. Similarly, there are numerous checklists, rating scales and observation schedules being developed to screen for ASDs in older children and adults, with variable success. In sum, no 'gold standard' for screening either very young children or older children and adults has yet emerged. The most reliable methods are those now used for screening but originally developed over many years as diagnostic procedures, for example the Autism Behaviour Checklist (ABC) and the Childhood Autism Rating Scale (CARS). Several methods of screening for Asperger syndrome have been reported with, again, only limited success.

The development, evaluation, modification and re-evaluation of many diagnostic and screening tests are actively proceeding, and there is no doubt that further improvements will be made.

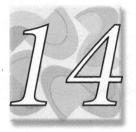

INTERVENTION

AIMS
••••
INTRODUCTION
••••
PRELIMINARY QUESTIONS
Why Intervene? The Goals of Interventions
Interventions for Whom, for What, and When?
••••
INTERVENTION METHODS
Preventing or Curing Autism
Changing Behaviour: Physical Interventions
Changing Behaviour: Non-physical Interventions
••••
EVALUATING INTERVENTIONS
Efficacy Studies: Why and How
Efficacy Studies of Physical Interventions for ASDs
Efficacy Studies of Non-physical Interventions
••••
SUMMARY

AIMS

The dual aims of this chapter are, first, to provide information about a representative sample of currently available interventions, broadly interpreted to include possibilities for prevention and cure as well as interventions designed to promote development and learning or to reduce unwanted behaviours; and, secondly, to establish a framework for thinking critically about interventions.

INTRODUCTION

There is currently no way of preventing or curing ASDs; nor is there any known medical, **psychosocial** or educational intervention that dramatically improves interaction and behavioural flexibility in all or even in most individuals across the spectrum. Nor is there any known intervention that invariably helps to control or alleviate any of the additional problems such as hyperactivity or sleep disturbance so often associated with autism. Nevertheless, there is a host of interventions on offer, and many of these help some individuals to a greater or lesser extent and in certain ways, for reasons that are not always well understood. For parents the choice must be bewildering. For practitioners prescribing medications or advising on other kinds of interventions, balancing the pros and cons of available treatments given the current uncertainties must also be daunting.

It is not possible here to cover the full range of available interventions meaningfully. This chapter aims instead to provide information about a representative sample of intervention methods that may have positive outcomes for people with ASDs. These summaries relate to the question of how to intervene. Before considering *how* to intervene, however, preliminary questions concerning *why* intervene, *for whom*, *for what*, and *when* will be considered.

PRELIMINARY QUESTIONS

Why Intervene? The Goals of Interventions

It is important to consider what the goals of interventions for people with ASDs might be, other than the common goal of having 'positive outcomes'. This common goal begs two important questions: 'What is a positive outcome?' and 'Positive for whom?' and answers to these questions vary according to whether an intervention aims to prevent or cure autism or bring about changes in behaviours (and possibly underlying brain structure and function) associated with autism.

Positive outcomes for whom? Prevention and cure

The aims of prevention and cure are to eliminate autistic spectrum disorders or at least to reduce their incidence. Prevention is designed to ensure that people with ASDs are not conceived; or, if conceived, not born; or, if conceived and born without incipient autism, then not exposed to whatever environmental factors might trigger autism. Cure is designed to ensure that the behaviours associated with autism are eliminated or reduced to 'normal' levels in people who have been diagnosed with an ASD, with associated changes of brain structure and/or function.

Preventing or curing autism might be assumed to be desirable from the point of view of individuals, even the unborn whose predictable suffering, it might be argued, can be prevented. It might also be assumed to be desirable for families who would be spared the sacrifices, stresses and strains associated with living with and caring for a person with an ASD. It might well be considered desirable for society in general, given the financial costs associated with providing for the health, educational, social and care needs of people with ASDs, especially the less able. Prevention or cure might, in sum, be judged to have positive outcomes for individuals, families, and society in general.

However, it would be wrong to assume that all people with ASDs would have preferred not to have existed or want to be 'cured', that is to say, changed; it would be wrong to assume that all families and other close carers experience living with and caring for a person with an ASD as a predominantly negative experience; and it would be wrong to assume that people with ASDs do not make contributions to society. It should not be assumed, therefore, that ridding the world of people with ASDs is the ultimate goal. At the same time the real suffering of many people with ASDs, the strains on families and other carers, and the needs of society must be recognised.

Positive outcomes for whom? Changing behaviour

The major aim of most interventions is to facilitate development and to increase an individual's competencies and control over their own lives. Interventions that aim to promote development often focus on those areas of behaviour in which people with ASDs are by definition less than averagely competent, and it is generally assumed that the goal of intervention is to normalise the individual's behaviour in these areas. It may be the case that being like the majority, being 'normal', is inherently desirable from all points of view. However, as is increasingly argued by the large and varied population of people with disabilities, including many articulate people with ASDs, being 'different' can have its own advantages and does not necessarily imply a need to be made less different (Mottron et al., 2008). It might also be argued that, especially for individuals with severe and multiple difficulties, enhancing quality of life (aiming for happiness) rather than straining towards unattainable goals of normality should be the pre-eminent aim of intervention (Florian, Dee, Byers, & Maudslay, 2000).

The major aim of some interventions is to eliminate or reduce behaviours that are patently distressing or disadvantageous to the individual with an ASD; and/or those that are particularly distressing or difficult for parents or carers to cope with; and/or those that place especially heavy burdens on society or may rank as antisocial or criminal. These aims might seem to be unquestionably desirable. Moreover, eliminating or reducing negative behaviours may free an individual to develop in more desirable ways, which must also be a positive good. So, for example, reducing hyperactivity may increase a child's ability to benefit from education.

Nevertheless, judgements as to what constitutes 'negative behaviour' are not always straightforward: an obsession with firearms might lead to antisocial behaviour, but might equally well provide a focus of interest and harmless activities (reading; visits to museums); temper tantrums in a non-verbal individual may be an effective communication signal. Moreover, judgements as to what constitutes a positive outcome are complicated by the fact that desirable outcomes for individuals, parents, and society do not always coincide. For example, medicating an adult with challenging behaviours may reduce demands on day-time State care but conflict with the wishes of relatives who manage the behaviours well at home.

In sum, answers to the questions 'What ranks as a positive outcome?' and 'For whom?' vary depending on a number of circumstances.

Interventions for Whom, for What, and When?

Intervention needs are never the same for any two individuals: as stressed in Chapter 3, people with ASDs are more different from each other than they are alike. Each individual's needs also vary according to the different contexts in which they are brought up and live their lives. There is, therefore, no prescription 'This is what you do for a person with an ASD': the first question is always 'For which person, in which family?' (or other context).

The immediate aims and targets of interventions (as opposed to the overall goals discussed in the previous section) are also enormously varied, reflecting the range of developmental problems and learning difficulties that people with ASDs may present, and the different intact abilities that may be built on, as described in Chapters 1–3. Especially in the case of individuals with multiple difficulties, not all their developmental needs and problem behaviours can be targeted at once, and decisions as to what aspects of behaviour and development should be targeted at any one time will have to take many factors into account. Having considered 'For whom?', therefore, the next question is 'For what?'

Age may help to decide 'For what?', because the priority needs of a two-year-old with an ASD clearly differ from those of an older child or adult. Age may also determine the appropriateness of a particular intervention. For example, play therapy using teddy bears and toy teacups is appropriate for preschool children, but not for teenagers; a particular medication may be tolerated by an adult but not by a child. In addition, there is a widespread view that early intervention targeting core problems may be more effective than later intervention (Howlin, 2003; Corsello, 2005). Having considered 'For whom?' and 'For what?', therefore, decisions about interventions must also take into account 'when' a particular intervention may be most useful and appropriate.

INTERVENTION METHODS

Preventing or Curing Autism

Regarding possibilities for preventing autism, genetic counselling can provide couples who are considering having a child, but who already have a child with an ASD or whose families include individuals with ASDs, with information about the statistical chances that they might conceive a child who develops an ASD. As more becomes known about the genes that constitute susceptibility factors for autism, DNA testing of parents will enable genetic counselling to be increasingly accurate and specific as to the probabilities. Genetic testing of unborn children offers a theoretical possibility for prevention. However, the detection of what are no more than susceptibility factors in the genes of an unborn child would be a questionable justification for preventing the birth by means of abortion.

Regarding possibilities for curing autism, gene therapy is foreseeable at least in theory. However, given the complexity of the genetic factors that may contribute to autism and the unknown environmental factors that influence the processes of brain-building and brain function set in motion by the genes, gene therapy effecting a complete cure is probably only a remote possibility. Equally, the complexity and variability of the neurobiological bases of autism suggest that completely curing all cases of autism by altering patterns of brain chemistry, growth and function is also only a remote possibility (but see Hu-Lince et al., 2005, for a more optimistic view).

Given that possibilities for the prevention or cure of ASDs are limited, at least for the foreseeable future, ways of changing behaviour 'for the better' become of pre-eminent importance. In the next two subsections, examples of physical treatments, and then examples of psychosocial and educational interventions, will be summarised and discussed. The coverage does not attempt to be exhaustive (fuller coverage can be found in Jordan, Jones, & Murray, 1998; and in the special issue of the *Journal of Autism and Developmental Disorders*, 2000, volume 30(5)).

Changing Behaviour: Physical Interventions

'Behaviours associated with autism' is used here to include the set of behaviours diagnostic of ASDs in their various forms, and also behaviours that are not specific to people with ASDs but that are commonly present, such as hyperactivity, self-injurious behaviours, and sleep disturbances. This section will not cover physical interventions for co-morbid or associated conditions such as immune system disorders or gastrointestinal problems, unless the treatment being discussed derives from a theory implicating such disorders as causes of autism itself.

Physical interventions for autism are those that seek to change the biological processes underlying the behaviours associated with autism. They may seek to do this by acting on biological processes directly, as in the case of medications, dietary supplements or brain stimulation. Alternatively, physical interventions may seek to change biological processes indirectly by, for example, exercise regimes or exposing the individual to specific sensory inputs.

Some physical treatments fall within the remit of conventional medicine. However, many physical treatments fall within the group of **complementary and alternative medicines (CAMs)**, defined as:

> A broad domain of healing resources that encompasses all health systems, modalities, and practices and their accompanying theories and beliefs, other than those intrinsic to the politically dominant health system of a particular society or culture in a given historic period. (Office of the Alternative Medicine Committee in Definition and Description, 1997)

There is no clear boundary between conventional and less conventional forms of physical interventions for autism. Many 'alternative' remedies in the autism field are developed and advocated by doctors or therapists working within the conventional medical system, although others are offered by practitioners working outside the conventional system, for example homeopaths. Some alternative remedies are advocated by parents and parent groups arguing from personal knowledge and experience.

However, CAMs are often excluded from treatments on offer in conventional medicine because they have not been proven to be safe and effective in the kind of well-controlled efficacy studies described later in the chapter. A complementary or alternative treatment that was exposed to testing and shown to be safe and effective would without doubt be quickly accepted into the armoury of conventional medical treatments. **Secretin** offers a good example (see Box 14.1, in the next main section). Following wide publicity in the CAMs literature, secretin was rigorously tested using conventional methods. Had it been shown to be effective, government watchdogs such as the Food and Drug Administration in the States and the National Institute for Clinical Excellence in England and Wales would undoubtedly have licensed it for general use.

In what follows, therefore, the dividing line used to discriminate conventional from complementary or alternative medicines is a pragmatic one based on how well a particular treatment has been tested (including ongoing, properly conducted testing). This dividing line recognises that what is today described as alternative might become tomorrow's conventional treatment of choice.

Conventional physical interventions

A summary of medications that have been used and reasonably well tested within the framework of conventional medicine is given in Table 14.1.

Table 14.1 Some conventional medical interventions

Biological systems targeted and mode of action	Type and generic name of medication	Behaviours for which treatment may be effective		Possible side-effects	Status
		Diagnostic behaviours	Associated behaviours		
Brain neurochemistry: Dopamine blocking agents	Atypical antipsychotics (AAPs): Risperidone Olanzapine	Repetitive behaviours especially stereotypies	Irritability, aggression, hyperactivity, self-injurious behaviours (SIBs)	Transient sedation, drowsiness; increased appetite, weight gain, drooling, and other	Risperidone is reasonably well authenticated (e.g., Chavez and Chavez-Brown, 2006). Olanzapine is less well authenticated but see Stachnik and Nunn-Thompson (2007)
Brain neurochemistry: Selective serotonin reuptake inhibitors (SSRIs)	Antidepressants: Fluvoxamine (adults)	Repetitive behaviours including repetitive language and motor stereotypies	Anxiety? Aggression?	Suicidal tendencies?	Not well authenticated at present, and carry significant risks (see reviews by Lewis & Lazoritz, 2005; Scahill & Martin, 2005)
	Fluoxetine (Prozac) (older children?)	As above, plus ?improved social interaction and language		Increased behavioural activity and irritability	
Brain neurochemistry: Increase production of dopamine	Stimulants: Methylphenidate (e.g., Ritalin)		Hyperactivity, inattention, impulsivity i.e., co-morbid ADHD	Irritability, weight loss and increased stereotypies	Disagreements in the literature concerning uses (see Lewis & Lazoritz, 2005; Scahill & Martin, 2005)

(Cont'd)

Table 14.1

Biological systems targeted and mode of action	Type and generic name of medication	Behaviours for which treatment may be effective		Possible side-effects	Status
		Diagnostic behaviours	Associated behaviours		
Brain neurochemistry: Opioid antagonist	Naltrexone	Social withdrawal? Stereotypies?	Self-injurious behaviours; hyperactivity?, agitation?, tantrums?	Drowsiness, decreased appetite, aggression	Only reliably useful for treatment of self-injurious behaviours (ElChaar et al., 2006)
Brain neurochemistry: Oxytocin peptide system	Oxytocin (infusion)	Repetitive behaviour		Unknown	One well-controlled study of adults (Hollander et al., 2003)
Brain chemistry: Promote neural inhibitory processes in various ways	Mood stabilisers Anticonvulsants Lithium		Epilepsy; may also alleviate aggression, mood lability	Cognitive slowing	Variable responses across individuals. No well-controlled studies (?)

Numerous reviews of pharmacological (drug) treatments are available (e.g., Scahill & Martin, 2005; Steingard, Connor, & Au, 2005; Broadstock, Doughty, & Eggleston, 2007; Moussavand & Findling, 2007). However, this is a fast-moving field and current reviews will soon be superseded. Interested readers should therefore search for updates.

Occupational therapists working within conventional medicine sometimes offer a form of treatment known as Sensory Integration Therapy that aims to change biological processes indirectly (as opposed to the direct effects of medications). The rationale underlying Sensory Integration Therapy is that neural organisation within the central nervous system can be strengthened by exposing the individual to various sensory inputs including touch and proprioceptive stimulation, in combination with appropriate motor outputs. Despite its quite widespread usage within the conventional medicine system, Sensory Integration Therapy has not, in fact, been rigorously tested. In his review of treatments, Francis (2005) describes it as 'plausible but unproven'.

Complementary and alternative physical interventions

Table 14.2 shows a sample of direct physical interventions falling in the CAMs category, using a similar set of headings as in Table 14.1 to facilitate comparison of the two groups of conventional and less conventional interventions.

Some indirect physical interventions fall in to the CAMs category. These include Auditory Integration Training (AIT) (briefly described in Levy & Hyman, 2005), which aims to retrain listening mechanisms in the ear; the Doman Delacato method, which uses sensory stimulation in all modalities combined with passive exercises designed to establish neural patterning in a damaged or immature brain (a rationale similar to that underlying Sensory Integration Training). The Doman Delacato method was developed for use with children with head injuries but is sometimes used as an intervention for autism. Dawson and Watling (2000) review the evidence for this type of intervention. Flexyx therapy, which uses electrical currents to stimulate neural activity, was also initially developed for use with individuals with brain injuries but is now occasionally used as an intervention for autism.

Changing Behaviour: Non-physical Interventions

Non-physical interventions, including psychosocial treatments and education methods, most often develop from the experience of 'what works' in increasing a particular competence or for reducing and replacing a particular form of unwanted behaviour. Thus, non-physical interventions have generally been developed 'bottom-up'. In this, they differ from physical interventions which are most often developed 'top-down' from theories of the causes of autism. Non-physical interventions are therefore most readily grouped according to the behaviours they are intended to effect, rather than in terms of underlying causal theory. This is the

Table 14.2 Some interventions within the group of complementary and alternative medicines

Biological system targeted; mode of action	Type of intervention	Behaviours and physical disorders for which the intervention may be effective			Possible side-effects	Status
		Diagnostic behaviours	Associated behaviours	Physical problems		
Various neurotransmitters and neuropeptides; various modes of action	*Dietary supplements:* Vitamin B6 (+magnesium)	Eye contact Speech/language	Hyperactivity, sleep problems, irritability, inattention		Peripheral neuropathy (tingling fingers, toes) if taken in excess	Widely used, but not well authenticated (Nye & Brice, 2002; Levy & Hyman, 2005)
	Dimethylglycine (DMG)	Social behaviour Speech	Inattention		None known (but see Baker, 2001)	
	Omega-3 fatty acids		Challenging behaviours		As above	Anecdotal reports
Immune system abnormalities < allergic reactions associated with abnormal neuropeptide metabolism	*Dietary restrictions:* Commonly omitted foods include cows' milk, wheat, sugar, citrus fruits and food additives		Generalised behaviour problems	Sweating, excessive thirst, red face, circles under eyes	(Care needed to ensure against overly narrow diet in already 'faddy' individuals)	Difficult to authenticate because different individuals may have different allergies
Immune system abnormalities < exposure to toxic metals, e.g., mercury, lead	*Chelation:* Chemical detoxification, e.g., dimercaptosuccinic acid (DMSA)	Diagnostic behaviours are targetted			Kidney and liver function must be monitored	Not authenticated

Table 14.2

Biological system targeted; mode of action	Type of intervention	Behaviours and physical disorders for which the intervention may be effective			Possible side-effects	Status
		Diagnostic behaviours	Associated behaviours	Physical problems		
Digestive system: malabsorption of ingested proteins ('leaky gut') > excess gut-brain opioids	Dietary restriction: Gluten-free/casein-free diet	Sociability	Challenging behaviours, SIBs		Care needed to ensure nutritionally adequate diet. Marked adverse effects on coming off the diet	Widely used; not well authenticated, but may well be useful (Francis, 2005)
Digestive system: excess yeast (candida) > effects on immune system and/or brain	Various: Yeast-free diet, antifungal agents, probiotics		Behaviour problems	Health problems, e.g., oral or vaginal thrush	Possible adverse effects of antifungal agents used long term	Very little evidence for or against

method of grouping interventions used in Table 14.3: behaviours listed in the left-hand column of the table are taken directly from the groupings that were used in characterising diagnostic, universal or common behavioural characteristics of people with ASDs in Part I of this book, and used again in the 'What has to be explained' headings in Chapters 8, 9, and 10 in Part II.

Psychosocial and educational interventions may also be grouped according to the life stage at which intervention is most needed or at which a particular intervention may be appropriate, as indicated in columns 2, 3 and 4 of Table 14.3.

In addition to 'behavioural change targeted' and 'life stage appropriateness', other contrasts exist between the various psychosocial and educational interventions available that may be relevant for understanding why particular forms of intervention are effective. These contrasts are indicated within the table, and include the following.

1 The broad approach used. Many interventions for people with ASDs use a *high level of structure*, reducing uncertainties and choices for the individual taking part. Interventions using a structured approach, including those based on behaviourist principles, resemble each other in that they are largely *adult-led,* in the sense that the content of the intervention is determined by the person carrying out the intervention, even where the aim of the intervention is to give an individual greater independence and autonomy. At the other end of the scale are interventions that are relatively *unstructured* and *child-led*.
2 A particular *medium* of intervention may be used to address many different targets, for example, learning through play or computer-based 'e-learning'. At the other end of the scale are highly specific forms of intervention that are narrowly targeted, for example, psychotherapy or sign-language instruction.
3 Interventions also vary according to where and by whom the intervention is carried out. They may be home-based, school-based, clinic-based, workplace-based or combinations of all or some of these, and carried out by parents and carers, siblings, peers, teachers, clinicians of various professions, therapists in the alternative medicine field, paid assistants, residential careworkers and many more. Interventions also vary according to whether the intervention is self-delivered or delivered one-to-one, or in formal or informal groups.

Table 14.3, unlike the two previous tables, does not include comments concerning how well authenticated the various treatments are. This is because so few of the interventions listed are well authenticated that the negative comments would be repetitive. The evaluation of interventions for ASDs is considered next.

EVALUATING INTERVENTIONS

Efficacy Studies: Why and How

Why are evaluative studies needed?

If a pharmaceutical company has developed a new treatment for, say, rheumatoid arthritis, that treatment will be tried out in efficacy studies involving

Table 14.3 Some psychosocial and educational programmes and methods

Behaviour targeted	Early childhood	Later childhood	Adulthood
Socio-emotional-communicative development	**Interactive approaches** *Parent-skilling*, e.g., Portage, Hanen, EarlyBird *Home-based; intensive; paid assistants:* Son-Rise (aka Option method) *Clinic-based; therapist and parent(s); individual/group:* Music interaction therapy, play therapies (various) *Playschool-based:* Interactive Curriculum, Playschool Curriculum **Behaviourist approaches** *Home-based; intensive; paid assistants:* Lovaas (aka Applied Behaviour Analysis – ABA); Early Intensive Behavioural Intervention (EIBI)	Several of the early childhood interventions are continued into, or started during, later childhood, including Son-Rise/Option, music interaction and various play therapies. Also ABA and EIBI **Other interventions** *Variously school, clinic, home-based; individual or group:* Music therapy; social skills training, e.g., Social Stories *Self-delivered:* Computer-based programmes	Depending on developmental level, the following may be used **Interactive** *Support-group or residence-based:* social skills training **Behaviourist/high structure** *Self-delivered:* Computer-based programmes, for e.g., emotion recognition *Residence or workplace-based:* Individualised behavioural programmes
Communication system acquisition		*Speech/language therapy + school + home, promoting:* Spoken language and/or Picture Exchange Communication System (PECS); Sign systems (e.g., Makaton; British/American Sign Language (BSL/ASL)); *Self-delivered:* Multimedia	For those with impaired language, any of the interventions in the cell to the left of this one

(Cont'd)

Table 14.3

Behaviour targeted	Early childhood	Later childhood	Adulthood
Creativity enhancement	**Interactive** *Home/clinic/playschool-based:* Play therapies; playschool curriculum programmes	*School-based, promoting creativity;* Art, drama, creative writing	Depending on developmental level: *Support group or residence-based:* Programmes to extend behavioural range; creative activities as in the cell to the left
Repetitive behaviour reduction and replacement	**Behaviourist/high structure** ABA or EIBA (as above) TEACCH approach	**Behaviourist** *School/clinic and home-based:* Behaviour modification programmes	**Behaviourist** *Residence or workplace-based:* Behaviour modification programmes
Mental health problems		*Clinic-based:* Psychotherapeutic play therapy; family therapy	*Clinic-based:* Counselling; psychotherapy; cognitive behavioural therapy (CBT)
Education for self-help/daily living, academic and vocational skills	**Behaviourist/high structure** ABA or EIBA (as above) TEACCH approach	**High structure** TEACCH approach Daily Life Therapy (Higashi) **Individual-led** Rudolph Steiner approach	**Non-specialised** College/university **Specialised/high structure** *College/residential-based:* Learning support programmes

hundreds of patients and large control or comparison groups. These studies will – or should – be carried out by researchers with no vested interest in study outcomes such as might introduce bias into the methods used or the interpretation or reporting of findings. The methods and results of these studies will be examined in depth by experts in the field, and the new treatment will be licensed for use only if the studies are judged to have been well-designed and carried out and to have produced reliable evidence that the new treatment is effective, safe, and cost-effective. In addition, patients treated with the drug will be monitored over several years to assess the long-term benefits and safety.

Unfortunately, this ideal has rarely if ever been realised in evaluations of interventions for people with ASDs, and there are instances when an intervention has been extensively used before there is any reliable evidence that it is either effective or safe. The media have much to answer for here, in that stories about 'miracle cures' help to sell newspapers and attract viewers for television programmes. Two rather different examples of 'miracle cures' that were highly publicised for a time, but subsequently shown to be largely ineffective, are described in Box 14.1.

BOX 14.1   Two 'cures' that failed to deliver

Secretin is a hormone produced in the small intestine that belongs to a group of biochemical substances also active in the brain. It has the potential, therefore, to provide a link between the gastrointestinal problems that have been hypothetically associated with autism and brain malfunctions associated with autism. In 1998 Horvath, Cataldo, Wachtel, Spurrier, Papadimitriou, and Tildon reported dramatic improvements in language and eye contact in three children with ASDs given intravenous injections of secretin as part of investigations of their gut problems. The findings were widely publicised in the media, and thousands of children with autism were expensively treated with secretin before there was any reliable evidence concerning its efficacy and safety. There was great excitement, also, amongst doctors responsible for treating people with ASDs, and several carefully designed efficacy studies were undertaken following publication of Horvath et al.'s paper. Disappointingly, these studies produced almost entirely negative results and it is now widely concluded that, as a treatment for autism, secretin is ineffective (e.g., Scahill & Martin, 2005; Levy & Hyman, 2005).

Holding therapy derived from the theory that autism results from disordered attachment relationships (Welch, 1984). It was believed that the child's defences against social contact could be broken down by forcing them into close physical contact with the mother (or other close carer) who was instructed to hold the child against their will until their struggle and rage subsided. At this point it was claimed

(Cont'd)

that the child became still, made eye contact, and accepted comfort from the mother, facilitating the bonding process. During therapy young children were held on the mother's lap, facing them; older children might be held on the floor with the mother lying on top of them. During the first phase of holding, whilst the child struggled, screamed and hit out, the mother was encouraged by the therapist to express her feelings about the child, whether of grief, anger, guilt or remorse.

No reliable evidence was ever presented concerning the efficacy of holding therapy for children with ASDs. The underlying theory was inconsistent with evidence that autism is biologically, not psychogenically, based. The ethics of the methods were questionable. When asked whether she considered that the claimed improvements resulted from holding the child or from the therapeutic effects of encouraging mothers to express their feelings about their child, one therapist replied emphatically that it was the latter (so holding the child was, presumably, incidental). Unfortunately, Welch's work was published in a book entitled *New Hope for a Cure*, and the therapy made for popular voyeuristic television.*

*It is essential to distinguish between methods of working with children with ASDs that, like holding therapy, coerce the child into physical contact as opposed to those that establish contact through activities the withdrawn child can tolerate and may enjoy, such as holding on the lap facing away, rocking and singing; gentle massage; rough and tumble play and tickling.

Many parents spent large sums of money to obtain secretin treatment for their children, and many children were subjected to holding therapy before it was generally discontinued. The two end columns of Table 14.1 show how often physical treatments that are largely ineffective have undesirable and sometimes dangerous side-effects, as revealed in well-controlled efficacy studies. Given that none of the CAMs interventions listed in Table 14.2 has been subjected to evaluation to the same standard, it is hardly surprising that many conventional practitioners express alarm as to the safety of many CAMs interventions (Baker, 2001), and at best retain an open mind as to their effectiveness (see the reviews cited in Table 14.2). Regarding non-physical intervention methods, although none of the interventions listed in Table 14.3 uses methods that might be unethical or harmful, some of them are costly not only financially but also in terms of commitment of time, effort and disruption of family life, even though the efficacy of these interventions remains controversial.

How should efficacy studies be carried out? Designs and methods

For all these reasons, it is important to understand the designs and methods that must be used if parents and practitioners are to be provided with reliable information about the efficacy, safety and cost-effectiveness of interventions for people with ASDs. Some principles of design and methodology in efficacy studies of conventional medical treatments are summarised in Box 14.2.

BOX 14.2   Designs and methods used in efficacy studies in general

Open or open label studies monitor the progress made by participants who are having a particular form of treatment. The participants (and/or their families or carers) know that they are having the treatment and they know the effects the treatment should have if successful.

Crossover designs as used to evaluate the effectiveness of physical interventions consist of a period when participants are on treatment and a period during which they receive a placebo. Behaviour at the beginning and end of each period is compared to assess behavioural change, and the behavioural change on-treatment and on-placebo is compared to test the prediction that more improvement will be seen over the treatment period than the placebo period. Half the group will start with a treatment phase, and half on placebo, and allocation to these subgroups should be randomised using an approved procedure. If neither the actively involved researchers nor the participants and their families know which individual is in which subgroup, this is a double blind trial. If the researchers know about subgroup membership but the participants and their families do not, this is a single blind trial.

Crossover designs used for the evaluation of non-physical interventions compare progress during periods of treatment with progress during periods of no-treatment (but this makes blind trials impossible) or alternative treatment (in which case, blind trials are possible but difficult to ensure).

Parallel designs are commonly used in the evaluation of both physical and non-physical interventions. In this type of design the progress of two groups of participants is compared, one of which receives the intervention that is being evaluated whilst the control or comparison group either receives a placebo (in studies of physical interventions; no treatment in studies of non-physical interventions) or a contrasting intervention. In either case, allocation to groups should be randomised. This type of design is referred to as a randomised control trial (RCT). Double blind trials should be used when evaluating physical interventions, but are less easy to achieve in studies evaluating non-physical interventions (as above).

The **open** or **open label design** constitutes an appropriate starting point for evaluating an intervention, in that it can produce suggestive evidence such as might be needed before embarking on a large-scale controlled study. However, open label studies cannot prove that any positive effects result from the intervention as opposed to **non-specific factors**. **Cross-over designs** can produce clearly interpretable and reliable findings when used to evaluate physical treatment methods, but are less satisfactory for the evaluation of non-physical interventions, because there is no exact equivalent to a placebo. **Parallel designs** may therefore be preferred in efficacy studies of non-physical interventions for people with ASDs, although using no-treatment control groups is ethically questionable.

More detailed points of method with particular relevance for efficacy studies of interventions for autism are outlined in Box 14.3. Fuller accounts of issues relating to design and methodology in the evaluation of interventions for autism can be found in Hollander et al. (2004) and in Smith et al. (2007).

BOX 14.3   Points of method in efficacy studies of interventions for autism

Participant groups should be:

- large enough to have statistical power;
- fully representative of the group targeted by the treatment, avoiding sampling bias;
- reasonably homogeneous in terms of diagnosis, sex, age, and ability; and, in the case of studies using parallel designs, groups should be matched on factors that might influence outcomes.

Interventions should be:

- delivered in the same way to all participants, for example in terms of drug dosage or in terms of the precise methods used in non-physical interventions (this is particularly important when several different people are involved in delivering a psychosocial or educational intervention, perhaps across several different schools or research centres: training may be required);
- delivered by more than one teacher/therapist working with different individuals (in non-physical interventions); and, in studies using a parallel design, the commitment of those delivering the intervention under study should be no greater than commitment to the comparison intervention.

Measures used to assess behaviour before and after intervention should:

- relate clearly to the behaviours targeted;
- be clearly defined and operationalised, so that different assessors all work to the same standard.

Assessors (those evaluating behaviour before and after treatment) should:

- not be involved in delivering the intervention;
- be trained in rating behaviour on the outcome measures and in the coding system used to enter ratings into a database; and assessor reliability should be systematically checked by having more than one assessor rating a proportion of the assessment sessions.

Efficacy Studies of Physical Interventions for ASDs

Conventional physical interventions

As can be seen from the two end columns of Table 14.1, quite a lot is known about the efficacy and safety of some of the drug treatments offered within conventional medicine. The information in these two columns comes from efficacy studies using, in the main, the designs and methods approved within the broader field of conventional medicine as outlined in Boxes 14.2 and 14.3. More studies are needed. However, the studies that have been carried out on the medications listed demonstrate that some drugs may be helpful for some individuals in modifying some behaviours; but none of the drugs that have been tested are helpful for all individuals in modifying core behaviours; and that all drugs have side effects, though not necessarily to the extent that use of that particular medication is contraindicated. At the time of writing, Risperidone is the only medication that has been reasonably well evaluated and shown to have some benefits outweighing any currently known side-effects (see Buitelaar, 2003, for discussion of why the search for drug treatments for ASDs has proved so difficult).

What is not apparent from Table 14.1 is that many other medications have been, and are being, tried out for use with people with ASDs. Some, such as the antipsychotic drug Halperidol, were quite widely used in the past until it was appreciated that their side-effects outweighed their benefits. Others are novel, and not well evaluated. Most reports of preliminary studies of novel medications stress the need for careful monitoring of those taking part, cautioning against use of the medication until more is known concerning efficacy and safety.

Complementary and alternative physical interventions

None of the CAMs intervention methods has been well evaluated (see the end column of Table 14.2). This is true by definition because, if any of these interventions had been rigorously evaluated and found to be safe and effective, they would be available as treatments within conventional medicine. Where an alternative or complementary treatment is (probably) harmless and low cost, lack of proven effectiveness is of no great importance, and there may be benefits for the particular individual being given the treatment. Where a CAMs treatment is either expensive or less certainly harmless, however, then the lack of proven effectiveness is of considerable importance. This suggests that parents should weigh up safety (first and foremost) and efficacy (second) against cost (last but not unimportantly) when considering any alternative or complementary therapy for their child, just as the official government bodies do for medicines that are licensed for use in the conventional field.

Efficacy Studies of Non-physical Interventions

Lack of reliable evidence concerning the efficacy and cost-effectiveness of the interventions listed in Table 14.3 (where safety is less of an issue) results mainly from the difficulties involved in evaluating these kinds of interventions. Some problems of design were mentioned in Box 14.2. Some problems relating to methodology are outlined next, relating to points listed in Box 14.3, followed by a section on problems of interpretation. After this is a summary of 'What works'.

Problems of method

It is difficult to recruit large, homogeneous groups of people with ASDs (often children with the co-operation of their families) willing to take part in the kinds of time-consuming studies that are needed. Collaboration across several research centres can mitigate this problem; multi-centre studies also have the advantage that sufficient numbers of people are working on the study to ensure that several individuals, rather than just one, are involved in delivering the intervention; also that assessment is carried out by individuals other than those delivering the intervention. Multi-centre collaborations do, however, exacerbate problems to do with standardising the methods used in delivering the intervention being studied (and any comparison intervention), and standardising assessment measures and coding criteria.

Because of the difficulties, and also the cost, of carrying out large-scale studies, small-scale efficacy studies predominate in this field. These have all the reverse advantages and disadvantages of large-scale studies. However, whereas the methodological problems that arise in large-scale studies can all be overcome with time and care, the problems inherent in small-scale studies are much harder to overcome.

In particular, many small-scale efficacy studies of non-physical interventions for autism are carried out by individuals strongly committed to the intervention being assessed. Lack of additional personnel to work on the study may mean that those delivering the intervention may also be involved in carrying out the before and after assessments, and possibly also in the data analysis and interpretation of the findings. Sometimes parents are asked to act as the before and after treatment assessors. However, they too, having agreed to participate in a study, may be committed to the intervention being investigated, and certainly hopeful of a positive outcome. The possibilities for unconscious bias can weaken small-scale studies irrevocably.

Problems of interpretation

The interpretation of findings from efficacy studies of non-physical interventions also present particular difficulties (Lord et al., 2005). Most of these are to do with the identification of the factors that are driving improvements in behaviour during treatment, if these occur. Key questions of interpretation are: did the improvement result from specific aspects of the intervention itself or from non-specific factors? And if the improvement resulted from specific aspects of the intervention itself, which aspects were most critical?

Many non-specific factors may be operating in the case of non-physical interventions for autism. For example, the personality and skill of the teacher or therapist delivering an intervention may be critical. Naturally gifted therapists, teachers and also parents often develop their own particular methods of working with individuals with ASDs, ways that are successful when they are the person carrying out the intervention, but not otherwise, because their own personality is the key factor. The one-to-one interaction involved in many psychosocial and educational interventions may itself be beneficial, regardless of the activities occurring within the one-to-one relationship. The time spent may be important: so intensive interventions may be effective *because* they are intensive, rather than because they involve particular activities or methods of intervention. For parents hopeful of successful outcomes for their child, small changes or improvements in behaviour may be greeted very positively, inflating the actual gains that have been made (see Levy & Hyman, 2005 for an account of striking **placebo** effects in some of the secretin trials). Simply knowing that their child is the focus of a treatment study may relieve parental anxieties with indirect positive effects for the child. For adults, the additional attention they are receiving as a participant in a research study may have positive effects, regardless of the intervention being studied (the so-called **Hawthorne effect**). Hawthorne effects and placebo effects are not, of course, unique to efficacy studies of interventions for ASDs: they are extremely common in efficacy studies in general.

Non-specific effects can be controlled to a considerable extent by tight design and methodology of the kinds itemised in Boxes 14.2 and 14.3, although this has rarely been done in studies of non-physical interventions for autism. Even when non-specific effects can be ruled out, however, there remains the difficulty of identifying which specific aspects of an intervention were driving the improvement: was it the high level of reward built into the interaction? – or the structured setting? – or the repetition used? – or the low demand for social interaction? Sometimes the factors driving improvement are not the explicit focus of an intervention. For example, if group play therapy sessions for recently diagnosed preschool children are also designed to provide an opportunity for parents to talk together over a cup of coffee, positive outcomes may owe as much to the therapeutic gains for parents (with positive effects for the children) as to the play therapy for the children. The release of feelings by mothers during holding therapy (described in Box 14.1) is another example where the explicit focus of the intervention was possibly neither useful nor ethical, whereas the secondary focus may have had some useful effects.

Because of the difficulties of design, method and interpretation associated with evaluative studies of non-physical interventions, and the resulting lack of reliable evidence, it is not possible to describe any of the psychosocial and educational methods listed in Table 14.3 as well authenticated (see Papps & Dyson, 2004; Howlin, 2005; Humphrey & Parkinson, 2006, for critiques of the evaluative research). This does not mean that the interventions are not effective, at least for certain individuals, in certain contexts, to achieve certain outcomes, at certain stages of development. The problem is to discriminate between the different interventions, and to understand why so many of them have at least some claim to success, despite their many differences.

So what works?

Interventions for young children   Strong claims have been made for the superior efficacy of early intervention based on a behaviourist model, as exemplified in the closely related Lovaas Method, Applied Behavioural Analysis (ABA), and Early Intensive Behavioural Intervention (EIBI). Early claims for a 'cure' for '47 per cent' of young children treated with these methods have not been substantiated (Howlin, 2003, 2005; Papps & Dyson, 2004; Shea, 2004). However, there is a consensus that these methods do produce some long-term gains, especially for children who are treated in the preschool years. For example, concerning EIBI, Francis (2005) concludes:

> [EIBI] clearly benefits children with autism and yields a high degree of parental satisfaction; however, the original effectiveness claim was overstated and its cost-effectiveness in terms of time, effort and money has not been adequately assessed. (Francis, 2005: 498)

However, it has not been proved that intensive behavioural intervention produces more favourable outcomes, either in the short or longer term, than, for example, attendance at a good specialist nursery school (Magiati, Charman, & Howlin, 2007). It is an open possibility, therefore, that the success of behavioural programmes such as Early Intensive Behavioural Intervention is at least partly due to non-specific factors. These might include any or all of the following.

The *intensive nature* of programmes such as Early Intensive Behavioural Intervention may be important. This non-specific factor is present in many of the other interventions offered for young children with ASDs, and for which there is at least anecdotal evidence of efficacy. For example, the Son-Rise/Option programme (see Table 14.3) is intensive, as is attendance at a nursery or playschool offering a specialist curriculum or the TEACCH (Treatment and Education of Autistic and related Communication handicapped CHildren) method. Interventions such as Portage, Hanen or EarlyBird (see Table 14.3) that aim to give parents the insights, skills and materials with which to promote social interaction, communication and language at home are also effectively intensive in that they can be applied in everyday situations and throughout the day.

Early intervention may also be important (Butter, Wynn, & Mulick, 2003; Corsello, 2005; but see Magiati & Howlin, 2001; McConachie & Diggle, 2007, for critiques of the evidence). This is, again, a non-specific characteristic shared by all the other interventions listed in column 2 of Table 14.3. A plausible argument for the beneficial effects of starting intervention early is that brain plasticity in the early years allows for intensive intervention to establish neural circuits that might not otherwise have been established (Dawson & Zanolli, 2003). However, this is unproven.

Family involvement may be a further non-specific factor that contributes to the success of many interventions for children with ASDs. Interventions carried out at home or carried across from clinic to home or from school to home, are more likely to be intensively practised than interventions carried out in the limited context of clinic or school. Interventions practised across varied environments are also more likely to have effects that **generalise** than treatments carried out only in one special place.

Structure is another characteristic that behavioural methods share with many other intervention methods or approaches, most notably the TEACCH approach, but also with educational programmes such as Daily Life Therapy (Higashi method) (see Table 14.3). It is also prioritised in the SPELL approach, used in the many schools run by the National Autistic Society in the UK (SPELL stands for the guiding principles of Structure, Positivity, Empathy, Low arousal, and Links with parents and mainstream education). If structure is important for successful outcomes, it might seem surprising that some relatively unstructured, child-led intervention methods such as Music Interaction Therapy or the Son-Rise programme, are reported to be successful for some children. In these programmes, however, the child to a large extent controls the interaction, reducing the unpredictability of others' behaviour and thus having an effect similar to adult-imposed structure.

In sum it may be concluded that, for young children at least, it may be the case that it is not so much the actual method of intervention that is important. Rather, it is that intervention should start early, be intensive, involve the family and be carried out in varied contexts, and either be delivered in a structured environment and in predictable ways, or in ways that give the young child control (Hurth, Shaw, Izeman, Whaley, & Rogers, 1999; Papps & Dyson, 2004).

Interventions for older children and adults Some social skills training materials and programmes have been shown to have some beneficial effects for older children and adults. The Social Stories materials (Gray, 1998) are widely used to promote a variety of specific social skills in people of varying ages and abilities, with variable success (see, for example, Crozier & Tincani, 2007; Sansosti & Powell-Smith, 2006). Interventions specifically designed to develop mindreading abilities or the ability to interpret emotional expression have also had some limited success, as reported in small-scale studies (Parsons & Mitchell,

2002; Golan & Baron-Cohen, 2006). A review of the kinds of strategies used to improve social interaction in higher-functioning individuals can be found in Attwood (2000).

Some of the methods of providing less able children and adults with a communication system have been evaluated in controlled, albeit small-scale, efficacy studies. In particular, the Picture Exchange Communication System (PECS), which provides the individual with a minimal 'vocabulary' of pictures that can be used to indicate needs and wants, has been shown to have some beneficial effects (Yoder & Stone, 2006; Howlin, Gordon, Pasco, Wade, & Charman, 2007). Facilitated Communication, however, in which an individual's use of a keyboard is supported by a facilitator, has not been shown to be effective in the most carefully controlled studies (Mostert, 2004). However, some parents remain convinced that it has helped their own child (Rubin & Rubin, 2005). Speech and language therapy is widely advocated to address the communication problems of children across the whole spectrum, as well as to provide communication systems for the less able. The efficacy of speech and language therapy of various kinds, provided at different ages, and to groups with different abilities and needs has not, however, been extensively investigated.

The effectiveness of therapies or school-based activities designed to foster creativity has not been scientifically tested. The poems and pictures displayed in schools and units that cater for children with ASDs suggest that capacities for creativity and imagination can be fostered and produce unexpectedly impressive results. However, as discussed at some length in Chapter 9, it is not clear exactly what unlocks these capacities, whether in autistic savants or more generally.

The efficacy of behavioural programmes for reducing unwanted behaviours is widely recognised (and not only for individuals with autism). It is important, however, that these programmes are based on an analysis of the function that an unwanted behaviour is serving for the individual, so that more appropriate ways for the individual to achieve that function are built into the programme (Whitaker, 2001).

Regarding the efficacy of non-physical interventions for mental health problems, especially anxiety and depression, psychotherapy is quite widely used but is notoriously difficult to evaluate (for an account of psychotherapy for people with AS, see Jacobsen, 2003). Most encouragingly, a relatively large-scale and well-controlled trial of Cognitive Behavioural Therapy (CBT) for treatment of anxiety in children with AS produced promising results, especially when parents were fully involved in the therapy programme (Sofronoff, Attwood, & Hinton, 2005). This type of intervention is based on the principle of setting small, achievable goals for each individual, designed to reinforce positive, anxiety-reducing modes of thought and action.

Less formally, young children may be helped to express their feelings through play, drawing or within the context of family therapy (Alvarez & Reid, 1999). Figure 14.1 illustrates how drawings may be used to externalise feelings

(a)

(b)

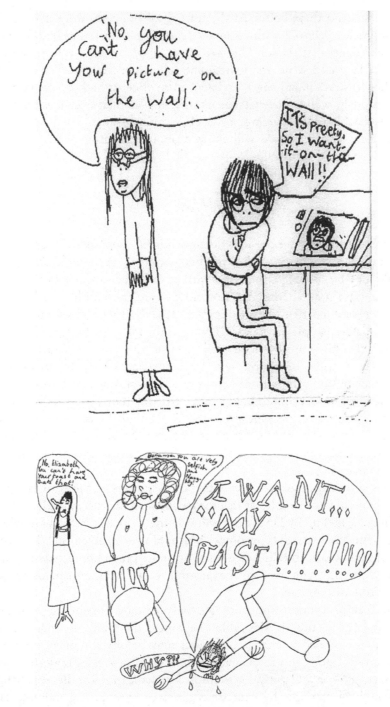

Figure 14.1 An illustration of how drawing may be used to externalise and understand feelings as a means of increasing behavioural self-control (with thanks to Lizzie and family)

and to understand them better. At the time these drawings were done, Lizzie was a bright ten-year-old with Asperger syndrome who found it difficult to control her temper at school. She was encouraged by an insightful support worker to draw and write about how she felt when frustrated, about what caused her frustration and anger, and about the effect it had on others. She is now a generally well-behaved teenager, thriving at mainstream school, and with considerable understanding of herself and her feelings.

In the next chapter, more will be said about educational provision and methods for people with ASDs.

SUMMARY

It is important to consider the justifications for intervening: whether to prevent or cure autism, or to change the behaviour of someone with an ASD. It should not be assumed that prevention, cure, or altering behaviour is always desirable; or that the views of individuals, the family, the State and other interested parties concerning the desirability of intervention will always coincide. People with AS/HFA, for example, are increasingly vocal in arguing that they are by no means in need of 'cure' or 'treatment'. By contrast, the families of people with complex and severe forms of ASDs clearly take the view that methods of prevention, cure or treatment are greatly needed. In addition to being aware that justifying intervention is not straightforward, it is important also to be aware that the appropriateness of any specific intervention depends on the person for whom the intervention is designed, their specific needs in specific contexts, and their age and developmental stage.

There is currently no way of preventing the occurrence of autism except by genetic counselling of couples at risk for having a child with an ASD. Genetic counselling backed up by DNA tests will become more accurate as knowledge of the genetic bases of ASDs becomes known. However, given the likely complexity of genetic susceptibility to autism, accurate prediction is only a remote possibility. For the same reason, the possibility of curing autism using gene therapy also looks remote.

Given that prevention and cure are only distant possibilities, changing behaviour, where this is desirable, becomes the goal of intervention. Interventions designed to change behaviour may be physical or non-physical. Physical interventions aim to change the biological processes underlying certain behaviours, either directly, for example by medications or dietary changes, or indirectly, for example by exercise regimes or by exposing individuals to specific sensory inputs. Physical interventions may also be divided into those offered within conventional medicine and those that fall into the category of complementary or alternative medicines (CAMs).

Conventional medicine has tried numerous forms of medication in attempts to reduce the prevalence or severity of autism-related behaviours, and to relieve some of the more negative behaviours often associated with autism, such as hyperactivity or self-injurious behaviours. These interventions are generally based on theories of the neurochemical bases of ASDs. To date, no treatment has been shown to have a significant and reliable effect on core behaviours. Only Risperidone has been found to reduce some unwanted behaviours without (at least as yet) any side-effects having been identified such as might contraindicate its use. Sensory Integration Therapy, an indirect form of physical intervention offered by occupational therapists, may be beneficial but has not been proved to be so.

Complementary and alternative medicines are more usually based on theories implicating immune system disorders or gastrointestinal disorders as the basis of ASDs. Correspondingly, there are a number of interventions using dietary supplements or restrictions, or methods such as ingestion of anti-fungal agents, to try to correct the hypothesised effects of these disorders. None of these interventions has been shown to be useful in rigorous evaluative studies. However, very many parents use the interventions and are convinced that they are helpful, and popular treatments such as vitamin B6 supplement and the gluten-free/casein-free diet are low cost with only minor risks of side-effects. Some other interventions falling under the heading of complementary or alternative medicines are, however, of doubtful safety.

Non-physical interventions are less often theory-based than physical interventions. More often they have been developed 'bottom-up' by teachers, therapists and parents who have experimented to find ways of teaching or promoting appropriate behaviours, and who have developed materials and methods that can be passed on to others to use for specific purposes. Non-physical interventions are therefore most conveniently grouped under headings relating to the behaviours they are designed to promote or change. They may also be grouped according to the age and developmental stage for which they are most appropriate. Of the many early intervention methods, none has been rigorously evaluated in large-scale studies, although numerous small-scale efficacy studies and personalised accounts have been reported. From these reports it seems most likely that early interventions which are intensive, involve families, are either structured or give the child control, and that promote the generalisation of behavioural gains, are most likely to have positive and lasting outcomes. The actual content and methods used may be less critical. Some interventions for older children and adults have some degree of proven success, in particular certain types of social skills training; some augmentative (computer-based) or alternative communication systems; behavioural methods of reducing and replacing unwanted behaviours; and behavioural approaches to anxiety reduction.

However, the proper evaluation of intervention methods in the autism field is only beginning to be undertaken. This is partly because of the numerous difficulties associated with the design and methodology required if robust and clearly interpretable findings are to emerge. Until data from carefully controlled evaluative studies become available, the safety, benefits and cost-effectiveness of any particular intervention remain uncertain.

CARE

AIMS
••••
INCLUSION
The Principle of Inclusion
Inclusive Care for People with ASDs: Ideals and Realities
••••
FAMILIES
Roles
Stressors and Responses to Stress
Families' Support Needs and Examples of Good Practice in Provision
••••
SUBSTITUTE OR OUT-OF-HOME CARE
Children
Adults
••••
ACCESSING RIGHTS AND SERVICES
••••
CONCLUSION AND PERSONAL VIEW
••••
SUMMARY

INCLUSION

The Principle of Inclusion

Inclusion is used in this chapter in the broad sense of the moral right of every person to be included as a valued member of their society and not discriminated against because of difference (Renzaglia, Karvonen, Drasgow, & Stoxen, 2003). According to the principles of **normalisation** (Nirje, 1969), from which the concept of inclusion has developed, people with disabilities should be enabled to have lives as similar as possible to those of people without disabilities; they should be enabled to achieve good quality of life; and they should have the same human rights as people without disabilities. Both the concepts of inclusion and normalisation take as their starting point that diversity is to be welcomed as enriching to communities, and provision should be made for this diversity in schools, workplaces and elsewhere.

Inclusive Care for People with ASDs: Ideals and Realities

In this chapter the principle of inclusion sets the standard for identifying the care needs and rights of people with ASDs, and for judging the quality of the provision made. According to current ideals in most developed countries, all members of society, including those with disabilities, should be provided with, or have access to, the following.

- Food, shelter, warmth, protection from harm.
- Emotional and social stimulation and support.
- Opportunities for physical, mental and social activity fostering the development and maintenance of capacities and skills.
- Health care, education, and employment or financial support as of right, and access to social services, financial and legal advice and representation as needed.

In addition, there should be recognition of the following rights.

- The right to self-determination in matters of care and daily living, and the right to be valued and respected on equal terms with others.

These ideas, however, have a very short history. Not so very long ago, children who were difficult to rear were often abandoned by parents who could not cope and who could not turn to the State for support. This is evident from the fact that rare children survived long enough to be rescued and subsequently described as 'wolf' or 'wild' children (see Chapter 1). Within living memory, parents of a Down syndrome baby (easy to detect at birth) were commonly advised to 'put him in a home'. In such 'homes' other children with learning disabilities, including those with autism, would also be placed in later child-hood or in adulthood. Basic care needs were provided for, but only those insti-tutions run by the most enlightened voluntary organisations would have perceived any needs for intervention, education or occupation, let alone any legal or moral right to self-determination or **advocacy**.

The ideal of 'equal value equal rights' applied to individuals with disabilities is also fragile, since it is only likely to be acted upon in societies that are not under survival pressure. When survival pressures increase as a result of war, famine, epi-demic or financial depression, the needs and rights of those least able to compete are increasingly discounted or ignored, even in so-called civilised societies (recent examples come easily to mind). In view of its recency and fragility, it is not sur-prising that the ideals of inclusion are rarely achieved in current provision of care for people with ASDs, even in developed countries (Volkmar, 2005).

In what follows, the provision of care for people with ASDs is considered under three main headings. First, support for families caring for someone with an ASD; secondly, substitute or out-of-home care for children, and forms of support or substitute care for adults; and, thirdly, access to those opportunities and services available to all members of society as of right. Generalisations are necessarily made, which may not hold true for all countries and regions. Terms such as 'government', 'State', 'local authority', 'public service' are used vari-ously and loosely to indicate the likely involvement of statutory authorities of one kind or another, whilst recognising that what is arranged and paid for by government-related authorities in one country or region may not be the responsibility of government-related authorities everywhere. For this reason, references to nation-specific laws or practices are avoided. The examples of good practice in caring for people with ASDs and their families that are quoted are, however, mainly examples of provision in the UK, because these are the services I know about, not because they do not exist elsewhere.

FAMILIES

Roles

Ensuring that an individual with an ASD receives the various sorts of care they need and to which they have a right is almost always critically dependent on members of the individual's family. The term 'family' is taken to include adoptive, long-term foster, and step-families; nuclear families, single-parent families, families based on long-term partnerships between same sex couples, and families in which grandparents or other non-parent family members are the major carers. This discussion will, however, use the terms 'parents', 'mother' and 'father' as conventionally understood when referring to research, most of which has focused on biological families.

Parents, or others in the parental role, directly provide for the survival needs of children, and sometimes also of dependent adults (first bullet point earlier). With other family members they also contribute directly and significantly to the provision of quality of life needs (second and third bullet points), although external agencies also have a role here. Health care, intervention and education, etc. (under the fourth bullet point) are generally provided by agencies outside the family, but parents are likely to be the channel through which these services are accessed and monitored. Parents and other family members may also be involved in delivering health care and intervention to children and dependent adults with ASDs, as initiated by themselves or under the direction of professionals. Finally, it is the parents who bear the brunt of the stigmatising attitudes of society and who fight the battles on behalf of their offspring for recognition of them as valued individuals.

If a family breaks down, the child's or dependent adult's access to all these forms of care is jeopardised. Having a child with an ASD introduces unusual sources of stress into a family. It is therefore important to identify these sources of stress and ways in which mothers, fathers, and siblings react and respond to them, so that appropriate support for families can be provided. Supporting families is thus a way of supporting individuals with ASDs and ensuring that their care needs are met.

Stressors and Responses to Stress

Parents

The period following diagnosis of any chronic childhood disability is one of particularly acute distress and family disturbance. A group of parents that included parents of children with ASDs reported that following their child's diagnosis they experienced 'depression, anger, shock, denial, fear, guilt, grief, confusion, and despair'. These feelings were associated with 'uncontrollable crying, sweating, headache and stomach-ache, trembling, and loss of appetite' (Heiman, 2002).

Although such acute distress decreases with time, many sources of stress remain. Some of these are common to all families caring for a disabled child.

- The time, attention, and energy needed to care for the disabled family member.
- Financial costs, often aggravated by loss of earning power.

- Loss of normal family life and leisure activities; changed and disrupted relationships amongst family members.

Caring for a child with an ASD has been shown to be more stressful than caring for children with other disabilities (Sanders & Morgan, 1997; Randall & Parker, 1999; Olsson & Hwang, 2002). Factors that may contribute to this include:

- behaviour problems and challenging behaviours (Gray, 2002; Hastings, 2003a);
- lack of emotional responsiveness and poor non-verbal communication (Tobing & Glenwick, 2002);
- confusion about the nature of autism and its causes, the unpredictability of its developmental course and outcome, and controversy concerning the efficacy of intervention methods (Marcus, Kunce & Schopler, 2005; Dale, Jahoda & Knott, 2006);
- the fact that autism falls somewhere between a mental health disorder and a learning disability, aggravating problems of access to provision (Barnard, Harvey, Potter, & Prior, 2001).

Despite the numerous sources of stress, many families adjust and cope well, showing great resilience in the face of problems associated with caring for a child with an ASD (Montes & Halterman, 2007). The experience of stress may diminish over time, as family members individually and jointly develop strategies for coping with care for the child with an ASD, and with changed family relationships (Gray, 2002). Some individuals with ASDs become easier to relate to as they get older, achieving a degree of understanding of others' needs and becoming able to give back not just by being themselves, but in intentional ways. I recall the relationship between a single mother and her adult, moderately learning-impaired, ASD son, which was in many ways reciprocal. He addressed her as 'dear', helped with the shopping and made cups of tea, telling her to put her feet up while he did so. In the long term, many parents report positively about the experience of bringing up a child with autism, saying that it had enriched their lives and provided challenges leading them to develop an inner strength and acceptance of life's setbacks they might not otherwise have developed (Krauss & Seltzer, 2000; Park, 2001).

Having said this, a proportion of parents succumb to the stresses, especially in the shorter term, becoming clinically depressed or anxious, or experiencing somatic disorders or burnout, partly in response to the difficulties inherent in caring for their child, but also because of the effects on other members of the family (Hastings, Kovshoff, Ward, degli Espinosa, Brown, & Remington, 2005a; Montes & Halterman, 2007). Mothers and fathers tend to develop different coping strategies, some of which are more successful than others in maintaining a sense of wellbeing (Hastings, Kovshoff, Brown, Ward, degli Espinosa, & Remington, 2005b). Factors that have been shown to be protective against the effects of stress include personality traits such as optimism and 'hardiness' (Weiss, 2002;

Greenberg, Krauss, Seltzer, Chou, & Hong, 2004); supportive partners, other family members and friendship groups (Boyd, 2002; Bromley, Hare, Davison, & Emerson, 2004; Hare, Pratt, Bruton, Bromley, & Emerson, 2004); and a feeling of being in control without having sole or main responsibility (Dale et al., 2006). Secure religious faith may also be protective (Tarakeshwar & Pargament, 2002).

Siblings

Siblings of children with ASDs are also significantly affected by having a child with autism in the family. The few studies of siblings that have been carried out suggest the experience can have both positive and negative effects (Kaminsky & Dewey, 2002; Hastings, 2003b). This is reflected in Box 15.1, which reproduces some of the verbatim responses of siblings to informal questioning about their experiences of having a brother or sister with an ASD. Several first-hand accounts of life with an ASD sibling can be found in the literature (for example, Konidaris, 2005; Barnhill, 2007), and some practical advice for parents concerning siblings can be found in Ives and Munro (2002). Ariel and Naseef (2005) bring together accounts of various family members, including parents, siblings, and grandparents, of their experiences of having someone with an ASD in the family.

BOX 15.1   Siblings' reactions to having a brother or sister with an ASD

Answers to the question 'What is the most difficult part of having a brother/sister with an ASD?' included the following:
'Trying to explain to other people what his problem is, 'cos he looks normal.'
'Because he's autistic I have to help my mum more than I might otherwise.'
'You try to play with her and she doesn't like it, and then she gets in a mood 'cos she doesn't get it. She gets angry with herself. And she gets angry with everybody else.'
'If you have a guest he won't take that into account. He'll just carry on shouting. It's quite embarrassing really. Quite often you don't want to have people around, 'cos when he's near, you just don't know what will happen.'
'If I could do something he doesn't like, like play sports or read, it would be all right. But he wants everything the way he likes it. If he's not interested in something, I have to stop it.'

Answers to the question 'What is the best part of having a sibling with an ASD?'
Four of the 14 siblings questioned could think of nothing.
Six mentioned the good nature of their brother or sister, describing them as 'fun', 'funny' or 'loving', or described playing and doing things together.
One said that she felt she had grown more mature and understanding as a result of having a sibling with an ASD.

(From Mascha & Boucher, 2006)

Families' Support Needs and Examples of Good Practice in Provision

Parents' support needs are universal and largely enduring in so far as there may be a continuing need for intervention for their child, for opportunities to discuss progress and problems, and for advice and practical help in accessing available resources and services.

The outstanding example of good practice in supporting families in the long-term care of individuals with ASDs is provided by Division TEACCH (Treatment and Education of Autistic and Related Communication handicapped CHildren) in North Carolina (Mesibov, Schopler, & Shea, 2004). The stated aim of the TEACCH approach to working with families is 'to help parents handle the special stressors that confront them and to support them in their efforts to deal effectively with their child's problems'.

Direct support for families includes provision of specialist diagnostic facilities, nursery school provision and preschool intervention programmes, advice on educational issues and approaches, parent counselling, and the facilitation of parent group activities. In addition, TEACCH programmes of intervention and education are designed explicitly to include parents as co-therapists. This ensures that the goals of intervention and education are dictated by the family's needs; that the broader needs and feelings of individual family members and of the family as a whole are taken into account; and that the techniques used can be carried through from the nursery, clinic, or classroom to the child's home.

In some respects, families' support needs change over time. Some examples of changing needs, and of good practice in responding to specific needs, are described below.

Support for families post-diagnosis

Families' needs for support are generally most acute in the period following diagnosis. Unfortunately, many parents feel abandoned at just this point, especially when diagnosis has been made by a medical practitioner who may see their role as limited to providing the diagnosis. As stated in Chapter 13, diagnosis should not be seen as an end in itself but as a tool for achieving things for people with ASDs, their families and other carers.

Following diagnosis, most families' immediate needs are for information, the chance to talk and to express feelings, and advice on practical strategies to solve problems and promote development (Randall & Parker, 1999). An example of good practice in responding to these needs is described in Box 15.2. This support package was designed and implemented by local government mental health and education agencies.

Ongoing support for families, including crisis care

During the years in which a child with an ASD is growing up within the family there are particular needs associated with enabling the family as a whole to prosper. The provision of occasional care for the affected child outside the family is particularly important, allowing the rest of the family respite from the caring role. Occasional care may take the form of after-school, weekend or school holiday play and activity groups, short-term residential **respite care,** or **befriending** schemes whereby a trusted individual undertakes to look after the child in the home or to take them out on a regular basis. Other family needs during this period include support groups for siblings. These are often organised by local groups of parents who have banded together to support each other, to lobby on behalf of their children, and to plug some of the gaps in formal provision.

Occasionally a family reaches breaking point, usually for an accumulation of reasons, and more radical help is required. An example of good practice in support for families in crisis is described in Box 15.3. The White Lodge Centre, whose practices are described, is a voluntary agency supported by charitable donations, but working in co-operation with, and sometimes under contract to, local government agencies. A wide range of services to individuals with disabilities and their families is provided by the Centre, some of which can be of particular benefit to families experiencing exceptional difficulties. Examples of the kinds of support that can help a family through a difficult patch are described in Box 15.3.

BOX 15.3   Support services that may be of particular benefit to families under stress

A *'parent to parent' scheme* whereby parents who are experiencing difficulties are supported by another parent, or parents, with successful experience of caring for a child with a severe disability.

Domiciliary support may be provided by a member of the Centre's staff on an occasional basis, or for a few hours each day or week, or by a team of staff offering home-based support on a 24-hour basis, depending on a particular family's needs. The support worker may assist with household tasks, share care of the child, advise on strategies that may help to alleviate acute difficulties such as challenging behaviours or severe sleep disturbance, and provide practical and emotional support for family members individually and jointly. A benefit of the domiciliary service is that staff are able to support families to develop routines and strategies at home that lead to them feeling more positive about the future and confident in their abilities to care for their child at home.

A *keyworker* may be appointed in collaboration with other agencies that may be involved. The keyworker might be a health visitor, Portage (early intervention) worker, social worker, member of the extended family or a member of the White Lodge Centre's staff. Their role is to co-ordinate services for the child and family, taking over the administration involved and thus removing what may be a major source of stress for parents.

A *family link scheme* is available under which the family is matched with another (unstressed) family or person in the neighbourhood who undertakes to share care of the child, providing respite care on an intensive basis, for example, three days a week.

(With kind permission of the White Lodge Centre, Chertsey, UK – www.whitelodgecentre.co.uk)

Support for parents caring for an adult with autism

Over half of all adults with ASDs, including many with a diagnosis of Asperger syndrome, continue to live at home on leaving school or college (Loynes, 2001;

Seltzer et al., 2003). When their child leaves school or full-time college education, the care role for parents with an ASD child living at home actually increases, because the child is no longer out for long periods of the day during term time, and the support offered by school and college staff is no longer available. As a result, parents' need for assistance to obtain work or day care for their son or daughter, and for regular respite care, becomes paramount (Hare et al., 2004).

Parents of adult children also need to plan for their move to out-of-home care, and to do this they need information and practical advice. Adults with ASDs need to learn how to live away from their parents because they are likely to have to do so at some time in the future, and this is best achieved gradually. However, the move from home may also be needed because older parents who have given decades of their lives to caring increasingly desire the freedom to live their own lives. Parents with adult children living at home and who are no longer earning may be in particular need of financial support, not least because lifelong caring has continuously drained resources. Finally, they may need advice about arrangements, financial and other, for safeguarding their children's future after they die (Hare et al., 2004).

Sources of support

Support for families at various stages across the lifespan comes from a range of sources, as is apparent from what has been said above. From the least to the most personal these include the following:

- governments and other national or regional bodies concerned with policy, laws and financial provision for services for people with disabilities;
- the administrative arms of specific agencies, such as health care providers, education providers, employment or social services;
- voluntary organisations, including national and local autism support groups, and churches;
- professionals providing various services (teachers, therapists, social workers, doctors, etc.);
- friends and friendship groups that may include others with a person with an ASD in the family;
- members of the extended family;
- close family members, pre-eminently partners.

There is evidence that the most valued support comes from the most personal, least formal sources, with the support provided by partners, family members (especially where there is an extended family), and friendship groups rated most highly (and in that order). However, family doctors, teachers and other professionals, especially those with specialist knowledge of ASDs, are also highly valued (Boyd, 2002; Bromley et al., 2004; Hare et al., 2004). This underlines the need for providing relevant professionals with information and training. Conversely, there is plentiful qualitative and anecdotal evidence suggesting that the impersonal, unspecialised agencies and organisations through which practical support must often be accessed are experienced negatively by many parents (Barnard et al., 2001). Hence the ongoing need for advocacy, whether provided by non-family members or by family members with relevant training and advice (Parsons, 2007).

SUBSTITUTE OR OUT-OF-HOME CARE

Children

Why substitute care may be desirable or necessary

Parents may be unable to care for a child with an ASD within the family home for a variety of reasons. These may include the fact that a child has complex disabilities (for example, co-morbid cerebral palsy or severe epilepsy) requiring exceptional levels of care. Parents themselves may have health problems that prevent them from looking after the child at home; or a family may have another child with a disability; or there may be intractable social, economic or emotional problems within the family, making care for the child with autism an intolerable additional undertaking. Children with profound learning difficulties additional to their autism may also require exceptional levels of care, especially if learning difficulties are accompanied by challenging behaviour. These children are frequently excluded from local schools that are not equipped to cope, putting even greater strain on the family.

Reasons of these kinds may lead parents to seek whole-year or term-time residential care and education for their children. The experiences of parents seeking residential care for their children through local government agencies are often negative. There is a perception that neither health care nor education nor social work agencies will take responsibility administratively or financially, and that cost-saving rather than their children's welfare is the priority (McGill, Tennyson, & Cooper, 2006). Parents may describe the process of obtaining appropriate residential education and care as 'a battle', and formal appeals against local education authority decisions are common (Loynes, 2001).

In rare cases an older child with an ASD may be compulsorily detained as a result of having committed an offence or because of a mental health problem that makes them a threat to themselves or others.

Occasionally a child with an ASD may be perceived as being at risk of neglect or abuse within a troubled or dysfunctional family, or simply because a family or family member reaches breaking point. Issues of child protection may arise in any family, but more especially in families caring for a child or dependent adult with a disability. Individuals with ASDs who cannot communicate, who are hyperactive, needing little sleep, or who have high levels of challenging behaviour may constitute an intolerable burden, and abuse may be the first sign that a family can no longer cope, even with the kinds of crisis support outlined in Box 15.3 in place. In such cases the child may be removed from family care by social services, either temporarily or permanently, and placed in substitute care, with a **guardian ad litem** appointed and a keyworker charged with co-ordinating the child's care, education, and access to other services in place of the parent(s).

A third common reason for a child's living away from home during school terms is the lack of appropriate educational provision locally. High-functioning children in particular may not thrive in their local mainstream school if no provision is made for their particular educational, social and other support needs (Jordan, 2005b).

Forms of substitute care for children

Whole-year care Residential homes offering whole-year care may cater specifi-cally for children with ASDs or for broader groups of children with special needs that include children with ASDs. For example, the combination of severe learning disability with challenging behaviour with or without autism is relatively common, and some care centres cater specifically for this group.

Children with exceptional needs require exceptional residential provision. Specialised provision may include high levels of security (for children with extreme forms of challenging behaviours), modified environments (for children with physical disabilities), on-site medical staff (for children with chronic medical problems), and almost always one-to-one levels of care staff. Whole-year residential provision for children with less complex difficulties, who can-not be looked after at home as a result of family circumstances, need not be so specialised. However, whole-year residential care for any child must provide not only for the child's basic needs but also for their emotional and social needs. Opportunities for physical, mental and social development must be provided, and access to appropriate education ensured either by locating resi-dential provision as part of a residential school, or by locating provision near to a school or schools able to cater for the children's educational needs. Finally, the children's human and legal rights must be respected.

Term-time care Residential schools offering term-time care and education should, like whole-year placements, cater for the full range of children's needs. However, links with families are more likely to be maintained when children are in termly, as opposed to whole-year, care, and major attachment figures and sources of emotional and social support are likely to come from the fam-ilies rather than the school.

Some residential schools offer education and care specifically for children with ASDs. Other residential special schools, for example, schools catering for children with language and communication problems, may offer appropriate education for children with Asperger syndrome for whom suitable provision cannot, or has not, been made by local government agencies. Occasionally a local education authority or similar government agency will fund a place for a child with Asperger syndrome in a privately run mainstream boarding school, but generally only if there are particular circumstances making it difficult for the child to live at home. Some parents who can afford to do so opt to send their high-functioning child to a private boarding school rather than accepting local provision. They may do this mainly for educational reasons. However, weekly or termly boarding has the additional advantage that it offers respite to other family members, while the holiday periods sustain relationships between the child and the family.

State provision for children at risk or detained   Children who are removed from their homes for their own or others' safety or because they have committed a significant offence, may be cared for under the auspices of local authorities in the following types of residential provision:

- foster home;
- residential care home or hostel;
- residential school;
- secure mental health unit;
- young offenders' institution.

Children with ASDs form a minority of the total population of 'looked after children' cared for by local authorities, where they are more likely to be placed in residential care homes or schools than in foster homes or other family-type provision (Meltzer, Gatward, Corbin, Goodman, & Ford, 2003). However, for some ASD children placed in foster care, a temporary placement evolves into a successful long-term placement, with the foster or adoptive family taking over the major family role.

Advantages and disadvantages of substitute care for children with ASDs

It is difficult to generalise about the advantages and disadvantages of substitute or out-of-home care because the reasons why a child is placed in such care, and the kinds of provision made and the quality of provision made, are so various.

Clearly, where substitute care offers specialised facilities a family is unable to provide, or where it relieves a family unable to cope for unavoidable reasons, or where it offers protection from neglect or abuse, it has immediate advantages over home care. For children with ASDs, the continuity and consistency of approaches to intervention and education made possible by residential schooling (the '24-hour curriculum') may be a further advantage. Termly placement in a residential school may not only benefit the child, but enable a family to stay together and to provide good home care during school holidays. At its best, residential care and education for children with ASDs can work well, for children and for families (McGill et al., 2006). Accreditation schemes run by organisations supporting families of children with ASDs can help to ensure this.

The major disadvantages of substitute care are cost (usually borne by the State); also the risk of loosening links with a supportive family, especially if substitute care is provided at a significant distance from the child's family home, which is all too often the case. There is also a risk that the care provided, if not conscientiously accredited and monitored, may fail to meet the child's needs in some way. In theory, children living away from home are protected by a raft of laws and government advice on good practice, supposedly enforced by regular monitoring and formal inspection by relevant agencies (health, education, and social services). However, a detailed study of monitoring procedures for children's homes in the UK found that these procedures were often inadequately carried out in practice (Morris, Abbott, & Ward, 2002). In particular, children were rarely consulted concerning their feelings about their care; parents were not supported financially to enable them to visit regularly; and, although inspection and monitoring was carried out for children placed in substitute care because of parental incompetence, where a child was in substitute care at the wish of parents, it was assumed that parents themselves would check on the adequacy of the placement.

Adults

Needs of those living away from home

Huge gaps may open up in the care of dependent adults when they leave home, for at least two reasons. First, the families of most children with ASDs have provided care in all its forms, as spelled out at the beginning of the chapter, and all these forms of care must eventually be taken over by other individuals and organisations working with and for the person with an ASD. Secondly, state provision for adults with ASDs generally lags behind provision for children. Educational authorities cease to have a statutory role; only a proportion of individuals with ASDs have clinically significant mental health problems such as might make them the responsibility of public health provision; and social service agencies in most countries and regions offer a generic service with no specialist autism expertise or facilities (Barnard et al., 2001).

Care needs are most acute for individuals with severe or complex forms of autism, including learning disability. However, even very high-functioning adults with AS who live independently have certain care needs. Many will require additional training and support if they are to find employment. Many are lonely or have troubled relationships, and are particularly vulnerable to depression and anxiety. They may therefore benefit from particular forms of social support (for example, meeting up with other high-functioning individuals for social events or holidays), and social skills training, relationship counselling or psychiatric care may be helpful. The short book by P.J. Hughes (2007), from which extracts were reproduced in Box 4.1, indicates the kinds of social and other support that can improve the quality of life for highly intelligent but vulnerable adults on the autistic spectrum.

Forms of substitute care for adults

Until the middle of the last century, adults with ASDs who were unable to care for themselves, and whose parents were not able to care for them at home, were looked after in long-stay hospitals alongside adults with a range of other developmental and mental health disorders. These establishments were generally large and impersonal, catering for basic needs and little else.

Full-time residential care for the most dependent or disturbed adults with ASDs is currently (in the UK) likely to be provided by specialist care homes or in homes or care villages catering for adults with a range of significant special needs. Individuals with some capacity or potential to care for themselves may live in small group homes or in sheltered housing located in the broader community. For example, a small group home might be located in a detached house in a suburban road, offering a home-like environment to six or eight individuals, who are supported by a resident warden and support staff.

Some public authorities offer supported living schemes, whereby individuals with disabilities that could include an ASD live in their own house or flat, either alone or with a partner or other companion, supported by visits from paid carers who may assist with daily living tasks, and by professionals from social service departments who provide assistance of other kinds. These forms of more individualised provision are likely to become increasingly common as legislation drives change from care within large-scale units, into which each individual has, to a greater or lesser extent, to 'fit', towards person-centred care in which support is customised to cater for the needs of each individual.

An example of good practice in the provision of out-of-home care within an integrated service for adults with ASDs is described in Box 15.4.

BOX 15.4   An example of good practice in the provision of out-of-home care for adults with ASDs

The National Autistic Society (UK) runs regionally based services for people with ASDs and their carers. Provision for adults in the county of Somerset includes residential care for the most dependent (described below). Other county-wide services include outreach support for adults with ASDs living independently, residential support services in the nearby community, and provision of a range of resources for lifelong learning, employment and therapeutic opportunities.

(Cont'd)

Full-time care is provided at Somerset Court, where residents live in purpose-built houses situated in extensive grounds. Each resident has their own room, with communal areas being shared with up to eight other residents in each house. There are facilities for lifelong learning and for sheltered employment on site, including a modern IT suite and facilities for woodwork, horticulture, creative arts and crafts, and cookery. On-site leisure facilities include a cycle track, trampolines, sensory gardens and an orienteering course, as well as a range of sports equipment, such as go-carts, bicycles, a fitness suite, and tennis and football equipment. Staffing levels are high, to cater for individually assessed needs, and all staff are specifically trained in methods of promoting communication, social interaction, and imaginative development.

The emphasis is on supporting individuals to become as independent as possible within a safe environment, using person-centred approaches. Each resident has a health and personal development plan that they have been involved in formulating, and they select their own learning and leisure activities as part of a weekly programme. Strong links with the local community have been built up over many years, and on-site residents regularly visit local shops and community-based leisure facilities. Some eventually transfer from the main residential site to live in small homes in the community or in their own flats with appropriate support from community-based staff within the regional network.

Somerset Court and other residential support services are inspected regularly by the local Social Services department and by independent assessors from the National Autistic Society.

Problems that can be associated with out-of-home care for adults

Every adult has the right to live as independently as is possible for them, and parents have the right to see their children living as independently as possible, with their needs well catered for, ensuring the best possible quality of life. The example of good practice given above demonstrates that this can be achieved for adults with ASDs, whether their needs are borderline, requiring minimal support, or they have complex needs requiring specialised residential care or intensive individualised support.

Many problems can and do, however, arise. There is the initial problem of identifying the right kind of out-of-home provision for any one individual, and finding where the needed provision exists, preferably close to the parental home or close to where a sibling or other involved family member lives. There is the inevitable problem of cost, and issues concerning who will bear costs, especially when specialised residential care is required. There is, as in the case of residential provision for children, the worrying problem that the prescribed processes of licensing and monitoring are not always fully adhered to.

Finally, quite often individuals themselves may not want to leave home, and this can make it difficult to achieve an acceptable balance between respecting an adult's right to self-determination and acting in ways agreed by responsible others to be in that adult's best interests. For parents also, and especially for mothers, separation from a dependent child after decades of caring in which a uniquely close type of relationship may have been established, can be difficult and painful (Krauss, Seltzer, & Jacobson, 2005). Sensitive management of the transition period, for both the individual and the parent, or parents, may be critical in determining that the move away from home is experienced positively in the longer term (for discussion of support during transition periods in general, see Smart, 2004).

ACCESSING RIGHTS AND SERVICES

Previous sections of the chapter have dealt with care in the sense of where the child or adult with an ASD lives (where is 'home'), and who provides for them there. Access to services and opportunities outside the home to which people with ASDs have a right, according to the principles of inclusion, is now considered.

Accessing health care

People with ASDs are more vulnerable to health-related problems than most people, including allergies and digestive disturbances, accidental or self-inflicted injury, anxiety and depression (Croen, Najjar, Ray, Lotspeich, & Bernal, 2006; Gurney, McPheeters, & Davis, 2006). Frequent visits to clinics and hospital stays have cost implications for families and independent adults, even in societies providing free medical care. Autism-related characteristics may cause additional problems of time and cost in accessing appropriate health care. For example, dental treatment for an individual with poor communication may involve travelling to a specialised clinic or dental hospital, rather than using local services. In addition, lack of up-to-date knowledge and understanding of ASDs by many health care workers can cause inappropriate interpretation of symptoms, misdiagnosis, and inappropriate treatment advice (Heidgerken, Geffken, Modi, & Frakey, 2005). This emphasises the need for training, a need that is – albeit belatedly – increasingly recognised and catered for in post-qualification courses (see, for example, the training package offered by National Health Service, Scotland, 2006). For a broad discussion of health care issues, see Morton-Cooper (2004).

Accessing education

Children with ASDs have the same right of access to education as any other child. However, for children with ASDs there is no clear division between education in the sense of providing a child with opportunities to acquire knowledge and skills (the goals of education as generally understood) and the provision of interventions designed to provide children with ASDs with the skills and strategies they uniquely lack as a consequence of their autism, and to modify non-adaptive behaviours associated with autism (Jordan, 2005b). The educational needs of children with ASDs are therefore 'special', or 'exceptional', even in the case of very clever children with Asperger syndrome or, indeed, highly able young adults with AS attending university or college.

Appropriate provision for children's and young adults' educational needs could include at least the following:

- modified environments and equipment (for example, small classroom(s); secure and specially equipped playgrounds; a sensory room; additional computers);
- modified curricula and individualised teaching programmes;
- modified teaching methods (see references to educational methods in Chapter 14);
- specialist training for teaching staff;
- parental or keyworker involvement to ensure continuity and consistency of educational and intervention approaches across home and school, playgroup or college (see Box 15.2).

Where and how these needs may best be catered for consistent with the principles of inclusion is a hotly debated issue, discussion of which goes beyond the scope of this book (see Jordan, 2008, for an account of the issues). However, the TEACCH principle that no one size fits all is useful to bear in mind. Each child with an ASD has different and changing educational/intervention needs. Each family has different needs, opinions and wishes for their child. Each playgroup or nursery, mainstream or special school, college or university differs in their motivation and capacity to welcome children or students with ASDs into their communities. Decisions as to where a child or young adult with an ASD should be educated must therefore be made on a case-by-case basis, often constrained by availability. Accessing appropriate education for their children is therefore frequently arduous and frustrating for parents (Batten, Corbett, Rosenblatt, Withers, & Yuille, 2006). However, where a range of autism-specific forms of provision is provided, parent satisfaction can be high (Department of Education and Science, Ireland, 2006).

Many adults with ASDs continue to benefit from education in the sense of intervention to help overcome autism-related limitations and problems or to increase daily living or vocational skills (as described, for example, in Box 15.4, earlier). Attendance at college courses or evening classes can provide more able adults with the kind of structured social event they are able to cope with, as well as providing stimulation and sometimes practical benefits.

Accessing employment

Examples of the kinds of employment or meaningful occupation that may be obtained by individuals with ASDs were described in the section on lifespan development in Chapter 4. By 'meaningful occupation' (as opposed to employment) is meant here unpaid, or nominally paid, work, for example household tasks carried out in a residential setting, work carried out on a voluntary basis or in a sheltered workshop or day care facility. The present section concerns the ability of people with ASDs to access paid employment, such as they have a right to expect (if they so wish) under the principle of inclusion.

Obtaining and keeping paid employment are both problematic for people with ASDs, from the least to the most able. Regarding access to employment for less able individuals and those with behavioural problems, the description of Nancy, in Box 4.3, provides an example of the kind of setting in which supported employment may be obtained, and the methods used to introduce the individual to a work environment and work practices so as to maintain the individual in their employment. A further example of how environmental modifications and specific task support may enable a less able person with an ASD to carry out paid work in a sympathetic setting is described by Hume and Odom (2007). These authors used TEACCH principles of structuring the work environment and providing a visual timetable to enable a young man, Mark, to stay on task and complete work assignments independently of external prompting.

Encouraging as they are, the descriptions of Nancy and Mark serve to underline the difficulties involved for less able individuals to access employment: at the least, it requires sympathetic employers and fellow employees, extensive and painstaking preparation and training, and continued support.

A somewhat different set of problems confronts more able individuals with ASDs in accessing and maintaining employment. These are vividly illustrated in quotes from people with AS who were interviewed about their experiences of employment (Hurlburt & Chalmers, 2004). For example, one woman reported:

> I have a degree in political science and am just trying to get a decent job with decent pay and benefits. I have cleaned cat cages, done janitorial work (which is boring, boring, boring), office work... [been] a telemarketer (which I hated, but I learned how to do public speaking!), and worked in a group home on the early morning shift. (Hurlburt & Chalmers, 2004: 218)

This woman attributed her inappropriate and changing employment to her difficulties in conforming socially. Another woman said that others in the office where she worked 'felt uncomfortable around her and tried to get rid of her'. A young man reported that he had just been laid off his job because of anxiety resulting from his inability to cope with changes in co-workers, supervisors and job coaches.

For reasons such as the above, only a small minority of high-functioning people with ASDs find paid employment in jobs for which they are well qualified. However, it has been shown that supported employment schemes for more able individuals can achieve a high level of success with significant benefits to individuals themselves and society in general in terms of cost savings (Howlin et al., 2005).

Accessing financial assistance, legal and financial advice, and other services

The financial costs to families rearing a child with an ASD are considerable (Järbrink & Knapp, 2001; Järbrink, Fombonne, & Knapp, 2003) and financial assistance to which a family may be legally entitled rarely if ever covers these costs. In addition, accessing the various forms of financial assistance to which a family, or an adult living independently, may be entitled is likely to involve seeking out somewhat inaccessible information, understanding regulations concerning eligibility, filling in complicated forms, and co-operating with intrusive assessments. Many families caring for a child or dependent adult with autism find the processes difficult and irksome, and adults living independently generally need assistance in making claims.

Assistance with obtaining financial benefits for which they are eligible is only one of numerous situations in which individuals with ASDs and their families need the assistance and advice of professionals such as lawyers or financial experts. Employing a professional can be just a further cost, and organisations that support people with ASDs and their families increasingly provide helplines, information packs, and day courses from which advice can be accessed. Some countries or regions have walk-in advice centres for people with legal or financial problems. However, specialist knowledge of autism is rarely if ever available in such centres.

Making social inclusion a reality

Achieving social inclusion, whether for children or adults, almost always involves breaking down barriers of ignorance and prejudice, for example amongst parents of neurotypical children in school, amongst fellow employees in the workplace, or amongst staff and clientele in supermarkets, restaurants, libraries, swimming pools, and other public places and spaces. Even something as apparently straightforward as using public transport to travel to school or to work or to see a friend or relative can be difficult and/or unpleasant for individuals and families, provoking hostile or humiliating comments. Genuine social inclusion, including freedom from abusive or discriminatory behaviour from others, can be achieved within small-scale environments in which others present become familiar with the person with an ASD. Hesmondhalgh & Breakey (2001), for example, provide a readable account of the struggle to achieve best practice educational and social inclusion for adolescents and young adults with ASDs in a mainstream school. In large or variable environments, however, full social inclusion is rarely achievable.

CONCLUSION AND PERSONAL VIEW

People with ASDs, their families and other carers travel a hard and often unending road in their attempts to obtain the inclusive care that is the right of all people, regardless of difference or disability. Much human misery would be avoided if current best practice in all the facets of care covered in this chapter could be spread more widely. So why is good inclusive care so unavailable or difficult to access?

The most obvious reason is cost. Järbrink and Knapp's estimate of the lifetime costs of supporting an individual with an ASD in the UK was £2.4 million (nearly $6 million) in 2001. Resources are finite, and providers have to make difficult decisions about their allocation. However, Järbrink and others have argued strongly that not providing resources to support people with ASDs and their families may be even more expensive in the long run, as it increases the risk of family breakdown and mental health disorders, costs of which are borne by the State. Equally, not providing the resources for early diagnosis, effective intervention, good health care and the assistance needed to enable people with ASDs to live independently and to work is all costly to taxpayers in the long term (Papps & Dyson, 2004).

Perhaps people with ASDs are poorly provided for because at some unacknowledged level the law of 'survival of the fittest' operates when it comes to allocating resources and prioritising provision. Autism itself, however, is a survivor: it does not die out of the gene pool. This is because people with pure autism have unique characteristics and abilities that make them valued contributors to society, and these people often have children, ensuring that their autism genes enrich future generations. The list of exceptional contributors who have been described as possibly having Asperger syndrome is long. It includes Archimedes, Socrates, Einstein, Wittgenstein, Isaac Newton, Marie Curie, Jane Austen, James Joyce, Glenn Gould, Eamon de Valera, Jeremy Bentham, General 'Stonewall' Jackson, Thomas Jefferson, Lewis Carroll, Mozart... the list could go on and on. These people may or may not have received a diagnosis of AS had they been alive today. However, what the retrospective evidence indicates is that certain personality traits that are associated with AS are often also associated with exceptional talents and achievements. Humanity would be significantly poorer without the genes contributing to these high achievements, and this must argue strongly for providing inclusive support for high-functioning individuals, as and however needed. It also argues strongly against preventing all cases of autism from occurring or 'curing' everyone who has an ASD.

At the other end of the spectrum, however, and in company with others with severe physical and mental disabilities, people with severe and complex forms of autism are not natural survivors, and the law of survival of the fittest would not prioritise their needs. Why, then, should they be valued and enabled to live good-quality lives? One reason is that precisely what separates humanity from other animals is our capacity to rule our actions on principles other than those of the jungle, and to appreciate that the weakest members of society are human beings like ourselves. Not to provide inclusive care demeans humanity. A stronger reason is that even the most disabled people with ASDs give back: it is not all give on our side and take on theirs. Those close to people with severe disabilities come to love them and those less close have much to learn from them and from the devoted caring of parents and others. Someone who has worked long-term as a carer of profoundly disabled individuals with autism writes:

> Working with people with special needs has enriched my life beyond measure. They have opened up my mind and heart to the beauty of the lost and the broken. They have taught me the value of listening and learning as opposed to talking and teaching. They have brought me laughter and left with me anecdotes to treasure for a lifetime. I have been both touched and humbled by their courage, patience, integrity and humility. I feel privileged to have been given insight into their unique perspective. (Isanon, 2001: 9)

This is not, of course, to say that Isanon or others like him would not wish for prevention or cure for the most severely disabled people with ASDs. But it is a vital argument for inclusion in that it says the more closely we know people with severe disabilities the less we fear them and the more we truly respect, value, and love them.

SUMMARY

Inclusion implies that people with disabilities should be enabled to have a good quality of life that is as similar as possible to 'normal', including recognition of their human rights. The concept of inclusion sets the standard for identifying the care needs and rights of people with disabilities, and for judging the degree to which they are met. Human needs include food, shelter and protection from harm; emotional and social stimulation and support, and opportunities for physical, mental and social development. Rights include access to health care, education and other services, and the right to self-determination and to be valued and respected.

Families are the major providers of care for people with ASDs. However, caring for someone with an ASD is demanding and stressful, involving unusual amounts of time, energy and money, and entailing loss of normal family life with disruption of within-family relationships. Support for families in their care roles is therefore important. Immediately following diagnosis, parents are often distressed and in need of information, emotional support, and practical advice. Later, the pre-eminent need is for support that enables the family as a whole to prosper. This includes making it possible for the family to spend time together on a regular basis without the affected child. Parent counselling and support for siblings may also be needed. Occasionally a family reaches a crisis point and more radical support is required to prevent family breakdown and deterioration of care for the affected child. In such situations a keyworker may be appointed to co-ordinate services, and a support worker placed in the home to provide practical assistance. Parents of adults with an ASD often have an increased care load when their child leaves full-time education, and the need for work opportunities, day care facilities and respite care for the dependent adult is then paramount. Throughout their lives, parents need advice and practical help in planning their children's future and in accessing available resources and services for them.

Substitute or 'out-of-home' care for children may be required for a variety of reasons. For example, a child may have exceptional needs that cannot be catered for at home; a family may be unable to cope for health reasons; appropriate educational provision may not be available locally. Occasionally a child is considered to be at risk within the family and is taken into care. Out-of-home care for children takes various forms, from foster care to term-time or whole-year residential care and education. The advantages and disadvantages of substitute care depend on the reasons why an individual has to be cared for out-of-home, and on the quality of the substitute provision. In all cases, provision is costly, and there is a risk of loosening links between the family and the affected child or adult.

Adults with ASDs who are not living at home may, at best, live completely independently. More commonly some degree of support is needed, either in the form of practical assistance to an individual living independently, or by residential carers in a small-scale community home, or intensively within a larger residential setting.

Many people with ASDs have exceptional lifelong needs for the kinds of care and opportunities provided by external agencies, including health care, education and intervention, employment, financial support and legal advice. Accessing appropriate services is often difficult because of the exceptional needs of people with ASDs, which are often poorly understood and catered for by relevant services. For example, it may be difficult to access appropriate health care because of a lack of specialist staff training; appropriate education for a child with an ASD may require modifications of standard environments, curricula, equipment and teaching methods and, again, specialist staff training. Finding and maintaining employment for an adult with an ASD may require considerable time and effort from support workers and, even so, may fail for personal or interpersonal reasons, even in the case of highly able people. Accessing much-needed financial benefits and advice is often, again, difficult and frustrating, although autism support networks increasingly provide helplines, written advice, and training in advocacy designed to help individuals and carers access services to which they have a right. In addition, people with ASDs have the right to social inclusion in the form of being enabled to access, and to be welcomed into, the same range of places and communities as anyone else, whether shops or schools, buses or swimming pools, pubs or clubs. For this, they are dependent on attitudes within society in general towards people who are perceived as different or disabled.

Many examples of good practice in care for people with ASDs of all the kinds referred to above can be cited. Nevertheless, provision is often inadequate, inappropriate, and difficult to access. The most obvious reason for inadequate provision is cost. Another likely reason is a deep-seated and probably evolutionarily old resistance to whole-hearted acceptance of the principles of inclusion. It is suggested that failure to adhere fully to the principles of inclusion fails to take account of the exceptional contributions that people with ASDs make to humanity in general and to the individuals with whom they come into contact.

GLOSSARY

Terms included in the Glossary are those indicated in bold typeface the first time they occur in the main text in the usage to be defined, plus some terms that occur in boxes but are not indicated in bold. Named assessment tests or intervention methods are not included, but can be identified via the index.

Absolute pitch (AP). The ability to recognise the pitch of any given note in music and give its name. Sometimes referred to as 'perfect pitch'.

Acquired autism. A term used to describe cases in which an older child or an adult develops behaviours characteristic of autism after an illness such as *herpes simplex encephalitis* that causes damage to certain areas of the brain. The autistic-like behaviours do not generally persist.

Action–outcome monitoring. The process of comparing the intended outcome of an action with the actual outcome of that action.

Adaptive behaviour. Behaviour that is appropriate and useful for the individual's survival and wellbeing. The opposite to *maladaptive*.

Advocacy. Work carried out by groups or individuals with the aim of advocating, or arguing for, the legal rights of individuals with disabilities. May take the form of lobbying for changes within society and the law or making the case for a specific individual's rights, for example to disability allowance or freedom from abuse. Also involved with providing information and advice to individuals and carers, and in training individuals and groups in self-advocacy.

Affect. A term used by psychologists to mean emotion/emotions/feelings. (See Box 3.1). Hence 'affective': to do with emotions and feelings.

Affective agnosia. Agnosia means 'not knowing'/'lack of knowledge'. In the current phrase, refers to the inability to perceive and interpret emotions. Synonymous with *emotion blindness*.

Affordances. In Gibson's theory of *perception*, the intrinsic properties or 'invitational possibilities' of items or situations: the uses or experiences they offer or the actions they invite.

Agency. A primitive form of self-awareness derived from the experience of intentionally altering one's *sensations* and *perceptions* by movement (e.g., turning the head; reaching to touch) or by *attention* (e.g., focusing on a particular sound).

Amniotic fluid. Fluid within the sac that encloses the developing *embryo/fetus* in the womb.

Amodal. Not confined to any one sensory *modality*: common to all the senses.

Amygdala. An almond-shaped structure in the interior of each *temporal lobe* containing several different *nuclei*. Part of the *limbic system*.

Animal model. Using an animal (commonly monkeys, rodents or fruit flies) to investigate issues in human biology and psychology on the assumption that animals and humans share features relevant to the issue in question, and that findings on animals will illuminate knowledge of humans. (See *modelling.*) (See also Box 7.1.)

Apoptosis. Death of a cell caused by a chemical signal that activates a genetic mechanism inside the cell.

Appearance–reality test. A test of the ability to understand that what an object looks like (appearance) may not coincide with what it actually is (reality); thought to be dependent on *metarepresentation*.

Apraxia. Loss of the ability to perform voluntary movements. Cf. *dyspraxia*.

Arousal. As used in neuropsychology and neurobiology, generally refers to the state of alertness or readiness of the nervous system to respond, as influenced by the activity of certain brain regions and *neurochemical* systems. (See *reticular activating system.*)

Articulation. Production of speech sounds (vowels and consonants) by bringing the moving parts of the speech apparatus (tongue, lips, soft palate) into contact with or proximity to other moving parts or non-moving parts (teeth, hard palate). Sometimes inaccurately used in place of *phonology*.

Asperger disorder. Synonymous with *Asperger syndrome* but less commonly used, although preferred in both DSM-IV and ICD-10.

Asperger syndrome (AS). The autistic spectrum disorder characterised by impaired social, emotional, and communicative interaction and by restricted, repetitive behaviour and lack of creativity, in people with normal language development and intellectual ability. Synonymous with *Asperger disorder* as defined in DSM-IV and ICD-10.

Attachment. An emotional tie involving mutual dependence in adults. In young children the term refers to the emotional *bond* between an infant and one or more adults with whom the infant feels secure and on whom s/he depends for the satisfaction of basic and emotional needs. (See Box 3.3.)

Attention. As used by psychologists this term refers to those processes that enable an organism to focus at any one moment on a certain feature or feature of their *sensory* or *perceptual* experience to the relative exclusion of other features. These processes include *selective attention, attentional bias,* and *attention switching.*

Attentional bias. An innate tendency to attend to certain kinds of stimuli; in particular the innate tendency of newborns and young infants to attend preferentially to faces and voices.

Attention deficit and hyperactivity disorder (ADHD). A disorder present from childhood involving distractibility, impulsivity, and excessive motor activity, often leading to academic failure and social difficulties.

Attention deficit disorder (ADD). Similar to *attention deficit and hyperactivity disorder* except that excessive motor activity is not present.

Attention switching/shifting. The process of disengaging *attention* from a stimulus or stimulus feature and focusing on a different stimulus or stimulus feature.

Atypical autism. A term used in ICD-10 (1992) synonymously with *pervasive developmental disorder not otherwise specified (PDD-NOS)* in DSM-IV.

Autism phenotype. The typical form(s) of autism.

Autistic continuum. This term was used for a short period synonymously with *autistic spectrum*, but is now rarely used.

Autistic disorder. The *autistic spectrum disorder* characterised by impaired social, emotional, and communicative interaction and by *behavioural inflexibility*, plus impaired or absent language development and intellectual disability, as defined in DSM-IV and ICD-10. Roughly synonymous with *classic autism* and *Kanner's autism/Kanner's syndrome*.

Autistic psychopathy. The term used by Asperger in his early descriptions of people with autism.

Autistic spectrum disorders (ASDs). The group of *developmental disorders* characterised by one or more of the *triad* of impairments diagnostic of autism, the disorders merging from one to the next with no clear boundaries between them.

Autoantibodies. Proteins in the blood that attack the body's own cells as if they were foreign invaders.

Autoimmune disorders. Disorders that occur when the immune system attacks normal body components as if they were foreign invaders.

Automatisation. The process by which an action carried out with some degree of conscious control becomes sufficiently practised to be carried out unconsciously.

Autonoetic awareness/autonoetic consciousness. Literally the 'self-knowing awareness' that accompanies memories of personally experienced events and involves knowing that the self recalling event is the same self that experienced the event originally.

Autonomic nervous system (ANS). That portion of the peripheral nervous system not under conscious control and concerned with vegetative functions, including digestion, circulation, and respiration.

Axon. A long threadlike structure leading from the main cell body and branched at the other end that carries information from one cell to other cells.

Basic emotions. Emotions that are universally experienced by humans regardless of race or culture: happiness, sadness, fear, anger, disgust, and surprise (though there is some controversy about including the latter). (See Box 3.1.)

Befriending. A method of supporting an individual, couple or family through a friendly relationship established specifically for the purpose of providing social and practical support.

Behavioural inflexibility/impaired behavioural flexibility. Terms sometimes used in the literature on autism, including in the present book, as a substitute for the lengthier 'repetitive and restricted behaviour, and lack of creativity and imagination'.

Behaviourism. The approach to psychology that argues that the only appropriate subject matters for scientific psychological investigation are observable, quantifiable, phenomena. Thus, stimuli external to an organism and the organism's observable responses to stimuli form the basic building blocks of *behaviourist* psychology.

Behaviourist model. A particular approach to conceptualising the nature, causes, and treatment of mental health disorders or behavioural disturbances that has its roots in *behaviourism*. Thus, the model conceives of disturbed behaviours as originating in *maladaptive* learning or conditioning, from which it follows that these behaviours can be unlearned by systematic de-conditioning and re-conditioning. The model is associated with a particular set of terms, such as 'stimulus', 'reinforcement' and 'association' and is sometimes equated with 'learning theory' (although this latter term has numerous other uses in psychology).

Blind trials.   A term used in *efficacy studies* to refer to trials (a set of studies or a sequence of tests within a single study) in which neither the actively involved researchers nor the participants (or their families) know whether the participant is receiving the treatment under investigation or a *placebo*. This is termed a *double blind* trial. If only the participants (and families) are unaware of whether they are on the treatment or on *placebo*, this is a *single blind* trial. (See Box 14.2.)

Body schema.   An abstract *representation* of one's own body parts and relations between them. Note: 'body image' is a non-abstract representation of one's own physical appearance.

Bonding.   The formation of a strong emotional tie, narrowly used in psychology to describe the relationship formed by the mother (or other very close primary carer) with her newborn infant: the counterpart of the infant's *attachment* to close carers. 'Bonding' is sometimes more loosely used to refer to the reciprocal emotional tie between infants and close carers.

Borna virus/Borna disease.   A viral disease that occurs in warm-blooded animals, including horses, cattle, sheep, dogs and foxes, producing mainly abnormalities of posture, movement, and other *motor* behaviours. However, experimental infection of rats produces altered social behaviour and learning impairments associated with abnormalities in the *limbic system* of the brain, hence the possible relevance for autism.

Bottom-up.   A term used in psychology to describe processes driven more by incoming *sensory* data than by higher-order principles, expectations or ideas. The opposite of *top-down.*

Brain-derived neurotropic factor (BDNF).   A *neurotrophin* important for brain growth and function, both pre- and post-natally.

Brain stem.   The stem of the brain leading from the spinal cord and including core structures of the evolutionarily old brain clustered round the liquid-filled spaces at the central interior of the brain. The most primitive part of the brain, and the earliest part to develop during gestation.

Brain system.   A term used loosely to describe a set of brain regions, structures or *nuclei* that are interconnected physically or functionally and jointly subserve some specific function, for example hearing, social interaction or memory.

Broader autism phenotype (BAP).   A term used to describe people who have clinically non-significant and partial forms of the behaviours diagnostic of clinically significant autism. Some of the behaviours associated with the BAP may be beneficial to the individual, contributing to superior academic achievement and career success. Synonymous with *lesser variant autism.*

Candidate genes.   Any gene thought likely to be involved in causing a disease (in this case autism), either because it is located in a particular chromosome region suspected of being involved or because the proteins produced by the gene suggest that it could be involved. (See Box 7.1.)

Catatonia/catatonic state.   A condition in which the individual remains in a fixed position for prolonged periods.

Categorical model. An approach to the classification of disorders that assumes there are qualitative differences between what is normal and what is pathological, or, disease-related; also that there are qualitative differences between different disorders or sub-types of a disorder.

Causal precedence criterion. See *primacy criterion*.

Central coherence. The tendency to look for meaning in experience. At the sensory-perceptual level this is manifested as a tendency to perceive wholes rather than parts (the whole barking, tail-wagging dog, rather than the sound of the bark or the movement of the tail alone). At the cognitive level the drive for coherence is manifested similarly as a tendency to interpret ongoing experience as wholes rather than as parts (the whole sentence, rather than individual words; the whole film, not just the moment when the boat sank). Cf. *global processing* and *local processing*; see also *weak central coherence*.

Central executive. Used narrowly, this term refers to the control system in the original model of *working memory* (see main text), later identified with the *supervisory attentional system* (see below). More broadly used, the term refers to a cognitive system subserving *executive functions*.

Central nervous system (CNS). That part of the nervous system comprised of the brain and spinal cord.

Cerebellar vermis. A 'wormlike' portion of the *cerebellum* that receives and transmits auditory, visual, tactile, and *kinaesthetic* sensory information.

Cerebellum. A structure situated at the back and lower part of the brain (above the nape of the neck), consisting of two cerebellar hemispheres and covered with cerebellar *grey matter*, or, cortex. Importantly involved in movement, and now known to contribute also to *attention, cognition, language*, and possibly emotion.

Cerebral cortex. The outermost layer of *grey matter* (cell bodies and their connections) of the *cerebral hemispheres*.

Cerebral hemispheres. The two (left and right) halves of the cerebrum, each consisting of a *frontal, temporal, parietal*, and *occipital* lobe, mediating most non-vegetative functions.

Challenging behaviour. 'Hard-to-handle' behaviours, such as hitting, biting or having a temper tantrum, that occur usually as a result of stress or frustration, and associated with inability to express needs, wants, and emotions in any other way.

Childhood disintegrative disorder. A rare degenerative disorder (sometimes known as Heller's syndrome) the clinical features of which closely resemble those of autism. However, age of onset is later than the typical age of onset for autism, usually being between the ages of three and five years, following a period of normal development. Most cases involve a severe loss of skills and a persistently low level of functioning.

Circadian rhythms. Biological rhythms in animals and some plants that have an approximate 24-hour cycle reflecting the day–night cycle experienced by the organism.

Circuit (brain circuit/neural circuit). A set of brain *nuclei*, or brain structures, and their neural connections, subserving a particular function or related set of functions. Analogous to an electrical circuit dedicated to a specific function or set of functions.

Classic autism. A term sometimes used to refer to autism as originally defined by Kanner and in other definitions of autism formulated before the existence of *Asperger* *syndrome/high-functioning autism* was recognised in the English language literature. Synonymous with *Kanner's syndrome/Kanner's autism*, and roughly synonymous with *autistic disorder* as defined in DSM-IV and ICD-10.

Clock genes.   Genes involved in establishing the physical foundations of the 24-hour, or *circadian, rhythms* that humans have in common with all other animals. May also be involved in establishing short-cycle rhythmic activity in the brain and other organs of the body.

Cognitive/cognition.   'To do with knowing, including *sensation* and *perception*, but excluding emotions, *volition*, and motivation' according to Chambers Dictionary. Commonly used by psychologists and some neuroscientists in place of 'psychological'/'psychology' despite the explicit exclusion of important facets of normal psychological functioning in the everyday usage of these terms.

Cognitive complexity and control (CCC) theory.   A theory concerning the cognitive requirements for success on *false belief tasks* that turn on the ability to represent and act on *embedded rules.*

Cognitive flexibility.   See *mental flexibility.*

Cognitivist model/cognitivism.   A model of psychological function driven by analogies between computers and the brain. Thus, the specific structures and circuits in the brain are equated with computer hardware, and brain functions and operations are equated with computer software or *computational programs.* According to the model, the adult brain consists of innately determined, *domain-specific modules* whose functions are overseen and co-ordinated by a *central executive.* Cf. *modularism.*

Common pathway.   A point at which the many causal routes leading to autism converge; a universal, shared causal factor.

Communication.   Something that humans and animals do, involving conveying, receiving and sharing information, thoughts and feelings non-verbally and, in the case of humans, verbally (i.e., utilising *language*). (See Box 3.5.)

Co-morbid/co-morbidity.   A medical term describing the co-occurrence in one individual of two or more identifiable conditions or disorders where one is not an integral component of the other.

Complementary and alternative medicines (CAMS).   A broad group of treatments, whether physical or non-physical, that are not considered within a particular culture to have any proven efficacy or to have any theoretical rationale recognised by that particular culture.

Complex emotions.   Emotions that are dependent on understanding how others see us, for example, pride, guilt, embarrassment. (See Box 3.1.)

Computational model.   The use of mathematical constructs and operations carried out using computers to investigate human behaviour, especially human learning. Based on an assumption that human behaviour operates in lawful ways that can be represented mathematically. (See *congnitivist model/cognitivism, connectionism, dynamic systems modelling.*)

Computerised axial tomography (CAT scan).   A method of assessing the status of bony tissue using radiation. (See Box 7.3.)

Conation.   See *volition.*

Concordance.   The occurrence of a particular trait or condition in both members of a twin pair. Cf. *discordance.*

Conjunctive search (test). A test involving searching for a stimulus that has a unique combination of features amongst a set of 'distractor' stimuli that have similar but not identical combinations of features. (See Figure 10.3.)

Connectionism/connectionist modelling. A type of *computational modelling* that assumes learning and behaviour emerge from experience that either strengthens or weakens connections between individual units in a network that may be explicitly seen as analogous to a *neural network*. For this reason, connectionism is sometimes referred to as 'neural network modelling'.

Connectivity. The structural and/or functional connections between individual *neurons*, *nuclei* or specific structures in the brain; the structural and/or functional connections within *neural circuits/systems*.

Constructivism – constructivist model. This term originally referred to a model of child development proposed by Piaget, according to which infants and young children construct their knowledge and skills on the basis of a minimal set of innate sensory, motor and learning capacities interacting with environmental inputs. However, the term is now more likely to be used synonymously with *neoconstructivisim*, a usage that must be carefully distinguished from the original Piagetian usage of the term. See also *emergence*.

Continuum. Literally, something that is continuous. When used to describe behaviours that may be associated with autism, the implication is that across individuals there is an unbroken range of ability or difference.

Corpus callosum. An extended band of *grey matter* consisting of *axons* connecting corresponding regions of the right and left *cerebral hemispheres*.

Correlate. Either of two factors or events that are systematically related to each other; that co-relate. Note: in statistics, 'significant correlation' refers to a relationship between two (or more) variables such that changes in one are reliably accompanied by changes in the other.

Cortex. *Grey matter* (predominantly cell bodies) forming the outer layers of both new and old brain structures, including the *cerebral hemispheres*, the cerebellar hemispheres (in the *cerebellum*), and structures within the *limbic system*.

Counterfactual reasoning. Reasoning based on a fictional/false supposition, for example, 'If the sky were yellow it would be the same colour as lemons'. Counterfactual reasoning in *false belief* tasks involves inhibiting one's own true belief and reasoning on the basis of a contrary supposition (e.g., that the marble is still in its original location, in the Sally and the marble task).

Critical cause. This phrase is used in the present book to refer to a *necessary* or *sufficient cause* of a particular facet of autism-related behaviour, as opposed to those causal factors that are neither *necessary* nor *sufficient*. Roughly speaking, the intended contrast is between 'essential/important' and 'inessential/less important' causal factors.

Crossover designs. A relatively tightly controlled design used in *efficacy studies* in which each participant has a period on the treatment being assessed and a period either off the treatment completely or on *placebo* treatment or a comparison treatment, and progress over the various periods is compared. (See Box 14.2.)

Crystallised intelligence. A form of intelligence that consists of accumulated knowledge and skills and depends on culture and learning opportunities. Cf. *fluid intelligence*.

Cytomegaloviral infections. Conditions caused by any one of a group of *herpes*-related viruses.

Declarative memory. Conscious or *explicit* forms of memory that can be reflected on and reported. Includes memory for personally experienced events (*episodic memory*) and factual memories/knowledge (*semantic memory*).

Dedicated system. Similar in meaning to *module* or *domain-specific* mechanism.

Default mechanism. A mechanism used in place of any more commonly used or more appropriate mechanism in the event that the latter is unavailable or inefficient; colloquially a 'fall-back' mechanism.

Deixis/deictic terms. A term used by linguists to refer to words the meaning of which is dependent on the identity of the speaker, and where and when they are speaking. Examples include 'you', 'here', and 'now'.

Dendrites. Branch-like structures attached to *neurons*, which receive information from the *axons* of other neurons.

Design fluency (test). A test of the ability to *generate* a varied range of patterns, shapes or representations of objects utilising a limited number of given constituents. (See *fluency.*)

Developmental. A term used by psychologists to mean 'childhood' and especially the changes that occur through childhood or, more widely, the changes that occur from infancy through the lifespan.

Developmental amnesia (DA). Congenital or early acquired loss of *declarative memory*, especially *hippocampally* mediated *episodic memory*.

Developmental disorder. A disorder or condition that manifests from infancy or early childhood, usually as a result of some organic rather than environmental cause.

Developmental dyslexia. Inability to learn to read to the expected standard in the absence of any obvious cause, such as significant visual impairment, *intellectual disability* or lack of learning opportunity. Often associated with poor spelling and writing, and sometimes with poor arithmetical ability.

Developmental trajectory. The passage or course of development and change over the lifespan.

Diagnosis. The identification by name of a particular disease, disorder, syndrome or condition. Identification is generally made on the basis of a set of symptoms or characteristics of a known disease, disorder, etc. At best, a diagnosis indicates the likely cause of the disease, its probable course and outcome (*prognosis*), and likely responses to different forms of treatment.

Diagnostic marker. A characteristic of any disease or disorder that is so reliably present in cases of the disease/disorder as to identify the disease/disorder. A 'trademark' sign; sometimes described as 'pathognomic' of the disease/disorder in which it occurs.

Differential diagnosis. Diagnosis that includes consideration not only of what a condition is but also what it is not: distinguishing one condition from another.

Dimension/dimensional model. A particular approach to conceptualising and describing certain developmental conditions that are manifested across a range of behaviours, and in which each facet of behaviour is conceptualised as a behavioural dimension. In the case of ASDs, relevant dimensions could include sociability, communication skills, and capacities for creative social imagination; also *language* ability, learning ability, *sensory* abilities, *adaptive* behaviours and *motor skills*. The dimensional model allows for each individual to be described in terms of a unique dimensional *profile*.

Discordance. The occurrence of a particular trait or condition in one member of a twin pair but not the other. Cf. *concordance*.

Dissociable/dissociation. If psychological or neuropsychological phenomenon A can occur independently of phenomenon B, then A and B can be described as dissociable. If B can also occur independently of A, A and B can be described as 'doubly dissociable' or constituting an example of a 'double dissociation'. Hearing impairment and visual impairment are doubly dissociable. Communication impairment and language impairment in autism, however, are merely dissociable (because communication impairment can occur without language impairment, but not vice versa).

Dizygotic (twins). Twins who develop from different fertilised eggs and who do not share identical *genotypes*. Cf. *monozygotic* twins.

Domain-specific. Pertaining to a particular area of knowledge and/or set of skills, for example *language*, mathematics, music or *mindreading/theory of mind*. Associated with *modularist* models of brain/mind organisation and development. See also *dedicated systems*.

Dopamine. A neurotransmitter with both excitatory and inhibitory functions, and involved in movement, attention, learning, and the experience of reward ('feel-good factor').

Double blind trial. See *blind trials*.

Down (Down's) syndrome. A developmental condition identified by Dr Langdon-Down in the nineteenth century, resulting from abnormal genetic material on chromosome 21. Characterised by a distinctive set of physical, psychological, and health anomalies, not all of which are present in all cases, allowing a broad range of developmental outcomes.

Dyad. Two of something that generally go together; a pair or 'twosome'. Used by social psychologists to refer to e.g., a 'mother–child dyad' or 'husband–wife dyad' (sometimes spelt 'diad').

Dyadic interaction. In social psychology, a face-to-face encounter or interaction between two people. In developmental psychology, closely similar in meaning to *primary intersubjectivity*, though with less emphasis on shared *affect* and awareness of *self–other correspondence*.

Dynamic systems modelling. A type of *computational*, or mathematical, *modelling* of brain–mind development, and of the organisation and control of ongoing behaviour, based on the assumption that development and behaviour emerge from the cumulative and ongoing effects of small changes in a multiplicity of components of the overall system. Compatible with the notion of *emergence* and *emergence models* of development.

Dysgenesis. Abnormal development.

Dyspraxia. Partial loss of the ability to perform voluntary movements. (Cf. *apraxia*).

Early-onset autism. A term used to refer to individuals with an ASD who showed signs of autism within the first year of life even if these signs were not noticed at the time, but only recalled retrospectively.

Echolalia.   Speech in which the words used by another person are repeated more or less exactly, with the same stress and inflexion, either immediately ('immediate echolalia', which is usually reflexive) or some time later ('delayed echolalia', which may be used communicatively). Cf. *echopraxia*.

Echopraxia.   Exactly imitated movements or facial expressions, usually considered to be reflexive and pathological (i.e., not under the individual's control). Cf. *echolalia*.

Ecological theory/model.   Used in psychology to refer to theories or models that stress the role of the environment in development and behaviour, seeing the organism–environment as constituting a *self-regulating* whole.

Efficacy study.   A scientific study of the effectiveness of a treatment or other form of intervention designed to cure or alleviate a medical condition or disorder. (See Box 14.2.)

Elective mutism.   See *selective mutism*.

Electroencephalography (EEG).   A method of recording electrical activity in the brain involving placing electrodes on the scalp that pick up changes in electrical potentials in underlying brain regions.

Embedded rules.   Conditional ('if') rules, often stating alternatives within a superordinate rule or precept, e.g., 'When it's raining [if walking, take an umbrella] but [if going by car, don't take an umbrella]. (See *cognitive complexity and control* (CCC)*theory.*)

Embodied/embodiment.   Terms used in theories based on the argument that the mind is shaped by bodily experiences, and that the organism and its environment constitute an interactive, *self-regulating*, organic whole. Similar to the concept of 'enactment' (cf. *enactive mind hypothesis*).

Embryo.   The developing organism in utero from two to eight weeks post-conception (in humans). Cf. *fetus*.

Embryogenesis.   Development of the embryo.

Emergence (model).   A model of development that emphasises the importance of interactions between body, environment, and mind in constructing brain/mind. Contrasts with *dedicated systems* models. Closely related to *(neo)constructivism*.

Emotion blindness.   Inability to perceive or understand emotions. Synonymous with *affective agnosia*.

Emotion contagion.   The involuntary sharing of others' basic emotions, consisting of physiological changes that may be accompanied by involuntary behaviours such as laughing or crying along with the laughter or tears of another person. This 'infectious behaviour' can occur in the absence of knowing what the other person is laughing or crying about. (See Box 3.1.)

Emotion detector (The Emotion Detector (TED)).   One of two components (see also *the empathising system*) subserving the *perception* and interpretation of *basic emotions* in the modified version of a *mindreading* system, according to Baron-Cohen's *extreme male brain theory*.

Empathising system (The Empathising SyStem (TESS)).   See *emotion detector*.

Empathy. Used here to mean the experience of emotion that includes physiological components (e.g., increased heart rate, sweating) combined with implicit knowledge of what the emotion is about in the sense of what has caused it. The combination of physiological emotion plus cognitive content is sometimes referred to by psychologists as a 'feeling' to distinguish the experience from contentless 'emotion'. Note: the terms 'empathy' and *sympathy* are used quite variously across specialist literatures and in everyday speech. (See Box 3.1.)

Enactive mind hypothesis. The theory that social impairments in autism result from the limited salience and reward value that social stimuli have for infants who will develop autism, and the consequent lack of everyday experience of social interaction such as becomes *embodied* in everyday social skills.

Enhanced discrimination–reduced generalisation theory. A theory proposed by Plaisted et al. based on the observation that, whereas unique combinations of features of a stimulus are discriminated better by individuals with ASDs than by non-autistic individuals, shared or similar features are less salient than for non-autistic individuals.

Enhanced perceptual function (EPF) theory. A theory proposed by Mottron and Burack, the main tenet of which is that superior low-level *perceptual* functioning leads to a restriction of interests in favour of preoccupation with perceptual processing within a selected domain.

Epidemiology. The study of the *incidence* and distribution of diseases.

Episodic memory. Memory for personally experienced events, including recall of some contextual information such as where and when the event took place, who one was with, and, crucially, a feeling of having been there oneself at the time (see *autonoetic awareness*). A subclass of *declarative memory*.

Epistemic. To do with knowledge and beliefs. Thus, epistemic *mental states* are conceived of as mental *representations* of knowing/believing/thinking/guessing/hypothesising/estimating, etc.

Etiology. The study of the initial or first causes of a disease or disorder. (Sometimes spelt 'aetiology'.)

Evoked response potential (ERP). A measure of the brain's response to a specific stimulus. (See Box 7.5.)

Exceptional children. The term used in the US to refer to any child whose educational needs cannot be met within the normal curriculum or utilising normal educational methods. Synonymous with *special educational needs* in UK usage.

Executive functions/dysfunctions. The set of cognitive processes that are involved in the organisation and control of mental and physical activity, including *attention, generativity,* inhibition, and *action monitoring*. Derives from an analogy with computers, in which a master programme controls and directs all the software programmes on the machine.

Explicit knowledge/memory. Memories (remembered episodes or facts) that can be consciously recalled, and about which there is a feeling of knowing/remembering (cf. *declarative memory)*. Contrasts with *implicit* (knowledge/memory), although the two terms refer to the ends of a *continuum* rather than being dichotomous.

Extra-dimensional (shift). A term used in tests of *mental flexibility* in which the ability to shift from a *mental set* to respond to stimuli within one dimension (e.g., colour) to respond to stimuli in a different dimension (e.g., shape). Cf. *intra-dimensional shift*.

Extreme male brain (EMB) theory. The theory that autism is associated with an extreme version of the typical male brain, including an abnormally strong capacity for *systemising* and an abnormally weak capacity for *empathising*.

Eye direction detection mechanism (EDD).   A hypothetical mechanism that enables infants of less than one year old to detect the direction in which another person is looking and to infer what they are seeing. A component of Baron-Cohen's *mindreading system* (see Figure 8.2).

False appearances test.   A test of the ability to understand that another person will assume that a familiar container (such as a matchbox) contains the expected content (matches), and to predict their behaviour accordingly, when it is known by the person being tested that the other person's assumption is incorrect.

False belief test/task.   Any test of the ability to understand that another person may believe something to be true that is in fact false, and to predict the other person's behaviour on the basis of their false belief.

False photograph test.   A test designed to assess whether the ability to *represent* a *mental state* differs from the ability to represent a physical state.

Familial.   Characteristic of a family. Inherited characteristics that are familial are those that tend to run in families, as opposed to those that occur as a result of *sporadic* variation or damage to genetic material.

Familiarity.   In memory theory this term refers to the feeling that what one is experiencing now e.g., a face, fact or event has been experienced before, although not accompanied by recall of contextual detail, such as when or where. Cf. *recollection*.

Feature binding.   A term used in the psychology of *perception* to refer to the integration of various different components of a stimulus. At the lowest level, this could refer to the colour, shape and size of a seen object; at an intermediate level it could refer to the various components of a complex scene; at the highest level it could refer to the ability to relate together the seen, heard, felt, etc. components of a personal experience or event. Cf. *neural binding*.

Fetus.   The developing organism in utero from the eighth week post-conception (in humans). Cf. *embryo*.

Fine cuts.   A term coined by Frith and Happé to refer to the phenomenon, which is striking in autism, of two closely related abilities being unimpaired and impaired, respectively. The phenomenon of unimpaired *protoimperative* communication and impaired *protodeclarative communication* provides an example.

Fine motor skills.   Those movements using selected body parts (often the hands and fingers) to carry out small-scale movements requiring subtle muscular co-ordination and control. Cf. *gross motor skills*.

Fluency.   As used by psychologists, this word generally means the ability to produce a number and variety of words, images or ideas in response to a prompt or cue. Synonymous with *generativity* in the sense of capacity to produce novel outputs.

Fluid intelligence.   A form of intelligence that involves the ability to perceive relationships between stimuli and to reason logically and abstractly. Thought to be genetically determined rather than critically dependent on culture or learning opportunities. Cf. *crystallised intelligence*. See also *general intelligence ('g')*.

Formulaic language.   Rigid, invariable phrases, expressions or grammatical 'frames'. For example: 'Many happy returns of the day'; 'Dead as a dodo'; 'Want (Mummy, Daddy, X, Y, Z) do it.'

Fragile-X (FRA-X) syndrome.   The most common inherited cause of mild to moderate *intellectual disability*, resulting from an abnormality on the X-chromosome and therefore manifesting differently in males and females (see *sex-linked*). Also characterised by a number of physical and behavioural anomalies, some of the latter resembling behaviours seen in autism.

Frontal lobe(s).   The lobe that lies at the front of each *cerebral hemisphere*. (See Figure 7.2.) The most recently evolved component of the *cerebral cortex*, involved in several higher-order or human-unique functions, including *language* and *theory of mind*.

Functional magnetic resonance imaging (fMRI).   See *magnetic resonance imaging*. (See also Box 7.5.)

Fundamental (causal factor).   Used here to refer to a causal factor at one or other level of explanation (*etiological, neurobiological* or psychological) that cannot itself be explained in terms of any other more fundamental factor at that level of explanation. Synonymous with *irreducible*.

Fusiform gyrus.   Sometimes referred to as the 'fusiform face area'. A region of the visual association cortex located in the inferior (lower) part of the *temporal lobes*. Involved in the perception of faces, and possibly other complex objects for which expertise in fine discrimination and identification can be developed.

'g'.   See *general intelligence*.

Gamma-amino-butyric acid (GABA).   The most important inhibitory *neurotransmitter* in the brain.

Gaze following.   The strong tendency amongst typically developing infants to turn to look in the same direction in which another person turns their head to look (see Figure 8.1). Sometimes referred to as 'gaze monitoring'.

General intelligence.   An innate capacity for learning, reasoning, problem solving and abstract thinking that makes a measurable contribution to performance on all tests of intelligence. Often referred to as 'g'. Sometimes equated with *fluid intelligence*.

Generalise/generalisation.   The process of extending knowledge or skills gained from a limited set of stimuli or life experiences to include other related, but non-identical, stimuli or experiences. The terms are sometimes used more narrowly in certain specialist areas within psychology.

General learning difficulty/disability/impairment.   A term sometimes used in the UK to describe individuals with overall *intellectual disability (mental retardation)* in contradistinction to individuals with *specific* (i.e., selective) *learning difficulty/disability*.

General-purpose mechanism.   In psychology, this refers to a psychological mechanism or process that is involved in many and varied facets of learning and behaviour, for example *short-term memory*, a *supervisory attention system*, conditioning, *self-regulation*. Contrasts with mechanisms and processes with *domain-specific* application, for example a *shared attention mechanism*, a grammar acquisition mechanism.

Generativity.   A term borrowed from linguistics, where it refers to the fact that an infinite number of different sentences can be generated from a finite set of words and grammatical rules. More loosely, 'productivity' and, in psychology, *fluency*.

Genetic linkage study.   See *linkage studies*. (See Box 7.1.)

Genetic screening.   The analysis of DNA samples to determine the genetic make-up of individuals or groups of individuals. (See Box 7.1.)

Genome.   The full set of genes of any individual organism.

Genotype.   The genetic constitution of an organism; a set of hereditary factors that influences, but does not fully determine, the development of an organism. Sometimes used to refer to the genetic make-up of a particular group of organisms/individuals. Cf. *phenotype*.

Glial cells/glia.   The supporting cells in the *central nervous system* that serve protective, nutritional and other 'housekeeping' functions for the information-carrying neurons and their projections.

Global network.   A neural network made up of the co-ordinated activity of several *local networks*, and mediating complex, multidimensional and multimodal experience.

Global processing.   A term used in the psychology of *perception*, referring to the tendency to perceive complex stimuli as wholes rather than to perceive individual parts of a stimulus. Cf. *local processing*; also *central coherence*.

Glutamate.   The most important excitatory *neurotransmitter* in the brain.

Grey literature.   Literature (in print or electronic form) within a field of study that has not been authoritatively *peer-reviewed* prior to publication.

Grey/gray matter. Brain tissue made up of cell bodies that are greyish-brown in colour. Cf. *white matter*.

Gross motor skills.   Those movements involving the whole (or most of the whole) body, such as walking, jumping or climbing stairs. Cf. *fine motor skills*.

Grounded.   Rooted in; having solid foundations in.

Guardian ad litem.   An individual with legal responsibility to care for the interests of another person who, for whatever reason, is deemed unable to do this for themselves.

Habituate/habituation.   The gradual loss of response to a repeated stimulus or experience as it becomes increasingly familiar.

Hack out.   An expression created to describe the process of consciously working out and reflecting on other people's *mental states*. A process widely thought to be used compensatorily by high-functioning individuals with ASDs in place of the usual intuitive *mindreading* capacity.

Hardwired.   Genetically determined. An expression used in computer-based models of brains and behaviour, based on an analogy between genetically determined brain structures and connections, and the unmodifiable hardware of a computer. Cf. *programmed*.

Hawthorne effect.   A term used in the literature on *efficacy studies* to describe changes in behaviour that result from an individual knowing that they are receiving a treatment and having positive expectations concerning the effectiveness of the treatment. Sometimes also used to refer to changes in behaviour resulting from the attention participants are getting from researchers, rather than from an intervention or treatment itself.

Herpes simplex encephalitis.   Inflammation in the brain, usually including regions of the *limbic system*, caused by one of the several herpes viruses.

Heterogeneity.   Variety or difference. The opposite of *homogeneous*.

Hippocampus.   A sea horse-shaped structure in the interior of each *temporal lobe*. Part of the *limbic system*.

Homogeneous – homogeneity. Similarity or overall sameness. The opposite of *heterogenous.*

Hyperacusia. Excessively sensitive hearing, sometimes restricted to certain sounds or groups of sounds, capable of causing actual distress.

Hyperlexia. A specific developmental condition in which the ability to read aloud with reasonable accuracy is significantly superior to reading comprehension. Cf. *mechanical reading.*

Hypersystemising. An extreme tendency to *systemise,* as used in Baron-Cohen's *extreme male brain* theory.

Hypertonia. Excessive muscle tone, i.e., tension or rigidity in the muscles. The opposite of *hypotonia.*

Hypothalamic-pituitary-adrenal axis (HPA). An interactive system comprising the hypothalamus and the pituitary gland in the brain, and the adrenal glands on the kidneys, that is a major part of the neuroendocrine system that controls reactions to stress and regulates various bodily processes.

Hypotonia. Lack of normal muscle tone, i.e., floppiness and lack of power in the muscles. The opposite of *hypertonia.*

Ideational fluency (test). A test of the ability to generate a varied range of functions or uses of a limited number of given constituents. (See *fluency.*)

Idiopathic. Describes any medical condition or disorder that arises from within the individual, or some part of the individual, in the absence of any known external factor. More loosely, the term is used to describe conditions the causes of which are unknown.

Immediate memory. The recall of something immediately after experiencing it, with no other stimulation intervening. Cf. *short-term memory.*

Implicit (knowledge/memory). Kinds of learning that cannot be consciously recalled and about which there is no feeling of knowing or remembering. Generally equated with *procedural* or 'non-declarative' memory in contrast to *declarative memory.* Contrasts with *explicit (knowledge/memory),* although the two terms refer to the ends of a *continuum* rather than being dichotomous.

Incidence. Refers to the number of new cases of a disease or disorder reported in a given period of time.

Inclusion. As used here, this term refers to the moral right of every person to be included as a valued member of their society and not discriminated against because of difference.

Information processing model. The information processing approach in psychology views the organism as an information processor not unlike a computer, which receives input from the environment; encodes, organises, and stores this information; and utilises it in various forms of output. The emphasis is on the acquisition and use of knowledge and skills via a sequence of processes that include *attention, perception,* memory, thinking, problem solving, *executive functions,* and actions.

Inner speech. The use of internalised language ('speech in the head') as an aid to memory, problem solving, self-control, etc. Less colloquially referred to as *verbal mediation* in psychology literature.

Intellectual disability (ID). The currently preferred term for what used to be referred to (and sometimes still is) as *mental retardation* or *general learning disability*. All these terms are defined in terms of a combination of subaverage intelligence (as measured on *standardised* tests) and poor day-to-day *adaptive*, or coping, abilities.

Intelligence quotient (IQ). The number derived either from a table (as in the Wechsler scales) or from dividing an individual's *mental age* as measured on an intelligence test by their chronological age and multiplying by 100. Note that in the Wechsler scales, 'IQ' is referred to as 'Full Scale IQ' (FS-IQ). (See Box 3.7.)

Intention detector (ID). A hypothetical, genetically determined mechanism that enables infants of less than one year old to detect the immediate goal of another person's action, e.g., that the other person intends/has the goal of reaching for the spoon. A component of Baron-Cohen's *mindreading system* (see Figure 8.2).

Intra-dimensional (shift). A term used in tests of *mental flexibility* meaning the ability to shift from a *mental set* to respond to one particular stimulus within a dimension (e.g., green, within the dimension of colour) to respond to a different stimulus within that dimension (e.g., yellow). Cf. *extra-dimensional shift.*

Irreducible. See *fundamental.*

Joint attention. A state of attention in which two (or more) individuals are not only attending to the same object, person or event, but also know that the other person is attending to it; thus they have knowledge of the other person's mental state. Synonymous with *shared attention.*

Kanner's syndrome/Kanner's autism. Terms used to refer to autism as originally defined by Kanner. Synonymous with *classic autism*, and roughly synonymous with *autistic disorder* as defined in DSM-IV and ICD-10.

Kinaesthesia/kinaesthetic. A feeling of movement; to do with the experience of one's own body movements. A specific component of *proprioception.*

Language. A system or code consisting of mainly arbitrary *symbols* (vocabulary) and rules for combining symbols (grammar) to convey meaning. Language can be spoken, signed, written or signalled in some other way. It is one of the means or methods used to *communicate*, and is unique to humans. (See Box 3.5.)

Late-onset autism. See *regressive autism.*

Lateralisation. The process by which different functions and processes become associated with one or the other side of the brain.

Learning disability. In UK usage, synonymous with *intellectual disability/general learning disability*. In US usage, refers to a selective impairment of learning, such as *developmental dyslexia* or *specific language impairment*. Synonymous with *specific learning impairment* in UK usage.

Lesion. Any impairment or flaw in body tissue produced by an injury, disease or surgery.

Lesser variant autism. See *broader autism phenotype.*

Limbic system. A set of evolutionarily old structures in the interior of the brain including the *amygdala* and *hippocampus*; important for emotion, motivation, and *declarative* memory.

Linkage studies.   A method of *genetic screening* that involves analysing genetic samples from two or more affected relatives in the same family to determine whether or not there are genetic anomalies held in common. (See Box 7.1.)

Local network.   A circuit involving relatively few *nuclei* situated close together in the brain.

Local processing.   A term used in the psychology of perception referring to the tendency to perceive the individual parts of a complex stimulus rather than to perceive wholes. Cf. *global processing* and *central coherence.*

Lumbar puncture.   A commonly used method of obtaining a sample of cerebro-spinal fluid for analysis. (See Box 7.4.)

Magnetic resonance imaging (MRI).   A method of assessing brain structure (sMRI) or brain function (fMRI) using a machine-generated magnetic field that is reflected back in specific ways and used to build up a detailed three-dimensional image of brain structure or activity. (See Boxes 7.3 and 7.5.)

Magnetoencephalography (MEG).   A method of assessing brain function by measuring magnetic fields produced by electrical activity in the brain in response to specific stimuli. (See Box 7.5.)

Maladaptive behaviour.   Behaviour that is inappropriate and ultimately not conducive to the individual's survival and wellbeing, though it may achieve immediate or short-term goals. Cf. *adaptive behaviour.*

Manifest behaviour.   Actual instances of any individual's day-to-day behaviour such as might come under generalised headings such as 'impaired social interaction' or 'restricted and repetitive behaviour'.

Maternal rubella.   German measles in a woman who is pregnant.

Mechanical reading.   Reading aloud with correct pronunciation. Superior to reading comprehension in *hyperlexia.*

Medial temporal lobe (MTL).   The interior part of the *temporal lobe* that includes the *amygdala, hippocampus*, and other *subcortical* structures.

Medical model.   A particular approach to conceptualising the nature, causes, and treatment of diseases, disorders or other conditions that has its roots in the practice of physical medicine. Sometimes referred to as the 'biomedical model' because of its emphasis on physical, or biological, processes. The model is associated with a particular set of terms (see Box 1.2) and entails a bias towards classifying diseases, etc. in terms of distinct categories and subcategories. When this bias predominates, the medical model may be equated with a *categorical* or *subtypes model.*

Mental age (MA).   Level of development or achievement expressed in terms of the chronological age (CA) at which this level would be average or prototypical. In a completely average child MA = CA; in a child with superior ability MA > CA; in a child with developmental delay MA < CA. Sometimes referred to as 'age equivalent'.

Mental flexibility.   The ability to switch or shift *attention* from one stimulus to another or to change *mental set*, involving the disengagement of attention, or abandonment of a mental set, so as to establish a new focus of attention, or a new mental set. Synonymous with *cognitive flexibility.*

Mentalising ability.   The ability to form *representations* of *mental states* and to think about one's own and others' mental states. Broader in meaning than *theory of mind* as originally defined, because it includes the ability to represent *perceptual* and *volitional* mental states as well as the ability to represent and reflect on *epistemic* mental states.

Mental retardation. See *intellectual disability*.

Mental set. A state of mind in which there is a preparedness to respond in a particular way (e.g., to press the buzzer when a circle (but not a square) appears; to perceive a particular face (not others) in a crowd).

Mental state. A perception, feeling, desire, thought, belief or other item of knowledge or feeling that, according to *representational* models (see Box 8.1), exists in the mind (and corresponds to a specific pattern of neural activity in the brain).

Mental time travel. The ability to project oneself mentally into the past to re-experience an event or to project oneself into the future to 'pre-experience' future events.

Meta-analysis. An analysis of the results of several research studies investigating a particular phenomenon.

Metabolic. To do with *metabolism*.

Metabolism. Chemical changes that mediate life processes within living organisms.

Metacognition. The ability to think about thinking; to reflect; to engage in human-unique, higher-order thought.

Metarepresentation. The ability to represent the relationship between something that is known/believed/imagined, etc. and the mental state of knowing/believing/imagining, etc. Necessary for higher-order thought (see *metacognition*).

Mindblindness (theory). Inability to *mindread;* the theory that impaired social interaction and *communication* in ASDs results from this inability.

Mindreading. Colloquially, the ability to 'read' other people's thoughts. In the psychological and especially the autism literatures, the term has the slightly broader meaning of an understanding of what minds are, and an ability to introspect about one's own mind as well as knowing and sometimes knowingly sharing the perceptions and thoughts of others.

Mirror neurons/mirror neuron system (MNS). A set of motor neurons that fire when an individual performs an action, and which are also active when the same action is seen to be performed by another individual of the same species (human or primate, according to current research).

Modality. One of the sensory systems, e.g., 'visual modality', 'auditory modality'.

Model. As used in, e.g., *medical model, behaviourist model, psychanalytic model*, refers to a particular way of envisaging the nature and causes of diseases or disorders, with a related set of approaches to treatment. As used in, e.g., *ecological model, computational model*, refers to a particular theoretical approach to describing and delineating structures and processes involved in development and behaviour.

Modelling. A method of investigating processes and behaviours indirectly using another organism (*animal model*) or mathematical constructs and operations (*computational model*) to simulate the process or behaviour under investigation.

Module/modular/modularism. Modularism is the theory that the brain/mind is largely organised in the form of discrete *domain-specific*, genetically specified processing systems (modules), associated with particular neural structures and *circuits* that are *programmed* to develop at a particular time and in a predictable sequence in all individuals of a particular species. Cf. *cognitivism, cognitivist model*. Contrasts with *(neo)constructivism*.

Monotropic attention.   Attention to *sensory* inputs from one modality only, to the exclusion of information from other sensory channels.

Monozygotic (twins).   Twins who develop from the same fertilised egg, and who have identical *genotypes*. Cf. *dizygotic* (twins).

Morpheme/morphemic/morphology.   Morphology is the study of the minimal components of a language comprising word stems (e.g., /run/, /her/) and the prefixes and suffixes that express grammatical contrasts (e.g., /-ing/, /re-/, /-'s/.

Motor (skills).   To do with bodily positioning and movement; the set of capacities and processes involved in the initiation, execution, and control of bodily posture and movement.

Myelin sheath.   The whiteish-coloured tube made up of *glial cells* that protects an *axon* and insulates it from other axons.

Necessary cause.   Any causal factor without which a particular effect cannot occur. Cf. *sufficient cause*.

Negative findings.   Those findings from research studies that do not support the hypothesis being tested. Such findings are important because they tend to disconfirm, or disprove, the hypothesis under investigation.

Neoconstructivism/neoconstructivist model.   (sometimes referred to as the *constructivist model*). A model of development that seeks to reconcile the older Piagetian *constructivist* model and the *modularist* model by maintaining that infants and young children construct their knowledge and skills on the basis of a set of genetically determined and often *domain-specific* biases and predispositions operating on environmental inputs. These biases and predispositions (for example, to attend to faces in preference to other visual stimuli) shape development in species-specific ways whilst allowing a substantial role for environmental influences and for variability in brain/mind development across individuals. See the closely related concept of *emergence*.

Neologism.   A made-up word; a newly invented expression.

Neural binding.   The co-ordination or integration of neural activity in diverse brain *nuclei* (cell clusters), *circuits* or regions. See also *feature binding* and *temporal binding*.

Neural circuit.   See *circuit*.

Neural network.   Any system of interconnected *neurons, nuclei* (cell clusters) or brain structures.

Neural network modelling.   See *connectionism*.

Neuroanatomy.   Study of the structure of the nervous system, usually in terms of named parts or regions identified by gross physical characteristics, by specific function or by cellular composition.

Neurobiology.   Branch of biology that deals with the structure and function of the nervous system.

Neurochemistry.   Study of the chemical constituents of the nervous system, their processes and functions.

Neurodevelopmental disordexr. Any brain-based condition that manifests from early childhood by disrupting normal psychological development, generally in ways that may be termed 'specific' or 'selective'. Thus, conditions such as *specific language disorder* or *attention deficit disorder* fall under the heading of 'neurodevelopmental disorder', whereas pervasive *intellectual disability* (*mental retardation*) is less likely to be so described.

Neuromodulator. A naturally secreted substance (usually a *neuropeptide*, e.g., *oxytocin, vasopressin*) that acts like a *neurotransmitter* except that its operates not only at *synapses* but also more widely, and often over whole *neural circuits/networks*.

Neurons. The information-processing and information-transmitting elements of the nervous system. Synonymous with 'nerve cell'.

Neuropeptides. *Peptides* that contribute to neural function.

Neurophysiology. Study of the chemical and electrical activity within the nervous system.

Neuropsychology. Study of the interface between brain and mind, where *fundamental*/irreducible psychological processes or behaviours can be identified with the structures and functions of the brain that subserve them. (See Figure 6.1.)

Neuroreceptors. Molecules within *neurons* that are selectively responsive to particular *neurotransmitters*.

Neurotic/neurotic disorder/neurosis. A personality or mental disturbance not resulting from any known biological cause. Sometimes equated with any mental health disorder in which an individual does not lose touch with reality (in contrast to *psychosis*).

Neurotransmitter. Chemical substances released by one *neuron* to stimulate or inhibit activity in other neurons.

Neurotrophins. Chemical substances that influence the growth of *neurons* and their connections.

Neurotypical. Neurobiologically normal, especially in terms of brain structure and function. (See Note under *typically developing*.)

Non-specific factors. Factors that may influence the outcome of a piece of research (e.g., an *efficacy study*) that are not controlled for in the research. Such factors are often ongoing, or background, factors, such as the motivation of an individual to participate or their expectations of the outcome.

Non-verbal abilities. See *non-verbal intelligence*.

Non-verbal communication. *Communication* achieved by means other than *language*, for example by facial expressions, body postures, orientation, and movement; body odours or odours of specially emitted body substances; by touch; electrical signals (some fish); vocalisation and other sounds. Not to be confused with *non-verbal abilities/non-verbal intelligence*.

Non-verbal intelligence (tests). Tests of reasoning and problem solving that are not dependent on the use of language, e.g., visual-spatial constructional skills, pattern perception and manipulation. Synonymous with Performance Scales in the Wechsler tests. Not to be confused with the use of 'non-verbal' in *non-verbal communication*. (See Box 3.7.)

Non-verbal learning disability (NLD/NVLD). A *neurodevelopmental disorder* characterised by poor *visuospatial* skills, clumsiness, and mild socio-emotional impairment, but with intact and sometimes superior verbal abilities. (See Box 2.1.)

Noradrenalin. Synonymous with *norepinephrine*.

Norepinephrine. A *neurotransmitter* that acts widely within the brain, also within the *autonomic nervous system*, and has important functions associated with *arousal* (alertness), sleep, and stress. (Note: epinephrine/adrenalin is a hormone with major functions within the *autonomic nervous system* but only minor functions as a *neurotransmitter* in the brain.)

Normalisation. The principle according to which people with disabilities should be enabled to have lives as similar as possible to those of people without disabilities; they should be enabled to achieve good quality of life; and they should have the same human rights as people without disabilities.

Nosology/nosological. The branch of medicine to do with the classification of diseases. (See Box 1.2.)

Nucleus. The central region of a cell, containing the chromosomes; or a cluster of neurons all of which are involved in transmitting and receiving the same information.

Nuclei. Plural of *nucleus* in either sense, but most commonly used to refer to clusters of neurons.

Obsessive-compulsive disorder (OCD). A specific form of anxiety disorder characterised by recurrent and persistent thoughts and compulsions to carry out repetititive and ritualised behaviours.

Occipital lobe(s). One of the lobes of the cerebrum, situated at the back of the skull (see Figure 7.2). Contains the primary visual cortex, where visual information is processed.

Open/open label designs. A relatively uncontrolled design used in *efficacy studies* in which the response to a particular form of ongoing treatment is monitored in a group of individuals without use of a comparison group. (See Box 14.2.)

Operationalise. As used here, this refers to the expansion of an abstract concept, instruction or precept by referring to the actual, or concrete, operations or procedures that are subsumed under the abstract term. So, for example, an instruction to assess an individual for 'improved mood' might be operationalised in terms of the number of positive statements the individual makes about themselves in the course of a structured interview. (See Box 14.3.)

Opioid peptides. A group of chemicals produced by the brain that act like opiate drugs, such as opium or morphine.

Orbitofrontal cortex. Part of the social brain situated in the part of the frontal lobe lying beneath the *prefrontal cortex*, and immediately above the bony cavities in which the eyes are set. Traditionally thought to be involved in personality traits such as social adjustment and the control of mood. More recently thought to be implicated in learned associations between stimuli and reward value.

Over-selective attention. Attention directed at a single feature of a stimulus when it would be more usual or appropriate to attend to a broader range of features. For example, focusing solely on the colour of an object instead of seeing the object as a whole, including colour, shape, size, texture, etc. Cf. *selective attention*.

Oxytocin. An *opioid* with direct effects on some reproductive organs, but that also acts as a *neurotransmitter* in the brain, modulating activity within brain *circuits* mediating pain perception, emotion, appetite, sexual and social behaviours, including social engagement and social reward. See also *vasopressin*.

Parallel design.   A relatively tightly controlled design used in *efficacy studies* in which the progress of two groups of participants is compared, one of which receives the intervention that is being evaluated, whilst the control or comparison group receives no treatment or a *placebo*. (See Box 14.2.)

Parietal lobe(s).   One of the lobes of the cerebrum situated behind the *frontal lobe*, above the *temporal lobe*, and in front of the *occipital lobe* (see Figure 7.2). The primary sensory areas for pain, pressure, and touch. Also involved in spatial orientation, *language* development, and *attention*.

Pathological Demand Avoidance Syndrome (PDA).   A suggested form of atypical ASD as common in females as males and characterised in particular by obsessive and sometimes manipulative avoidance of demands/requests from other people.

Peer review.   The process by which scholarly articles are critically assessed by other experts in the same field when submitted for publication. Determines whether or not an article is accepted for publication, and acceptance is often subject to conditions designed to improve the work reported or the report itself, as suggested by the reviewers.

Peptides.   Chains of amino acids linked together by peptide bonds (giving their name to the amino acid chain). Most *neuromodulators* are peptides.

Perception.   The processes that give coherence and meaning to sensory input.

Perceptual memory.   Memory for *unimodal*, single-item percepts that may, however, be complex (e.g., a street scene viewed as a whole).

Performance quotient (PQ).   The number derived either from a table (as in the Wechsler scales) or from dividing an individual's *mental age* as measured on a 'Performance scale' by their chronological age and multiplying by 100. (See Box 3.7.)

Peripheral vision.   Vision using the peripheral parts of the retina (colloquially, seeing things out of the corners of the eyes).

Perirhinal cortex.   A region of 'old brain' cortex within the *temporal lobe*, which receives highly processed information from all sensory regions. Thought to be important for memory in addition to complex sensory processing.

Perseveration/perseverative.   The tendency to continue to do something or continue in a particular line of thought, with the implication that the persistence or repetition is non-*adaptive*/pathological. Cf. *stuck in set*.

Pervasive developmental disorders (PDDs).   A group of five disorders characterised by delays in the development of multiple basic functions including socialisation and *communication*. According to the *Diagnostic and Statistical Manual* (4th edition) the group consists of *autistic disorder, Asperger syndrome, pervasive developmental disorder not otherwise specified, Rett syndrome*, and *childhood disintegrative disorder*.

Pervasive developmental disorder not otherwise specificied (PDD-NOS).   A diagnostic term used in DSM-IV to describe individuals with mild, partial or atypical forms of autism-related behaviours. Synonymous with *atypical autism* in ICD–10.

Pervasive mutism.   A poorly understood and little-researched condition in which an individual understands at least some language but is unable to produce any voluntary and intentional form of communicative output.

Phenotype.   The outcome of the interaction between a *genotype* and environmental factors in an individual, as manifested in the structure, function and behaviour of the individual. Sometimes used to refer to outcomes characteristic of a particular group of individuals, e.g., *autism phenotype, broader autism phenotype*.

Phenylketonuria (PKU). An inherited disorder of protein *metabolism* that, if untreated, arrests brain development and causes *intellectual disability*.

Phonological loop. One of the *slave systems* in the original model of *working memory*, with the role of holding *phonological* information in memory whilst manipulating or otherwise operating on it.

Phonology. Knowledge of, or study of, the sound system of a language, i.e., the phonemes (e.g., in English /ch/, /ee/, /z/, etc.) and the rules for combining phonemes into syllables and words.

Pica. A compulsion to eat non-edible substances, e.g., grass, earth, paper.

Placebo. A substance with no medicinal properties, administered as a control condition in efficacy studies of drug or dietary treatments. (See Box 14.2.)

Place-holder. In mathematics, a symbol (e.g., 'x' or 'y') representing a missing element in an equation. Analogously, a term (e.g., *'central executive', 'shared attention mechanism'*) having a temporary role within a theory or model, until such time as the missing element in the theory can be more fully specified.

Plasticity. A term used in *neurobiology* to refer to the adaptability of the brain in terms of which *nuclei/circuits/*regions carry out specific functions.

Polydipsia. Excessive thirst; a pathological compulsion to ingest liquids.

Polygenic. A pattern of inheritance involving many genes that applies to characteristics which vary continuously, such as height, gender orientation, intelligence.

Positive findings. Those findings from research studies that support the hypothesis being tested. Cf. *negative findings*.

Positron Emission Tomography (PET scan). A method of assessing brain function using a radioactive tracer injected into the bloodstream to assess levels of activity in specific *neurochemical* brain systems. (See Box 7.4.)

Prader-Willi syndrome. An inherited condition manifesting from birth and characterised by *intellectual disability*, immature physical development, emotional instability, *hypotonia*, and excessive appetite.

Pragmatic (language) impairment (PLI/PI). A *neurodevelopmental disorder* characterised by a selective impairment of *pragmatics* and therefore of the use of language in conversation/discourse. (See Box 2.1.)

Pragmatics. Knowledge of the rules and conventions governing the choice of words and word forms used in any instance of actual conversation. Cf. *pragmatic language impairment*.

Predictive value. A measure of the efficacy of a screening test based on the accuracy with which a particular test predicts the proportion of individuals in the general population who have a particular disease or disorder as compared to the proportion who do not. (See Box 13.5.)

Prefrontal cortex (PFC). The front of the frontal lobes (lying approximately behind the forehead). Subdivisions include *ventromedial PFC*, which is part of the *social brain*. Other subdivisions are important for *executive functions*, including *working memory*.

Prepotent response. The most powerful response; the response most likely to be made unless explicitly inhibited.

Prevailing model. Any theoretical *model* that is the most influential in its field over a particular period of time.

Prevalence. The total number of cases of a disease or disorder in a specified population at a particular point in time.

Primacy criterion. A yardstick for assessing the validity of a theory/hypothesis concerning the causes of a disorder or a particular facet of a disorder based on the fact that cause always precedes effect. Synonymous with *causal precedence criterion*.

Primary intersubjectivity. The earliest forms of one-to-one co-ordinated interaction between infants and carers, in which infants indicate some awareness of the sameness between themselves and other people (self-equivalence). Similar to *dyadic interaction,* but with greater emphasis on emotion sharing. See also *secondary intersubjectivity.*

Priming. In memory theory, this term refers to the unconsious influence of a prior experience on a current response. A component of *procedural memory*.

Procedural memory. Covers various kinds of learning that take place unconsciously, laying down knowledge, associations and skills that cannot be reflected on or reported and the details of which cannot be consciously recalled although importantly influencing behaviour (e.g., how to ride a bike; the rules of English grammar). The opposite of *declarative memory*, and sometimes referred to as 'non-declarative memory' or *implicit* memory.

Profile/profiling. Terms associated with the *dimensional model* that describes an individual's autism-related behaviour in terms of a profile of behavioural strengths and weaknesses.

Prognosis. The predicted course and eventual outcome of a particular disease or disorder (see Box 1.2).

Programmed. Genetically determined to occur at a certain time in a certain sequence. An expression used in discussions of development and behaviour, based on an analogy between brains and computers. Cf. *hardwired*.

Proprioception/proprioceptive. A general term used to refer to all those *sensory* systems that are involved in providing information about position, location, orientation, and movement of one's own body/body parts.

Prosody. The use of pitch, loudness, tempo and rhythm in spoken language, with the functions of enhancing meaning, conveying emotion, and co-ordinating conversational interactions.

Protoconversation. Conversation-like, turn-taking exchanges of vocalisations and other *non-verbal communication* signals between prelinguistic infants and carers, often initiated as well as maintained by the infant. (See Box 8.2.)

Protodeclarative (pointing). *Communication* for the sake of sharing something of interest with another person, often by pointing at the object or event of interest; but it can also involve bringing something to show another person or drawing attention to something using language. Associated with *joint/shared attention*.

Protoimperative (pointing). *Communication* designed to obtain something an individual needs or wants, sometimes by pointing, sometimes by asking, sometimes by taking another person towards a wanted object or guiding their hand towards it.

Pruning. See *synaptic pruning*.

Pseudo-autism. A term used to describe cases in which an individual has the behaviours characteristic of autism or resembling those of autism, but where the causes of those behaviours are believed to be significantly different from the kinds of causal factors that more usually lead to autism-related behaviours. So, for example, 'autism' or 'autistic-like behaviours' associated with blindness or with extreme deprivation in early childhood, may be described as cases of pseudo-autism. Synonymous with *quasi-autism*.

Psychic akinesia. A rare neurological condition characterised by extreme passivity, apathy, and profound generalised loss of self-motivation, affected individuals describing themselves as having a complete mental void or blank. However, complex physical and mental tasks can be carried out under instruction, and with prompts to continue. Cf. *self-activation*.

Psychoanalysis. A method of treatment of certain types of mental disorder associated originally with the theories and methods of Sigmund Freud. In-depth 'talking out' therapy involving the exploration of childhood and experiences and unconscious mental processes. Derives from the *psychoanalytic model*.

Psychoanalytic model (more broadly referred to as the 'psychodynamic model'). A particular approach to conceptualising the nature, causes, and treatment of mental health disorders that has its roots in the basic tenet of Freudian theory, namely that mental health disorders are rooted in unresolved emotional conflicts from childhood, which have been repressed into the unconscious. It follows that treatment involves bringing these experiences into consciousness and eventual resolution.

Psychogenic autism A term used to describe cases of autism that, according to one particular theory, result from adverse experiences in very early childhood.

Psychosocial (interventions). Interventions in which social interaction is the main vehicle for changing behaviour.

Psychotic/psychotic disorder/psychosis. A severe personality or mental disturbance usually of biological origin though precipitating experiences may also be involved. Sometimes equated with any mental health disorder in which an individual loses touch with reality (in contrast to *neurosis*).

Purkinje cells. Large branching neurons found in the *cortex* of the *cerebellum*.

Quantitative trait loci (QTL) study. A method of *genetic screening* involving a search for gene abnormalities that may be associated with specific behaviours, such as (in the case of autism) 'desire for sameness' or 'age of speech onset'. (See Box 7.1.)

Quasi-autism. See *pseudo-autism*.

Randomisation. A term used in *efficacy studies* to refer to the process by which participants are allocated to treatment or non-treatment groups so as to avoid *sampling bias*. (See Box 14.2.)

Recollection. In memory theory, this term refers to the recall of contextual associations to a target item (e.g., a face, novel word or fact or an event), such as time and place of a previous experience of the target item. Cf. *familiarity*.

Reelin. A protein with a critical role in brain development.

Regressive autism. A diagnostic or descriptive term used to describe cases in which behaviours associated with autism appear in children usually after the age of three years, and following ostensibly normal early development. (Synonymous with *late-onset autism*.)

Relational memory.   Memory for complex, multimodal stimuli and events, including contextual information. Cf. *recollection*.

Reliable.   When used to describe an assessment procedure or diagnostic test, implies that the test in question produces consistent results when used under different conditions, for example, when administered to an individual by different testers or to an individual on different occasions. Various aspects of test reliability can be assessed statistically. Cf. *valid*.

Representation.   A construct used in philosophical and some psychological theories concerning the mind, its properties and functions. Such theories envisage the mind as furnished with images or *symbols* that represent, or stand for, things in the external world, experienced feelings, abstract ideas, etc. Thus, representations may be roughly equated with 'the stuff of thought'. Most representational theories of the mind envisage a hierarchy of at least three levels of representation (see Box 8.1).

Respite care.   Care of an individual by someone or some organisation outside the family (or other full-time carer(s)), for a period of time, often on a regular basis (e.g., one night a week for a child). Provides carers with some respite from their responsibilities to the individual, and provides the individual with opportunity to extend their social relationships and life experiences.

Response inhibition.   Stopping oneself from making a response, especially if there is a strong tendency to make that response. Cf. *prepotent* response.

Reticular activating system.   A structure within the *brain stem* that modulates *arousal* levels amongst other functions.

Rett (Rett's) syndrome.   A rare degenerative disorder occurring only in girls, and which at various stages in its course involves hand stereotypies resembling those that occur in some people with autism, and also loss of language and some degree of social withdrawal.

Reversed asymmetry.   Used here to refer to any reversal of the usual asymmetry between two paired structures in the brain (e.g., the *cerebral hemispheres*, the *frontal lobes*, the right and left *amygdala*e). So, for example, the right prefrontal cortex is larger in volume than the left in most *neurotypical* individuals, but the reverse is true for many individuals with language-related impairments who may thus be described as having 'reversed asymmetry'.

Rote memory.   The recall of items of information (e.g., words, numbers, musical phrases) in sequential order and regardless of meaning.

Sampling bias.   A term widely used in research to refer to bias introduced into a study or experiment by the selection of participants (or other entities under investigation) that are not representative of the population being studied, thus producing findings that are not reliably applicable to that population. (See Box 14.2.)

Savant abilities.   Abilities that are outstanding by comparison with those of members of the general population, and even more striking because they occur in individuals with modest or low intellectual ability and, frequently, autistic features of behaviour. Examples of savant abilities have been documented in the fields of arithmetical calculation, drawing, musical memory and improvisation, foreign language learning, and poetry writing.

Savant. Someone with *savant abilities.* (Note: the term 'idiot savant' is now rarely used.)

Schizoid personality disorder. A mental health disorder characterised by emotional coldness and impaired reciprocal social interaction, abnormalities of verbal and non-verbal *communication,* and obsessive interests. (See Box 2.1.)

Screening. A process of administering clinical tests either to whole populations or to selected populations with the purpose of either making a firm diagnosis of the presence/absence of a particular disease or disorder in individuals within the population tested or to estimate the probability that certain individuals within the population have, or may later be found to have, a particular disease or disorder. (See Box 13.5.)

Sculpting. A figurative term used to describe the processes of *programmed* cell death and *synaptic pruning* that help to shape the structure and *connectivity* of the brain following the period of intensive growth during infancy.

Secondary intersubjectivity. A form of early developing social interaction in which two (or more) individuals attend to a third person, object, action or event and are aware that the person with whom they are interacting is having a similar perceptual/cognitive/emotional experience to their own. Essentially synonymous with *triadic relating,* but with greater allowance for the role of emotion sharing. Cf. *primary intersubjectivity.*

Second-order belief. A belief that someone believes (knows/assumes, etc.) that x, y or z is the case, e.g., Othello believed [first-order belief] that Iago knew [second-order belief] that Desdemona was deceiving him.

Secretin. A peptide hormone produced in the gut that can penetrate the blood–brain barrier and stimulate peptide receptors in the brain.

Selective attention. The process involved in situations involving complex stimuli from which a single stimulus or stimulus feature is selected as the attentional focus. Cf. *over-selective attention.*

Selective mutism. A rare condition in which an individual who understands and can use language normally is inhibited (usually by pathological anxiety) from speaking to particular individuals or in particular locations or contexts, whereas they speak normally in other situations. Synonymous with *elective mutism.*

Self-activation. The motivation, and capacity to act on the motivation, to perform a particular action or to embark on a particular activity. Impaired self-activation occurs in a range of neurological and psychiatric disorders, when it is sometimes referred to as *psychic akinesia.*

Self-injurious behaviours (SIBS). Behaviours in which an individual inflicts injury on themselves, often repetitively and compulsively.

Self-monitoring. The process of comparing one's intended action with the actual ongoing action one is carrying out. Differentiate from *action–outcome monitoring.*

Self–other equivalence/correspondence. The equation of oneself as a person/member of the human species with other persons/members of the species (in contrast to lack of equivalence between oneself and inanimate objects or oneself and members of other species).

Self-regulation/self-regulatory system. In psychology and physiology, a *general-purpose mechanism* operating to maintain an organism or some facet of an organism's functions in *adaptive* equilibrium with its environment.

Semantic memory.   Memory for factual information accompanied by a feeling of knowing/of confidence in the knowledge. A subclass of *declarative memory*.

Semantics.   Knowledge of, or the study of, linguistic meaning, whether at the level of individual words, phrases or sentences.

Sensation/sensory processing.   The processing of raw data from the senses prior to the processes associated with *perception*.

Sensitivity   (as used in the context of *screening* tests). A measure of the efficacy of a screening test based on the proportion of those tested who are correctly identified as having the disease or disorder being screened for, relative to the proportion who have the disorder but are not identified. High sensitivity (i.e., a high proportion) is desirable. (See Box 13.5.)

Sensory modulation.   Variation of the impact of incoming experience on the senses, e.g., increasing or decreasing sensitivity to a particular sound or class of sounds. Partly physiologically determined by states of *arousal*, but may be partly controlled by attentional processes.

Serotonin.   A *neurotransmitter* with important roles in the regulation of mood and of pain, and in the control of eating, sleeping, and *arousal* (alertness). Synonymous with '5-hydroxytryptamine (5-HT)'.

Sex-linked.   A characteristic, disease or disorder (partly) determined by the presence/absence/variation of genes located on the sex chromosomes (i.e., the X- and Y-chromosomes).

Shared attention.   See *joint attention*.

Shared attention mechanism (SAM).   A hypothetical genetically determined mechanism that enables infants approaching their second year to engage in acts of *shared attention* with another person. A component of Baron-Cohen's *mindreading system* (see Figure 8.2).

Short-term memory (STM).   Memory for something very recently experienced, usually with no other stimulation occurring before the memory is recalled and therefore synonymous with *immediate memory*. However, the term is used in a number of slightly different ways within various psychological theories.

Shutdown.   A self-explanatory term often used by high-functioning people with ASDs to describe the defence mechanism they use to avoid over-*arousal* by excessive sensory-perceptual stimulation (see Box 3.2).

Signal-to-noise ratio.   The relationship between a wanted signal conveying information in some form, and unwanted accompanying stimuli, referred to metaphorically as 'noise'.

Simulation.   The capacity to imagine oneself as someone else, with that other person's knowledge, beliefs, feelings, past experiences, etc. Colloquially 'to put oneself in another person's shoes'. Considered by some philosophers and psychologists to offer a better explanation of the acquisition and operation of mindreading abilities than an explanation in terms of representational abilities and theory formation.

Single blind trial.   See *blind trials*.

Single-factor theory/hypothesis.   As used here, any theory or hypothesis concerning the origins of autism that seeks to explain the whole of autism or a named subtype of autism in terms of a single causal factor at one or other level of explanation.

Single Photon Emission Computed Tomography (SPECT). Assesses blood flow using a radioactive 'tracer', from which to infer relations between brain activity and specific behavioural functions. (See Box 7.5.)

Slave system. A subordinate system controlled by a superordinate system or mechanism. In memory theory, used to refer to the *phonological loop* and the *visuospatial sketchpad* in the original model of *working memory* (see main text).

Social brain. A brain system subserving social behaviour that includes the *amygdala*, the *fusiform gyrus*, the *superior temporal sulcus*, the *ventromedial prefrontal cortex*, and *orbitofrontal cortex*.

Social orienting. The innate bias of neonates and very young babies to attend preferentially to social stimuli, in particular to human faces and voices.

Spatial working memory. That aspect of *working memory* that holds and operates on spatial information (e.g., holding in mind the spatial arrangement of furniture in a room whilst mentally rearranging it).

Special educational needs (SEN). A term used in the UK to refer to the needs of individuals who, for whatever reason, are unable to benefit from teaching content and methods designed for typically developing individuals. Those with SENs may include exceptionally gifted individuals, as well as those with a range of problems that interfere with the capacity to learn. Synonymous with *exceptional children* in US usage.

Specificity (as used in the context of *screening* tests). A measure of the efficacy of a screening test based on the proportion of those tested who are correctly identified as having the disease or disorder being screened for relative to the proportion who are incorrectly identified as having the disorder. High specificity is desirable. (See Box 13.5.)

Specificity criterion. A yardstick for assessing the validity of any theoretical explanation of a *neurodevelopmental disorder* or facet of a disorder, e.g., autism. The criterion states that, if a theory proposes that a particular causal factor is both *necessary* and *sufficient* for autism or a particular facet of autism to occur, then that factor must occur only in individuals with autism (or the facet of autism identified in the theory).

Specific language impairment (SLI). Significant delay or anomaly in the acquisition of a first language system that cannot be explained by intellectual disability, sensory impairment, environmental deprivation, autism or other obvious cause.

Specific learning disability/difficulty. The term used in the UK to refer to individuals (usually children) whose learning abilities overall are within the normal range, but in whom one facet of learning ability (often relating to language, literacy or maths) is impaired. Synonymous with *learning disability* in US usage.

Spectrum. A term used in the autism literature based on an analogy between the range of forms, or *dimensional profiles*, in which autism may be manifested and the spectrum of light. The analogy turns on the fact that colours in the light spectrum vary from red to violet with five other identifiable colours in between, but with no clear boundaries between adjacent colours. Similar to *continuum* but with greater emphasis on the breadth of variation within the (autistic) spectrum.

Speech. The output channel for spoken language (just as writing is the output of written language). (See Box 3.5.)

Sporadic. A term used to differentiate between genetic disorders that are inherited via chance abnormality or variation of genetic material in eggs or sperm, as opposed to genetic disorders that are *familial*, i.e. that run in families.

Standardised (as in 'standardised tests'). A formal test (usually of some psychological capacity, i.e., a 'psychometric' test) that has been carried out in rigorous conditions and with large groups of individuals, and the results statistically analysed to yield norms for the population being studied. The test will also have been shown to produce results that are *reliable* and *valid*.

Statistical power. A technical term that refers to the probability, in statistical terms, that a research study fails to detect evidence in support of a hypothesis when that hypothesis is in fact correct. Various factors affect this probability, including the number of participants (or other entities to be examined) included in a study, and how common or marked are the phenomena predicted by the hypothesis (i.e., how easy they are to detect). (See Box 14.3.)

Structural language. Refers to *language* as a system of items and combinatorial rules, knowledge of which is stored in the brain or written down in dictionaries and textbooks on grammar and linguistics. Contrasts with the use of language for *communication*.

Structural magnetic resonance imaging (sMRI). A method of assessing the *neuroanatomy* of the brain at gross structural, volumetric or cellular levels by utilising *magnetic resonance imaging*. (See Box 7.3.)

Stuck in set. A form of *perseveration* in which an individual maintains a *mental set* beyond the point at which it is *adaptive* and appropriate to do so.

Subcortical. Parts of the brain that are not part of the *cerebral cortex*. Evolutionarily older than much of the cerebral cortex and subserving vital but 'lower-order' processes.

Subtypes model. An approach to the classification of diseases and disorders relying on the assumption that there are qualitative differences between different disorders or subtypes of a disorder. Cf. *categorical model*.

Sufficient cause. Any causal factor, or set of causal factors, that, if present, will invariably cause a particular effect/disorder/condition to occur.

Superior temporal sulcus (STS). One of the grooves or fissures lying between two convolutions ('gyri') on the external surface of each *temporal lobe*; that part of the *social brain* involved in processing biological motion.

Supervisory attentional system (SAS). A system comparable to the *central executive* in the original model of *working memory*. Hypothetical components of the system generate goals of activity, maintain these goals in working memory, and make decisions concerning the focus of attention and action necessary to achieve the goals. Cf. *central executive*.

Susceptibility genes. Genes that increase the likelihood of an individual developing a particular characteristic or condition.

Symbol/symbolic/symbolise. A symbol is something that stands for, or represents, something else. The relationship between a symbol and what it stands for can be arbitrary, e.g., most words and what they stand for, or meaningfully linked to what it stands for, e.g., a crucifix and the Christian religion, the storm in *King Lear* and the state of Lear's mind, a blue cloth and a pretend 'river'.

Sympathy. Literally 'feeling with', and sometimes used by psychologists with the same meaning as *emotion contagion*. However, because the term has a much wider and looser meaning in common usage, 'emotion contagion' is preferred in the present book.

Synaesthesia. A neurological condition in which inputs from the different senses become confused, for example, a sound triggering the experience of a particular colour.

Synapse. The junction between the end point of an *axon* from one *neuron* and the *dendrites* of another neuron, across which information is transmitted in the form of electrical impulses.

Synaptic pruning. Loss of less-used connective fibres (*axons* and *dendrites*) and their synapses following early proliferation of fibres. See (brain) *sculpting.*

Synaptogenesis. The formation and development of *synapses.*

Syndrome. A cluster of often seemingly unrelated symptoms or characteristics that may be psychological physical or health-related and are sometimes, but not always, assumed to have a single ultimate cause (as in, for example, the case of *Down syndrome*).

Systemise/systemising mechanism. A tendency (and the hypothetical mechanism underlying this tendency) identified in Baron-Cohen's *extreme male brain* theory, to look for lawful regularities in experience that can be used to predict or calculate outcomes, occurrences, events, etc. Stronger in males than in females, as a general rule. (See also *hypersystemising.*)

Temporal binding. Neural binding that is achieved by the synchronisation of neural activity in diverse brain circuits or regions.

Temporal lobe(s). One of the lobes of the cerebrum, situated below the *frontal* and *parietal lobes* within the lower sides of the skull (see Figure 7.2). Involved in hearing, the integration of information from several senses, and memory processing.

Teratogen. Any environmental agent that causes damage to the *embryo* or *fetus* in utero.

Thalidomide. A drug presecribed for morning sickness until its *teratogenic* effects became known.

Theory of mind (ToM). A coherent understanding of the nature of minds that includes the ability to attribute *mental states* to oneself and others, to understand others have mental states different from one's own, and to reflect on one's own and others' mental states.

Thimerosal. A substance containing mercury that was for a time used as a vaccine preservative.

Top-down. A term used in psychology to describe processes driven more by higher-order principles, expectations or ideas than by incoming sensory data. The opposite of *bottom-up.*

Tourette's syndrome. A neurological disorder characterised by uncontrolled tics, body movements, and vocalisations or other utterances (often obscenities).

Triad. A threesome; any set of three things. As used in the autism literature, the term generally refers to a triad of impairments considered to be diagnostic of autism. However, the term is also used (in the autism literature and elsewhere) in the phrases *triadic relating* or *triadic social interaction* (see *joint/shared attention; secondary intersubjectivity*).

Triadic relating/triadic social interaction. See *secondary intersubjectivity.*

Trichotillomania. Compulsive pulling out of one's own hair.

Tuberous sclerosis. A rare genetic disorder in which benign growths occur in various organs of the body, including the brain. It is frequently associated with seizures, *intellectual disability*, and autistic features of behaviour.

Turner's syndrome. An inherited condition manifesting in females and caused by the absence or abnormality of one of the X-chromosomes. Numerous and variable characteristics include physical anomalies, absence or underdevelopment of female reproductive organs and secondary sexual characteristics and functions, and in some cases mild *intellectual disability* and autistic tendencies.

Typically developing. Used to describe children or adolescents who would be termed 'normal' in everyday speech. (Note: 'typical' is widely preferred to 'normal' in much of the autism literature because the converse of 'typical' is 'non-typical' or 'different', whereas the converse of 'normal' is 'abnormal' or 'subnormal', which is a stigmatising term when applied to people. Cf. *neurotypical*.)

Unimodal. In a single *modality*/sensory channel.

Unitary/unitary disorder. A disorder or condition resulting from a single cause or set of closely related causes with generally *homogeneous* and predictable symptoms, course, outcome and response to treatment.

Universality criterion. A yardstick for assessing the validity of any theoretical explanation of a disorder, or facet of a disorder, e.g., autism. The criterion states that if a theory proposes a particular causal factor is a *necessary* cause of autism, or of some facet of autism, then that causal factor must occur universally in all individuals with autism (or with the facet of autism identified in the theory).

Validity. The property of being true, correct, in conformity with reality. Thus, a valid theory is one that fits well with what is seen in practice or with the findings from research. A valid test or assessment is one that measures what it purports to measure. This can only be judged by comparing the outcomes of a particular test or procedure with the outcomes of other *reliable* tests or procedures used to measure the same thing.

Valproic acid. An anticonvulsant medication, with *teratogenic* effects.

Vasopressin. An *opioid* that acts in association with *oxytocin* to modulate activity within brain circuits mediating various vegetative functions and also social engagement and social reward.

Ventromedial prefrontal cortex. The area that lies towards the front and underside of the *prefrontal cortex*, and that forms part of the *social brain*. May have a role in representing the self.

Verbal abilities. See *verbal intelligence*.

Verbal fluency (test). A test of the ability to generate as many words as possible in reponse to a given cue, such as an initial letter or named category (flowers, animals). (See *fluency*.)

Verbal intelligence. Those aspects of intelligence measured using tests that assess knowledge of language directly; or that require the use of language in the form of *verbal mediation* (*inner speech*) or response output; or that assess the kinds of knowledge obtained via language-mediated learning.

Verbal mediation. See *inner speech*.

Verbal quotient (VQ). The number derived either from a table (as in the Wechsler scales) or from dividing an individual's *mental age* on a verbal intelligence test by their chronological age and multiplying by 100. (See Box 3.7.)

Visual search (tests).   Tests used by psychologists to assess aspects of visual *attention* and *perception* in which a target stimulus (or stimuli) has to be identified within an array of non-target stimuli or other form of visual distraction, often at speed.

Visuospatial sketchpad/scratchpad.   One of the *slave systems* in the original model of *working memory* with the role of maintaining visuospatial information in memory whilst manipulating or otherwise operating on it.

Volition.   The conscious, voluntary selection of a particular action or course of action; a mental decision preceding the initiation of a conscious voluntary action. Synonymous with *conation*.

Volitional.   To do with wanting and willing (see *volition)*. Thus, volitional *mental states* may be conceived of as mental *representations* of various forms of motivation and desire.

Weak central coherence (WCC).   An unusual degree of weakness in the normal drive for *central coherence*, resulting in a tendency to process complex perceptual stimuli as parts rather than as wholes, and a failure to integrate the component parts of higher-order experience, such as narratives or events, into meaningful wholes.

White matter.   Brain tissue consisting of concentrations of *axons*, each covered in a whiteish-coloured *myelin sheath* made up of *glial cells*.

Williams syndrome.   A rare genetic disorder characterised by 'elfin' facial features and other physical anomalies, and generally accompanied by intellectual disability but relatively spared social interaction and language.

Working memory.   A *short-term memory* system in which information is held, and can be maintained by rehearsal, whilst the information is operated on or manipulated. See also *central executive; slave systems; phonological loop; visuospatial sketchpad, spatial working memory*.

Zoom in, zoom out.   Descriptive terms referring, respectively, to the narrowing and broadening of one's focus of *attention*, for example, from looking at the whole of a picture to focusing on a detail, then refocusing back on the whole picture.

REFERENCES

Adrien, J.L., Lenoir, P., Martineau, J., Perrot, A., Hameury, L., Larmande, C., & Sauvage, D. (1993). Blind ratings of early symptoms of autism from family home movies. *Journal of the American Academy of Child and Adolescent Psychiatry, 32*, 617–627.

Ainsworth, M., Blehar, M., Waters, E., & Wall, S. (1978). *Patterns of Attachment*. Hillsdale NJ: Erlbaum.

Allen, G. & Courchesne, E. (2003). Differential effects of developmental cerebellar abnormality on cognitive and motor functions in the cerebellum: An fMRI study of autism. *American Journal of Psychiatry, 160*, 262–273.

Allison, C., Williams, J., Scott, F., Stott, C., Bolton, P., Baron-Cohen, S., & Brayne, C. (2007). The Childhood Asperger Syndrome Test (CAST): Test–retest reliability in a high scoring sample. *Autism, 11*, 173–186.

Alvarez, A. & Reid, S. (1999). *Autism and Personality: Findings from the Tavistock Autism Workshop*. London: Routledge.

Ameli, R., Courchesne, E., Lincoln, A., Kaufman, A., & Grillon, C. (1988). Visual memory processes in high functioning individuals with autism. *Journal of Autism and Developmental Disorders, 18*, 601–615.

American Psychiatric Association (1980). *Diagnostic and Statistical Manual of Mental Disorders*, (3rd edition) (DSM III). Washington, DC: APA.

American Psychiatric Association (1987). *Diagnostic and Statistical Manual of Mental Disorders*, (3rd edition revised) (DSM III-R). Washington, DC: APA.

American Psychiatric Association (1994). *Diagnostic and Statistical Manual of Mental Disorders*, (4th edition) (DSM-IV). Washington, DC: APA.

American Psychiatric Association (2000). *Diagnostic and Statistical Manual of Mental Disorders*, (4th edition, text revised) (DSM-IV-TR). Washington, DC: APA.

Anagnostou, E., Soorya, L., Stamper, K., & Hollander, E. (2006). fMRI for the study of response inhibition, and face and linguistic processing in autism. *Neuropediatrics, 37*, DOI:10.1055/s-2006–945806.

Anderson, G. (2005). Serotonin in autism. In M. Bauman & T. Kemper (Eds.), *The Neurobiology of Autism* (2nd edition) (pp. 303–318). Baltimore: The Johns Hopkins University Press.

Anderson, G. & Hoshino, Y. (2005). Neurochemical studies of autism. In F. Volkmar, R. Paul, A. Klin, & D. Cohen (Eds.), *Handbook of Autism and Pervasive Developmental Disorders, Vol. 2* (3rd edition) (pp. 453–472). Hoboken, NJ: John Wiley & Sons.

Anns, S., Bigham, S., Mayes, A., & Boucher, J. (2008). Development and test of discriminating between the contributions of recollection and familiarity to declarative memory in young or learning disabled individuals with ASDs. Poster presented at the *International Meeting for Autism Research, London, May 2008*.

Ariel, C. & Naseef, R. (2005). *Voices from the Spectrum: Parents, Grandparents, Siblings, People with Autism and Professionals Share their Wisdom*. London: Jessica Kingsley Publishers.

Arndt, T., Stodgell, C., & Rodier, P. (2005). The teratology of autism. *International Journal of Developmental Neuroscience, 23*, 189–199.

Ashwood, P. & Van de Water, J. (2004). Is autism an autoimmune disease? *Autoimmunity Reviews, 3*, 557–562.

Asperger, H. (1944/1991). 'Autistic psychopathy' in childhood. Translated in U. Frith (Ed.), *Autism and Asperger Syndrome* (pp. 37–92). Cambridge: CUP.

Aston, M. (2001). *The Other Half of Asperger Syndrome*. London: National Autistic Society.

Atance, C. & O'Neill, D. (2001). Episodic future thinking. *Trends in Cognitive Sciences, 5*, 533–536.

Atance, C. & O'Neill, D. (2005). The emergence of episodic future thinking in humans. *Learning and Motivation, 36*, 126–134.

Attwood, T. (2000). Strategies for improving the social integration of children with Asperger syndrome. *Autism, 4*, 85–100.

Bachevalier, J. (1991). An animal model for childhood autism. In C. Tamminginga & S. Schultz (Eds.), *Advances in Neuropsychiatry and Psychopharmacology, Vol 1.* (pp. 129–140). New York: Raven Press.

Bachevalier, J. (1994). Medial temporal lobe structures and autism: A review of clinical and experimental findings. *Neuropsychologia, 32*, 627–648.

Bachevalier, J. (2008). Temporal lobe structures and memory in non-human primates: Implications for autism. In J. Boucher & D.M. Bowler (Eds.), *Memory in Autism.* Cambridge: CUP.

Bachevalier, J. & Loveland, K. (2006). The orbitofrontal-amygdala circuit and self-regulation of socio-cmotional behaviour in autism. *Neuroscience Behavioural Review, 30*, 97–117.

Baddeley, A.D. (2000). The episodic buffer: A new component of working memory? *Trends in Cognitive Science, 4*, 417–423.

Baddeley, A.D. (1986). *Working Memory.* Oxford: OUP.

Baieli, S., Pavone, L., Meli, C., Fiumara, A., & Coleman, M. (2003). Autism and phenylketonuria. *Journal of Autism and Developmental Disorders, 33*, 201–204.

Bailey, A., Le Couteur, A., Gottesman, I., Bolton, P., Simonoff, E., Yuzda, E., & Rutter, M. (1995). Autism as a strongly genetic disorder: Evidence from a British twin study. *Psychological Medicine, 25*, 63–77.

Bailey, A., Luther, P., Dean, A., Harding, B., Janota, I., Montgomery, M. et al. (1998). A clinicopathological study of autism. *Brain, 121*, 889–905.

Bailey, A., Phillips, W., & Rutter, M. (1996). Autism: Towards an integration of clinical, genetic, neuropsychological, and neurobiological perspective. *Journal of Child Psychology and Psychiatry, 37*, 89–126.

Baird, G., Charman, T., Baron-Cohen, S., Swettenham, J., Wheelwright, S., & Drew, A. (2000). A screening instrument for detecting autism at 18 months of age: a six-year follow-up study. *Journal of the American Academy of Child and Adolescent Psychiatry, 39*, 694–702.

Baird, G., Simonoff, E., Pickles, A., Chandler, S., Loucas, T., Meldrum, D., & Charman, T. (2006). Prevalence of disorders of the autism spectrum in a population cohort of children in South Thames: The Special Needs and Autism Project (SNAP). *The Lancet, 368*, 210–215.

Baker, S. (2001). Unregulated dietary supplements: Bitter medicine for children. *Journal of Pediatric Gastroenterology, 33*, 439–441.

Baranek, G. (1999). Autism during infancy: A retrospective video analysis of sensory-motor and social behaviours at 9–12 months of age. *Journal of Autism and Developmental Disorders, 29*, 213–224.

Barnard, J., Harvey, V., Potter, D., & Prior, A. (2001). *The Reality for Adults with Autistic Spectrum Disorders.* London: National Autistic Society.

Barnhill, A. Clinard (2007). *At Home in the Land of Oz: My Sister, Autism, and Me.* London: Jessica Kingsley Publishers.

Baron-Cohen, S. (1989a). Do autistic children have obsessions and compulsions? *British Journal of Clinical Psychology, 28*, 193–2000.

Baron-Cohen, S. (1989b). The autistic child's theory of mind: A case of specific developmental delay. *Journal of Child Psychology and Psychiatry, 30*, 285–298.

Baron-Cohen, S. (1991). Do people with autism understand what causes emotion? *Child Development, 62*, 385–395.

Baron-Cohen, S. (1995). *Mindblindness: An Essay on Autism and Theory of Mind.* Cambridge, MA: The MIT Press.

Baron-Cohen, S. (1999). The evolution of a theory of mind. In M. Corballis & S. Lea (Eds.), *The Descent of Mind* (pp. 261–277). Oxford: OUP.

Baron-Cohen, S. (2000). Is Asperger syndrome/high-functioning autism necessarily a disability? *Development and Psychopathology, 12*, 489–500.

Baron-Cohen, S. (2005). The Empathizing System: A revision of the 1994 model of the Mindreading System. In B. Ellis & D. Bjorklund (Eds.), *Origins of the Social Mind* (pp. 468–492). New York: Guilford Press.

Baron-Cohen, S. (2006). Two new theories of autism: Hyper-systemising and assortative mating. *Archives of Diseases of Childhood, 91*, 2–5.

Baron-Cohen, S., Baldwin, D., & Crowson, M. (1997). Do children with autism use the speaker's direction of gaze (SDG) strategy to crack the code of language? *Child Development, 68*, 48–57.

Baron-Cohen, S., Cox, A., Baird, G., Swettenham, J., Nightingale, N., Morgan, K., Drew, A., & Charman, T. (1996). Psychological markers in the detection of autism in infancy in a large population. *British Journal of Psychiatry, 168*, 158–163.

Baron-Cohen, S., Hoekstra, R., Knickmeyer, R., & Wheelwright, S. (2006). The Autism-Spectrum Quotient (AQ) – Adolescent version. *Journal of Autism and Developmental Disorders, 36*, 343–350.

Baron-Cohen, S., Knickmeyer, R., & Belmonte, M. (2005). Sex differences in the brain: Implications for explaining autism. *Science, 310* (5749), 819–823.

Baron-Cohen, S., Leslie, A., & Frith, U. (1985). Does the autistic child have a 'theory of mind'? *Cognition, 21*, 37–47.

Baron-Cohen, S., Ring, H., Wheelwright, S., Ashwin, C., & Williams, S.C.R. (2000). The amygdala theory of autism. *Neuroscience and Biobehavioural Reviews, 24*, 355–364.

Baron-Cohen, S., Wheelwright, S., Skinner, R., Martin, J., & Clubley, E. (2001). The Autism Spectrum Quotient (AQ): Evidence from Asperger syndrome/high functioning autism, males and females, scientists and mathematicians. *Journal of Autism and Developmental Disorders, 31*, 5–18.

Bartak, L., Rutter, M., & Cox, A. (1975). A comparative study of infantile autism and receptive developmental language disorder: I. The children. *British Journal of Psychiatry, 126*, 127–145.

Barth, C., Fein, D., & Waterhouse, L. (1995). Delayed match-to-sample performance in autistic children. *Developmental Neuropsychology, 11*, 53–69.

Bartlett, C., Flax, J., Logue, M., Brett, J., Smith, D., Vieland, J., Tallal, P., & Brzustowicz, L. (2004). Examination of potential overlap in autism and language loci on chromosomes 2, 7, and 13 in two independent samples ascertained for specific language impairment. *Human Heredity, 57*, 10–20.

Bartolucci, G., Pierce, S., Streiner, D., & Tolkin-Eppel, P. (1976). Phonological investigation of verbal autistic and mentally retarded subjects. *Journal of Autism and Childhood Schizophrenia, 6*, 303–315.

Bates, E. (1990). Language about me and you: Pronominal reference and the emerging concept of self. In D.C. Cicchetti & M. Beeghly (Eds.), *The Self in Transition: Infancy to Childhood.* Chicago, IL: The University of Chicago Press.

Batten, A., Corbett, C., Rosenblatt, M., Withers, L., & Yuille, R. (2006). *Make School Make Sense*. London: National Autistic Society.

Bauman, M.L. & Kemper, T.L. (2003). The Neuropathology of Autism spectrum disorders: What have we learned? In G. Bock & J. Goode (Eds.), *Autism: Neural Bases and Treatment Possibilities* (pp. 112–128). Chichester, UK: John Wiley & Sons for the Novartis Foundation.

Bauman, M.L. & Kemper, T.L. (2005a). Structural brain anatomy in autism: What is the evidence? In M. L. Bauman & T.L. Kemper (Eds.), *The Neurobiology of Autism* (pp. 121–135). Baltimore: The Johns Hopkins University Press.

Bauman, M.L. & Kemper, T.L. (2005b). *The Neurobiology of Autism*. Baltimore: The Johns Hopkins University Press.

Bauminger, N. & Shulman, C. (2003). The development and maintenance of friendship in high-functioning children with autism: Maternal perceptions. *Autism, 7*, 81–97.

Bee, H. & Boyd, D. (2007). *The Developing Child* (11th edition). New York: Pearson Education.

Belmonte, M., Allen, G., Beckel-Mitchener, A., Boulanger, L., Carper, R., & Webb, S. (2004b). Autism and abnormal development of brain connectivity. *The Journal of Neuroscience, 24*, 9228–9231.

Belmonte, M. & Carper, R. (2006). Monozygotic twins with Asperger syndrome: Differences in behaviour reflect variations in brain structure and function. *Brain and Cognition, 61*, 110–121.

Belmonte, M., Cook, E., Anderson, G., Rubenstein, R., Greenough, W., Beckel-Mitchener, A., Courchesne, E., Boulanger, L., Powell, S., Levitt, P., Perry, K., Jiang, Y., DeLory, T., & Tierney, E. (2004a). Autism as a disorder of neural information processing: Directions for research and targets for therapy. *Molecular Psychiatry, 9*, 646–663.

Bender, L. (1956). Schizophrenia in childhood: Its recognition, description and treatment. *American Journal of Orthopsychiatry, 26*, 499–506.

Bennett, H., Wood, C., & Hare, D.J. (2005). Providing care for adults with autistic spectrum disorders in learning disability services: Needs-based or diagnosis-driven? *Journal of Applied Research in Intellectual Disabilities, 18*, 51–64.

Bennetto, L., Pennington, B., & Rogers, S. (1996). Intact and impaired memory functions in autism. *Child Development, 67*, 1816–1835.

Ben Shalom, D. (2000a). Autism: Emotions without feelings. *Autism, 4*, 205–207.

Ben Shalom, D. (2000b). Developmental depersonalisation: The prefrontal cortex and self-functions in autism. *Consciousness and Cognition, 9*, 457–460.

Ben Shalom, D. (2003). Memory in autism: Review and synthesis. *Cortex, 39*, 1129–1138.

Berk, L. & Ashkenaz, J. (2006). *Child Development* (7th edition). Boston, MA: Pearson Education.

Bespalova, I., Reichert, J., & Buxbaum, J. (2005). Candidate susceptibility genes for autism. In M. Bauman & T. Kemper (Eds.), *The Neurobiology of Autism*. Baltimore: The Johns Hopkins University Press.

Betrand, J., Mars, A., Boyle, C., Bove, F., Yeargin-Allsop, M., & Decoufle, P. (2001). Prevalence of autism in a United States population: The Brick Township, New Jersey, investigation. *Pediatrics, 108*, 1155–1161.

Bettelheim, B. (1967). *The Empty Fortress: Infantile Autism and the Birth of Self*. New York: The Free Press.

Beversdorf, D., Manning, S., Hillier, A., Anderson, S., Nordgren, R., Walter, S., Nagaraja, H., Cooley, W., Gaelic, S., & Bauman, M. (2005). Timing of prenatal stressors and autism. *Journal of Autism and Developmental Disorders, 35*, 471–478.

Bigham, S. (2008). Comprehension of pretence in children with autism. *British Journal of Developmental Psychology, 26*, 265–280.

Biro, S. & Russell, J. (2001). The execution of arbitrary procedures by children with autism. *Development and Psychopathology, 13*, 97–110.

Bishop, D.V.M. (1989). Asperger's syndrome and semantic-pragmatic disorder: Where are the boundaries? *British Journal of Disorders of Communication, 24*, 107–121.

Bishop, D.V.M. (1998). Development of the Children's Communication Checklist (CCC): A method for assessing qualitative aspects of communicative impairment in children. *Journal of Child Psychiatry and Psychology, 39*, 879–891.

Bishop, D.V.M. (2006). Developmental cognitive genetics: How psychology can inform genetics and vice versa. *Quarterly Journal of Experimental Psychology, 59*, 1153–1168.

Bishop, D.V.M. & Norbury, C. (2002). Exploring the borderlands of autistic disorder and specific language impairment: A study using standardised diagnostic instruments. *Journal of Child Psychology and Psychiatry, 43*, 917–929.

Blatt, G. (2005). The GABAergic system in autism. In M. Bauman & T.Kemper (Eds.), *The Neurobiology of Autism* (2nd edition) (pp. 319–330). Baltimore: The Johns Hopkins University Press.

Bloom, P. (2000). *How Children Learn the Meanings of Words.* Cambridge, MA: MIT Press.

Boger-Megiddo, I., Shaw, D.W., Friedman, S., Sparks, B., Artru, A., Giedd, J., Dawson, G., & Dager, S. (2006). Corpus callosum morphometrics in young children with autism spectrum disorder. *Journal of Autism and Developmental Disorders, 36*, 733–739.

Boggs, K., Gross, A., & Gohm, C. (2006). Validity of the Asperger Syndrome Diagnostic Scale. *Journal of Autism and Developmental Disorders, 36*, 163–182.

Bolton, P., Murphy, M., Macdonald, H., Whitlock, B., Pickles, A., & Rutter, M. (1997). Obstetric complications in autism: Causes or consequences of the condition? *Journal of the American Academy of Child and Adolescent Psychiatry, 36*, 272–281.

Bonara, E., Beyer, K., Lamb, J., Par, J., Klauk, S., Benner, A., Paolucci, M., Abbott, A., Ragoussis, I., Poustka, A., Bailey, A., & Manaco, A. (2003). Analysis of reelin as a candidate gene for autism. *Molecular Psychiatry, 8*, 885–892.

Bott, L., Brock, J., Brockdorff, N., Boucher, J., & Lamberts, K. (2006). Perceptual similarity in autism. *Quarterly Journal of Experimental Psychology, 59*, 1237–1254.

Botting, N. & Conti-Ramsden, G. (2003). Autism, primary pragmatic difficulties, and specific language impairment: Can we distinguish them using psycholinguistic markers? *Developmental Medicine and Child Neurology, 45*, 515–524.

Boucher, J. (1976). Articulation in early childhood autism. *Journal of Autism and Childhood Schizophrenia, 6*, 297–302.

Boucher, J. (1977). Alternation and sequencing behaviour, and response to novelty in autistic children. *Journal of Child Psychology and Psychiatry, 18*, 67–72.

Boucher, J. (1981a). Immediate free recall in early childhood autism: Another point of behavioural similarity with the amnesic syndrome. *British Journal of Psychology, 72*, 211–215.

Boucher, J. (1981b). Memory for recent events in autistic children. *Journal of Autism and Developmental Disorders, 11*, 293–302.

Boucher, J. (1988). Word fluency in high functioning autistic children. *Journal of Autism and Developmental Disorders, 18*, 637–645.

Boucher, J. (1996a). The inner life of children with autistic difficulties. In V. Varma (Ed.), *The Inner life of Children with Special Needs* (pp. 81–94). London: Whurr Press.

Boucher, J. (1996b). What could possibly explain autism? In P. Carruthers & P.K. Smith (Eds.), *Theories of Theory of Mind* (pp. 223–241). Oxford: OUP.

Boucher, J. (2000). Time-parsing, normal language acquisition, and language-related developmental disorders. In M. Perkins & S. Howard (Eds.), *New Directions in Language Development and Disorders* (pp. 13–23). London: Kluwer Academic/Plenum Publishers.

Boucher, J. (2001). Lost in a sea of time: Time-parsing and autism. In C. Hoerl & T. McCormack (Eds.), *Time and Memory* (pp. 111–135). Oxford: Clarendon Press.

Boucher, J. (2003). Language development in autism. *International Journal of Pediatric Otorhinolaryngology, 67S1,* S159–S164.

Boucher, J. (2006). Is the search for a unitary explanation of autism justified? *Journal of Autism and Developmental Disorders, 36,* 289.

Boucher, J. (2007). Memory and generativity in very high functioning autism: A firsthand account and an interpretation. *Autism, 11,* 255–264.

Boucher, J., Bigham, S., Mayes, A., & Muskett, T. (2008). Recognition and language in low-functioning autism. *Journal of Autism and Developmental Disorders, 38,* 1259–1269.

Boucher, J., Cowell, P., Howard, M., Broks, P., Farrant, A., Roberts, N., & Mayes, A. (2005). A combined clinical neuropsychological and neuroanatomical study of adults with high-functioning autism. *Cognitive Neuropsychiatry, 10,* 165–214.

Boucher, J. & Lewis, V. (1989). Memory impairments and communication in relatively able autistic children. *Journal of Child Psychology and Psychiatry, 30,* 99–122.

Boucher, J. & Lewis, V. (1992). Unfamiliar face recognition in relatively able autistic children. *Journal of Child Psychology and Psychiatry, 33,* 843–860.

Boucher, J., Mayes, A., & Bigham, S. (2008). Memory, language, and intellectual ability in low functioning autism. In J. Boucher & D.M. Bowler (Eds.), *Memory in Autism.* Cambridge: CUP.

Boucher, J., Pons, F., Lind, S., & Williams, D. (2007). Temporal cognition in children with autistic spectrum disorders: Tests of diachronic thinking. *Journal of Autism and Developmental Disorders, 37,* 1413–1429.

Boucher, J. & Warrington, E. (1976). Memory deficits in early infantile autism: Some similarities to the amnesic syndrome. *British Journal of Psychology, 67,* 73–87.

Bowlby, J. (1953). *Child Care and the Growth of Love.* London: Pelican Books.

Bowlby, J. (1973). *Attachment and Loss, Vol. 2. Separation and Anxiety* (pp. 292–312). New York: Basic Books.

Bowler, D.M. (2001). Autism: Specific cognitive deficit or emergent end point of multiple interacting systems? In J. Burack, T. Charman, N. Yirmiya, & P.R. Zelazo (Eds.), *The Development of Autism: Perspectives From Theory and Research* (pp. 219–236). Mahwah, NJ: Lawrence Erlbaum Associates.

Bowler, D.M. (2007). *Autism Spectrum Disorders: Psychological Theory and Research.* Chichester: John Wiley & Sons.

Bowler, D.M., Briskman, J., Gurvidi, N., & Fornells-Ambrojo, M. (2005). Understanding the mind or predicting signal-dependent action? Performance of children with and without autism on analogues of the false-belief task. *Journal of Cognition and Development, 6,* 259–283.

Bowler, D.M., Gardiner, J., & Berthollier, N. (2004). Source memory in adolescents and adults with Asperger syndrome. *Journal of Autism and Developmental Disorders, 34,* 533–542.

Bowler, D.M., Gardiner, J., & Grice, S. (2000). Episodic memory and remembering in adults with Asperger syndrome. *Journal of Autism and Developmental Disorders, 30,* 295–304.

Bowler, D.M., Matthews, N., & Gardiner, J. (1997). Asperger syndrome and memory: Similar to autism but not amnesia. *Neuropsychologia, 35,* 65–70.

Boyd, B. (2002). Examining the relationship between stress and lack of social support in mothers of children with autism. *Focus on Autism and Other Developmental Disabilities, 17,* 208–215.

Broadstock, M., Doughty, C., & Eggleston, M. (2007). Systematic review of the effectiveness of pharmacological treatments for adolescents and adults with autism spectrum disorder. *Autism, 11,* 335–348.

Brock, J., Brown, C., Boucher, J., & Rippon, G. (2002). The temporal binding deficit hypothesis of autism. *Development and Psychopathology*, *14*, 209–224.

Bromley, J., Hare, D., Davison, K., & Emerson, E. (2004). Mothers supporting children with autistic spectrum disorders: Social support, mental health status and satisfaction with services. *Autism*, *8*, 409–423.

Brothers, L. (1990). The neural basis of primates' social communication. *Motivation and Emotion*, *14*, 81–91.

Brothers, L. (1997). *Friday's Footprint: How Society Shapes the Human Mind*. Oxford: OUP.

Buitelaar, J. (2003). Why have drug treatments been so disappointing? In G. Bock & J. Goode (Eds.), *Autism: Neural Basis and Treatment Possibilities* (pp. 235–44). Chichester: John Wiley & Sons for the Novartis Foundation.

Butter, E., Wynn, J., & Mulick, J. (2003). Early intervention critical to autism treatment. *Pediatric Annals*, *32*, 677–684.

Campbell, J. (2005). Diagnostic assessment of Asperger's disorder: A review of five third-party rating scales. *Journal of Autism and Developmental Disorders*, *35*, 25–37.

Capps, L., Yirmiya, N., & Sigman, M. (1992). Understanding of simple and complex emotions in non-retarded children with autism. *Journal of Child Psychology and Psychiatry*, *33*, 1169–1182.

Cardy, O., Flagg, E., Roberts, W., Brian, J., & Roberts, T. (2005). Magnetoencephalography identifies rapid temporal processing deficit in autism and language impairment. *NeuroReport*, *16*, 329–332.

Carlson, N.R. (2007). *Physiology of Behaviour*. New York: Pearson Education.

Carpenter, P., Just, M., Keller, T., Cherkassky, V., Roth, J., & Minshew, N. (2001). Dynamic cortical systems subserving cognition: fMRI studies with typical and atypical individuals. In J. McClelland & R. Siegler (Eds.), *Mechanisms of Cognitive Development: Behavioral and Neural Perspectives* (pp. 353–383). Mahwah NJ: Lawrence Erlbaum Associates.

Carruthers, P. (1996). Autism as mindblindness: An elaboration and partial defence. In P. Carruthers & P.K. Smith (Eds.), *Theories of Theory of Mind* (pp. 257–273). Cambridge: CUP.

Carter, A.S., Volkmar, F., Sparrow, S., Wang, J-J., Lord, C., Dawson, G., Fombonne, E., Loveland, K., Mesibov, G., & Schopler, E. (1998). The Vineland Adaptive Behaviour Scales: Supplementary norms for individuals with autism. *Journal of Autism and Developmental Disorders*, *28*, 287–302.

Carter, C.S. (2007). Sex differences in oxytocin and vasopressin: Implications for autism spectrum disorders? *Behavioural Brain Research*, *176*, 170–186.

Casanova, M., Van Kooten, I., Switala, A., Van Engeland, H., Heinsen, H., & Steinbusch, H. (2006). Minicolumnar abnormalities in autism. *Acta Neuropathologica*, *112*, 287–303.

Cesaroni, L. & Garber, M. (1991). Exploring the experience of individuals through first-hand accounts from high-functioning individuals with autism. *Journal of Autism and Developmental Disorders*, *21*, 303–314.

Chakrabati, S. & Fombonne, E. (2000). Pervasive developmental disorders in preschool children. *American Journal of the American Medical Association*, *285*, 3093–3099.

Chandana, S., Behen, M., Juhasz, C., Muzik, O., Rothermel, R., Thomas, J., Mangner, T., Chakraborty, P., Harry, T., Chugani, H., & Chugani, D. (2005). Significance of abnormalities in developmental trajectory and asymmetry of cortical serotonin synthesis in autism. *International Journal of Developmental Neuroscience*, *23*, 171–182.

Charman, T. (2002). The prevalence of autistic spectrum disorders. *European Child and Adolescent Psychiatry*, *11*, 249–256.

Charman, T., Swettenham, J., Baron-Cohen, S., Cox, A., Baird, G., & Drew, A. (1997). Infants with autism: An investigation of empathy, pretend play, joint attention, and imitation. *Developmental Psychology*, *33*, 781–789.

Chavez, B. & Chavez-Brown, M. (2006). Role of risperidone in children with autism spectrum disorder. *The Annals of Pharmacotherapy, 40*, 909–916.

Chen, W., Landau, S., Sham, P., & Fombonne, E. (2004). No evidence for links between autism, MMR and measles virus. *Psychological Medicine, 34*, 543–553.

Chess, S. (1971). Autism in children with congenital rubella. *Journal of Autism and Childhood Schizophrenia, 1*, 33–47.

Chess, S. (1977). Follow-up report on autism in congenital rubella. *Journal of Autism and Childhood Schizophrenia, 7*, 69–81.

Chugani, D.C. (2002). Role of altered brain serotonin mechanisms in autism. *Molecular Psychiatry, 7*, S16–S17.

Churchill, D.W. (1972). The relation of infantile autism and early childhood schizophrenia to developmental language disorders of childhood. *Journal of Autism and Childhood Schizophrenia, 2*, 182–197.

Clark, A. (1997). *Being There: Putting Brain, Body and World Together Again*. Cambridge, MA: MIT Press.

Cline, T. & Baldwin, S. (2004). *Selective Mutism in Children*. London: Whurr Press.

Collacott, R.A., Cooper, S.A., Branford, D., & McGrother, C. (1998). Epidemiology of self-injurious behaviour in adults with learning disabilities. *The British Journal of Psychiatry, 173*, 428–432.

Coltheart, M. & Langdon, R. (1998). Autism, modularity and levels of explanation in cognitive science. *Mind and Language, 13*, 138–152.

Coonrod, E. & Stone, W.L. (2005). Screening for autism in young children. In F. Volkmar, R. Paul, A. Klin, & D. Cohen (Eds.), *Handbook of Autism and Pervasive Developmental Disorders, Vol. 2* (3rd edition) (pp. 707–729). Hoboken, NJ: John Wiley & Sons.

Corbett, B., Mendoza, S., Abdullah, M., Wegelin, J., & Levine, S. (2006). Cortisol circadian rhythms and response to stress in children with autism. *Psychoneuroendocrinology, 31*, 59–68.

Corsello, C. (2005). Early intervention in autism. *Infants and Young Children, 18*, 74–85.

Courchesne, E. (2004). Brain development in autism: Early overgrowth followed by premature arrest of growth. *Mental Retardation and Developmental Disabilities Research Reviews, 10*, 106–111.

Courchesne, E. & Pierce, K. (2005). Why the frontal cortex in autism might be talking only to itself: Local over-connectivity but long-distance disconnection. *Current Opinion in Neurobiology, 15*, 225–230.

Creak, M. (1961). Schizophrenic syndrome in childhood: Progress report of a working party. *Cerebral Palsy Bulletin, 3*, 501–504.

Croen, L., Najjar, D., Ray, G., Lotspeich, L., & Bernal, P. (2006). A comparison of health-care utilization and costs in children with and without autism spectrum disorders in a large-group model health plan. *Pediatrics, 118*, 1203–1211.

Crozier, S. & Tincani, M. (2007). Effects of social stories on prosocial behaviour of preschool children with autistm spectrum disorders. *Journal of Autism and Developmental Disorders, 37*, 1803–1814.

Curcio, F. (1978). Sensorimotor functioning and communication in mute autistic children. *Journal of Autism and Childhood Schizophrenia, 2*, 264–287.

Dakin, S. & Frith, U. (2005). Vagaries of visual perception in autism. *Neuron, 48*, 497–507.

Dale, E., Jahoda, A., & Knott, F. (2006). Mothers' attributions following their child's diagnosis of autistic spectrum disorder: Exploring links with maternal levels of stress, depression and expectations about their child's future. *Autism, 10*, 463–479.

Damasio, A. & Maurer, R. (1978). A neurological model for childhood autism. *Archives of Neurology, 35*, 777–786.

Dapretto, M., Davies, M.S., Pfeifer, J., Scott, A.A., Sigman, M., Bookheimer, S.Y., & Iacoboni, M. (2006). Understanding emotions in others: Mirror neuron dysfunction in children with autism spectrum disorders. *Nature Neuroscience, 9*, 28–30.

Dawson, G. (1989). *Autism: Nature, Diagnosis and Treatment.* New York: Guilford Press.

Dawson, G. (1991). A psychobiological perspective on the early socioemotional development of children with autism. In S. Toth & D. Cicchetti (Eds.), *Rochester Symposium on Developmental Psychopathology, Vol. 3* (pp. 207–234). Hillsdale, NJ: Erlbaum.

Dawson, G., Estes, A., Munson, J., Schellenberg, G., Bernier, R., & Abbott, R. (2007). Quantitative assessment of autism symptom-related traits in probands and parents: Broader Autism Phenotype Symptom Scale. *Journal of Autism and Developmental Disorders, 37*, 523–536.

Dawson, G. & McKissick, F.C. (1984). Self-recognition in autistic children. *Journal of Autism and Developmental Disorders, 14*, 383–394.

Dawson, G., Meltzoff, A., Osterling, J., & Rinaldi, J. (1998a). Neuropsychological correlates of early autistic symptoms. *Child Development, 69*, 1247–1482.

Dawson, G., Meltzoff, A., Osterling, J., Rinaldi, J., & Brown, E. (1998b). Children with autism fail to orient to naturally occurring social stimuli. *Journal of Autism and Developmental Disorders, 28*, 479–485.

Dawson, G., Munson, J., Estes, A., Osterling, J., McPartland, J., Toth, K., Carver, L., & Abbott, R. (2002). Neurocognitive function and joint attention ability in young children with autism spectrum disorder versus developmental delay. *Child Development, 73*, 345–358.

Dawson, G., Osterling, J., Meltzoff, A., & Kuhl, P. (2000). Case study of the development of an infant from birth to two years of age. *Journal of Applied Developmental Psychology, 21*, 299–313.

Dawson, G., Osterling, J., Rinaldi, J., Carver, L., & McPartland, J. (2001). Recognition memory and stimulus-reward associations: Indirect support for the role of the ventromedial prefrontal dysfunction in autism. *Journal of Autism and Developmental Disorders, 31*, 337–341.

Dawson, G., Toth, K., Abbott, R., Osterling, J., Munson, J., Estes, A., & McPartland, J. (2004). Early social attention impairments in autism: Social orienting, joint attention, and attention to distress. *Developmental Psychology, 40*, 271–283.

Dawson, G. & Watling, R. (2000). Interventions to facilitate auditory, visual, and motor integration in autism: A review of the evidence. *Journal of Autism and Developmental Disorders, 30*, 415–421.

Dawson, G., Webb, S.J., & McPartland, J. (2005). Understanding of the nature of face processing in autism: Insights from behavioural and electrophysiological studies. *Developmental Neuropsychology, 27*, 403–424.

Dawson, G., Webb, S., Schellenberg, G., Aylward, E., Richards, T., Dager, S., & Friedman, S. (2002). Defining the broader phenotype of autism: Genetic, brain, and behavioural perspectives. *Development and Psychopathology, 14*, 581–611.

Dawson, G. & Zanolli, K. (2003). Early intervention and brain plasticity in autism. *In Autism: Neural Basis and Treatment Possibilities* (pp. 266–280). Chichester: John Wiley & Sons for the Novartis Foundation.

Dawson, M., Soulières, I., Gernsbacher, M.-A., & Mottron, L. (2007). The level and nature of autistic intelligence. *Psychological Science, 18*, 657–662.

DeLong, G.R. (1978). A neuropsychological interpretation of infantile autism. In M. Rutter & E. Schopler (Eds.), *Autism* (pp. 207–218). New York: Plenum Press.

DeLong, G.R. (1992). Autism, amnesia, hippocampus, and learning. *Neuroscience and Biobehavioural Reviews, 16*, 63–72.

DeLong, G.R. (2007). GABA(A) receptor alpha5 subunit as a candidate gene for autism and bipolar disorder: A proposed endophenotype with parent-of-origin and gain-of-function features, with or without oculocutaneous albinism. *Autism, 11*, 135–147.

DeLong, G.R. & Heinz, E. (1997). The clinical syndrome of early-life bilateral hippocampal sclerosis. *Annals of Neurology, 43*, 687.

Deonna, T., Ziegler, A.-L., Moura-Serra, J., & Innocenti, G. (1993). Autistic regression in relation to limbic pathology and epilepsy: Report of two cases. *Developmental Medicine and Child Neurology, 35*, 158–177.

DeMyer, M., Alpern, G., Barton, S., DeMyer, W., Churchill, D., Hingten, J., Bryson, C., Pontius, W., & Kimberlin, C. (1972). Imitation in autistic, early schizophrenic, and non-psychotic subnormal children. *Journal of Autism and Developmental Disorders, 2*, 264–287.

DeMyer, M., Barton, S., Alpern, G., Kimberlin, C., Allen, J., Yang, E., & Steele, R. (1974). The measured learning abilities of autistic children. *Journal of Autism and Childhood Schizophrenia, 4*, 42–60.

Department of Education and Science (Ireland) (2006). *An Evaluation of Educational Provision for Children with Autistic Spectrum Disorders.* www.education.ie/servlet/blobservlet/des_autismreport_foreword.htm

De Villiers, J. (2000). Language and theory of mind: What are the developmental relationships? In S. Baron-Cohen, H. Tager-Flusberg, & D. Cohen (Eds.), *Understanding Other Minds: Perspectives from Developmental Cognitive Neuroscience* (2nd edition) (pp. 83–123). Oxford: OUP.

DiCiccio-Bloom, E., Lord, C., Zwaigenbaum, L., Courchesne, E., Dager, S., Schmitz, C., Schultz, R., Crawley, J., & Young, L. (2006). The developmental neurobiology of autism spectrum disorder. *The Journal of Neuroscience, 26*, 6897–6906.

Dickerson-Mayes, S. & Calhoun, S. (2003). Analysis of WISC-III, Stanford-Binet IV, and Academic Achievement Test scores in children with autism. *Journal of Autism and Developmental Disorders, 33*, 329–342.

Dietz, C., Swinkels, S., van Daalen, E., van Engeland, H., & Buitelaar, J.K. (2006). Screening for autistic spectrum disorder in children aged 14–15 months. II: Population screening with the Early Screening of Autistic Traits questionnaire (ESAT). Design and general findings. *Journal of Autism and Developmental Disorders, 36*, 713–722.

Dissanayake, C., Sigman, M., & Kasari, C. (1996). Long-term stability of individual differences in the emotional responsiveness of children with autism. *Journal of Child Psychology and Psychiatry, 37*, 461–468.

Dobbinson, S. (2000). Repetitiveness and productivity in the language of adults with autism. Unpublished PhD thesis, University of Sheffield, UK.

Doja, A. & Roberts, W. (2006). Immunizations and autism: A review of the literature. *Canadian Journal of Neurological Sciences, 33*, 431–436.

Dykens, E. (2002). Are jigsaw puzzle skills 'spared' in persons with Prader-Willi syndrome? *Journal of Child Psychology and Psychiatry, 43*, 343–352.

Dykens, E., Sutcliffe, J., & Levitt, P. (2005). Autism and 15q11-q13 disorders: Behavioural, genetic, and pathophysiological issues. *Mental Retardation and Developmental Disabilities Research Reviews, 10*, 284–291.

Dziuk, A., Larson, J.G., Apostu, A., Mahone, E., Denkla, M., & Mostofsky, S. (2007). Dyspraxia in autism: Association with motor, social, and communicative deficits. *Developmental Medicine and Child Neurology, 49*, 734–739.

Ehlers, S. & Gillberg, C. (1993). The epidemiology of Asperger syndrome. *Journal of Child Psychology and Psychiatry, 34*, 1327–1350.

Ehlers, S., Gillberg, C., & Wing, L. (1999). Screening Questionnaire for Asperger Syndrome. *Journal of Autism and Developmental Disorders, 29*, 129–141.

Eigsti, I., Bennetto, L., & Dadlani, M. (2007). Beyond pragmatics: Morphosyntactic development in autism. *Journal of Autism and Developmental Disorders, 37*, 1573–3432.

ElChaar, G., Maisch, N., Augusto, L., & Wehring, H. (2006). Efficacy and safety of Naltrexone use in pediatric patients with autistic disorder. *The Annals of Pharmacotherapy, 40*, 1086–1095.

Elia, M., Ferri, R., Musumeci, S., Del Gracco, S., Bottitta, M., Scuderi, C., Miano, G., Panerai, S., Bertrand, T., & Grubar, J. (2000). Sleep in subjects with autistic disorder: A neurophysiological and psychological study. *Brain Development, 22*, 88–92.

Elman, J., Bates, E., Johnson, M., Karmiloff-Smith, A., Parisi, D., & Plunkett, K. (1996). *Rethink-ing Innateness: A Connectionist Perspective on Development*. Cambridge, MA: MIT Press.

Erickson, C., Stigler, K., Corkins, M., Posey, D., Fitzgerald, J., & McDougle, C. (2005). Gastrointestinal factors in autistic disorder: A critical review. *Journal of Autism and Developmental Disorders, 35*, 713–727.

Faran, Y. & Ben Shalom, D. (2008). Possible parallels between memory and emotion processing in autism: A neuropsychological perspective. In J. Boucher & D.M. Bowler (Eds.), *Memory in Autism*. Cambridge: CUP.

Fatemi, S. ((2005). The role of reelin in autism. In M. Bauman and T. Kemper (Eds.), *The Neurobiology of Autism* (2nd edition) (pp. 349–361). Baltimore: The Johns Hopkins University Press.

Fay, W. & Schuler, A.L. (1980). *Emerging Language in Autistic Children*. London: Edward Arnold.

Feldman, R. (2007). Parent-infant synchrony and the construction of shared timing; physiological precursors, developmental outcomes, and risk conditions. *Journal of Child Psychology and Psychiatry, 48*, 329–354.

Ferster, C.B. (1961). Positive reinforcement and behavioural deficits of autistic children. *Child Development, 32*, 437–456.

Fisher, N., Happé, F., & Dunn, J. (2005). The relationship between vocabulary, grammar, and false belief task performance in children with autistic spectrum disorders and children with moderate learning difficulties. *Journal of Child Psychology and Psychiatry, 46*, 409–419.

Fisher, S. (2006). Tangled webs: Tracing the connections between genes and cognition. *Cognition, 101*, 270–297.

Florian, L., Dee, L., Byers, R., & Maudslay, L. (2000). What happens after the age of 14? Mapping transition for pupils with profound and complex learning difficulties. *British Journal of Special Education, 27*, 124–128.

Folstein, S. & Rutter, M. (1977). Infantile autism: A study of 21 twin pairs. *Journal of Child Psychology and Psychiatry, 18*, 297–321.

Folstein, S.E., Santangelo, S.L., Gilman, S.E., Piven, J., Landa, R., Lainhart, J., Hein, J., & Wzorek, M. (1999). Predictors of cognitive test patterns in autism families. *Journal of Child Psychology and Psychiatry, 40*, 1117–1128.

Fombonne, E. (1999). The epidemiology of autism: A review. *Psychological Medicine, 29*, 769–787.

Fombonne, E. (2002). Ask the Editor: Is exposure to alcohol during pregnancy a risk factor for autism? *Journal of Autism and Developmental Disorders, 32*, 243.

de Fossé, L., Hodge, M., Makris, N., Kennedy, D., Caviness, V., McGrath, L., Steele, S., Ziegler, D., Herbert, M., Frazier, J., Tager-Flusberg, H., & Harris, G. (2004). Language-association cortex asymmetry in children with autism and specific language impairment. *Annals of Neurology, 56*, 757–766.

Fotheringham, J. (1991). Autism and its primary psychological and neurological deficit. *Canadian Journal of Psychiatry, 36*, 686–692.

Francis, K. (2005). Autism interventions: A critical update. *Developmental Medicine and Child Neurology, 47*, 493–499.

Freeman, B., Ritvo, E., Yokota, A., & Ritvo, A. (1986). A scale for rating the symptoms of patients with autism in real life settings. *Journal of the American Academy of Child Psychiatry, 25*, 130–136.

Frith, C. (1992). *The Cognitive Neuropsychology of Schizophrenia*. Hove: Lawrence Erlbaum Associates.

Frith, C. (2003). What do imaging studies tell us about the neural basis of autism? In G. Bock and Jamie Goode (Eds.), *Autism: Neural Basis and Treatment Possibilities* (pp. 149–176). Chichester: John Wiley & Sons for the Novartis Foundation.

Frith, U. (1989). *Autism: Explaining the Enigma* (2nd edition, 2003). Oxford: Blackwell.

Frith, U. (2004). Confusions and controversies about Asperger syndrome. *Journal of Child Psychology and Psychiatry, 45*, 672–687.

Frith, U. & Happé, F. (1994a). Autism: Beyond theory of mind. *Cognition, 50*, 115–132.

Frith, U. & Happé, F. (1994b). Language and communication in the autistic disorders. *Philosophical Transactions of the Royal Society, series B, 346*, 97–104.

Frith, U. & Happé, F. (1998). Why specific developmental disorders are not specific: On-line and developmental effects in autism and dyslexia. *Developmental Science, 1*, 267–272.

Frith, U. & Happé, F. (1999). Theory of mind and self-consciousness: What is it like to be autistic? *Mind and Language, 14*, 1–22.

Frith, U. & Snowling, M. (1983). Reading for meaning and reading for sound in autistic and dyslexic children. *Journal of Developmental Psychology, 1*, 329–342.

Frye, D., Zelazo, P.D., & Palfai, T. (1995). Theory of mind and rule-based reasoning. *Cognitive Development, 10*, 483–527.

Fyffe, C. & Prior, M. (1978). Evidence for language recoding in autistic, retarded and normal children: A re-examination. *British Journal of Psychology, 69*, 393–402.

Gadone, K., DeVincent, C., & Pomeroy, J. (2006). ADHD symptom subtypes in children with pervasive developmental disorder. *Journal of Autism and Developmental Disorders, 36*, 271–283.

Gaigg, S. & Bowler, D. (2007). Differential fear conditioning in Asperger's syndrome: Implications for an amygdala theory of autism. *Neuropsychologia, 45*, 2125–2134.

Gallese, V., Keysers, C., & Rizzolatti, G. (2004). A unifying view of the basis of social cognition. *Trends in Cognitive Sciences, 8*, 396–403.

Gallese, V. & Stamenov, M. (2002). *Mirror Neurons and the Evolution of Brain and Language*. Philadelphia: John Benjamins Publisher.

Gallistel, C.R. (1993). *The Organisation of Learning*. Cambridge, MA: MIT Press.

Garcia, J., Zhang, D., Estill, S., Michnoff, C., Rutter, J., Reick, M., Scott, K., Diaz-Arrastia, R., & McKnight, S. (2000). Impaired cued and contextual memory in NPAS2-deficient mice. *Science, 288*, 2226–2230.

Gepner, B., Deruelle, C., and Grynfeltt, S. (2001). Motion and emotion: A novel approach to the study of face processing in young autistic children. *Journal of Autism and Developmental Disorders, 31*, 37–45.

Gepner, B. & Mestre, D. (2002). Rapid visual motion integration deficit in autism. *Trends in Cognitive Sciences, 6*, 255.

Gervais, H., Belin, P., Boddaert, N., Leboyer, M., Coez, A., Sfaello, I., Barthélémy, C., Brunelle, F., Samson, Y., & Zilbovicious, M. (2004). Abnormal cortical voice processing in autism. *Nature Neuroscience, 7*, 801–803.

Geschwind, D. & Levitt, P. (2007). Autism spectrum disorders: Developmental disconnection syndromes. *Current Opinion in Neurobiology, 17*, 103–111.

Ghaziuddin, M. & Butler, E. (1998). Clumsiness in autism and Asperger syndrome: a further report. *Journal of Intellectual Disability Research, 42*, 1365–2788.

Ghaziuddin, M., Tsai, L.Y., Eilers, L., & Ghaziuddin, N. (1992). Autism and herpes simplex encephalitis. *Journal of Autism and Developmental Disorders, 22,* 107–114.

Gibson, J.J. (1979). *The Ecological Approach to Visual Perception.* Boston, MA: Houghton-Mifflin.

Gillberg, C. (1986). Onset at age 14 of a typical autistic syndrome. A case report of a girl with herpes simplex encephalitis. *Journal of Autism and Developmental Disorders, 16,* 369–375.

Gillberg, C. (1995). Endogenous opioids and opiate antagonists in autism: Brief review. *Developmental Medicine and Child Neurology, 37,* 239–245.

Gillberg, C., Gillberg, C., Rastam, M., & Wentz., E. (2001). The Asperger Syndrome (and high-functioning autism) Diagnostic Interview (ASDI): A preliminary study of a new structured clinical interview. *Autism, 5,* 57–66.

Gilliam, J. (2001). *Gilliam Asperger's Disorder Scale.* Austin, TX: ProEd.

Golan, O. & Baron-Cohen, S. (2006). Systemising empathy: Teaching adults with Asperger syndrome or high-functioning autism to recognise complex emotions using interactive multimedia. *Development and Psychopathology, 18,* 591–617.

Goldberg, W., Osann, K., Filipek, P., Laulhere, T., Jarvis, K., Modahl, C., Flodman, P., & Spence, M.A. (2003). Language and other regression: Assessment and timing. *Journal of Autism and Developmental Disorders, 33,* 607–617.

Goldman, S., Salgado, M., Florance, N., Wang, C., Kim, M., & Greene, P. (2006). Longitudinal prevalence of stereotypies in autistic vs. non-autistic developmentally disabled children. *Neuropediatrics, 37,* DOI: 10.1055/s-2006-945809.

Gomot, M., Bernard, F., Davis, M., Belmonte, M., Ashwin, C., Bullmore, E., & Baron-Cohen, S. (2006). Change detection in children with autism: An auditory event-related fMRI study. *Neuroimage, 29,* 475–484.

Goodman, R. (1989). Infantile autism: A syndrome of multiple primary deficits? *Journal of Autism and Developmental Disorders, 19,* 409–424.

Gopnik, A., Capps, L., & Meltzoff, A. (2001). Early theories of mind: What the theory can tell us about autism. In S. Baron-Cohen, H. Tager-Flusberg & D. Cohen (Eds.), *Understanding Other Minds: Perspectives from Developmental Cognitive Neuroscience.* Oxford: OUP.

Gowen, E. & Miall, R.C. (2005). Behavioural aspects of cerebellar function in adults with Asperger syndrome. *The Cerebellum, 4,* 1473–4222.

Grandin, T. & Scariano, M. (1986). *Emergence Labelled Autistic.* Novato, CA: Arena Press.

Gray, C. (1998). Social stories and comic strip conversations with students with Asperger syndrome and high functioning autism. In E. Schopler, G. Mesibov, & L. Kunce (Eds.), *Asperger's Syndrome or High Functioning Autism?* (pp. 167–199). New York: Plenum.

Gray, D. (2002). Ten years on: A longitudinal study of families of children with autism. *Journal of Intellectual and Developmental Disability, 27,* 215–222.

Green, D., Baird, G., Barnett, A., Henderson, L., Huber, J., & Henderson, S. (2002). The severity and nature of motor impairment in Asperger's syndrome: A comparison with Specific Developmental Disorder of Motor Function. *Journal of Child Psychology and Psychiatry, 43,* 655–668.

Greenberg, J., Krauss, M., Seltzer, M., Chou, R., & Hong, J. (2004). The effect of quality of the relationship between mothers and adult children with schizophrenia, autism, or Down syndrome on maternal well-being: The mediating role of optimism. *American Journal of Orthopsychiatry, 74,* 14–25.

Grigorenko, E., Klin, A., Pauls, D., Senft, R., Hooper, C., & Volkmar, F. (2004). A descriptive study of hyperlexia in a clinically referred sample of children with developmental delays. *Journal of Autism and Developmental Disorders, 32,* 2–12.

Gross, T.F. (2004). The perception of four basic emotions in human and non-human faces by children with autism and other developmental disabilities. *Journal of Abnormal Child Psychology, 32,* 469–480.

Grossman, J.B., Klin, A., Carter, A.S., & Volkmar, F.R. (2000). Verbal bias in recognition of facial emotions in children with Asperger syndrome. *Journal of Child Psychology and Psychiatry, 41*, 369–379.

Gurney, J., McPheeters, M., & Davis, M. (2006). Parental report of health care conditions and health care use among children with and without autism. *Archives of Pediatrics and Adolescent Medicine, 160*, 825–830.

Gustafsson, L. & Papliński, A. (2004). Self-organisation of an artificial neural network subjected to attention shift impairments and familiarity preference characteristics studied in autism. *Journal of Autism and Developmental Disorders, 34*, 189–198.

Gutierrez, G., Smalley, S., & Tanguay, P. (1998). Autism in tuberous sclerosis complex. *Journal of Autism and Developmental Disorders, 28*, 97–104.

Hadjikhani, N., Joseph, R., Snyder, J., & Tager-Flusberg, H. (2006). Anatomical differences in the mirror neuron system and social cognition network in Autism. *Cerebral Cortex, 16*, 1276–1282.

Hala, S., Pexman, P., & Glenwright, M. (2007). Priming the meaning of homographs in typically developing children and children with autism. *Journal of Autism and Developmental Disorders, 37*, 329–340.

Happé, F. (1994). *Autism: An Introduction to Psychological Theory*. London: UCL Press.

Happé, F. (1999). Autism: Cognitive deficit or cognitive style? *Trends in Cognitive Sciences, 3*, 216–222.

Happé, F. & Frith, U. (2006). The weak coherence account: Detail-focused cognitive style in autism spectrum disorders. *Journal of Autism and Developmental Disorders, 36*, 5–23.

Happé, F., Frith, U., & Briskman, J. (2001). Exploring the cognitive phenotype of autism: Weak 'central coherence' in parents and siblings of children with autism: I. Experimental findings. *Journal of Child Psychology and Psychiatry, 42*, 299–307.

Happé, F., Ronald, A., & Plomin, R. (2006). Time to give up on a single explanation for autism. *Nature Neuroscience, 9*, 1218–1220.

Hare, D.J., Gould, J., Mills, R., & Wing, L. (1999). *A Preliminary Study of Individuals with ASDs in Three Special Hospitals in England*. London: National Autistic Society.

Hare, D.J., Jones, S., & Evershed, K. (2006). A comparative study of circadian rhythm functioning and sleep in people with Asperger syndrome. *Autism, 10*, 565–575.

Hare, D.J. & Malone, C. (2004). Catatonia and autistic spectrum disorders. *Autism, 8*, 183–195.

Hare, D.J., Pratt, C., Burton, M., Bromley, J., & Emerson, E. (2004). The health and social care needs of family carers supporting adults with autistic spectrum disorders. *Autism, 8*, 425–444.

Harris, G.L., Chabris, C., Clark, J., Urban, T., Aharon, I., Steele, S., McGrath, L., Condouris, K., & Tager-Flusberg, H. (2006). Brain activation during semantic processing in autism spectrum disorders via functional magnetic resonance imaging. *Brain and Cognition, 61*, 54–68.

Harris, P.L. (1989). *Children and Emotion*. Oxford: Blackwell.

Harris, P.L. (1991). The work of the imagination. In A. Whiten (Ed.), *Natural Theories of Mind*. Oxford: Blackwell.

Harris, P. (1994). Understanding pretence. In C. Lewis & P. Mitchell (Eds.), *Children's Early Understanding of Mind* (pp. 235–260). Hove: Lawrence Erlbaum Associates.

Hastings, R. (2003a). Child behaviour problems and partner mental health as correlates of stress in mothers and fathers of children with autism. *Journal of Intellectual Disability Research, 47*, 231–237.

Hastings, R. (2003b). Behavioural adjustment of siblings of children with autism. *Journal of Autism and Developmental Disorders, 33*, 99–104.

Hastings, R., Kovshoff, H., Ward, N., degli Espinosa, F., Brown, T., & Remington, B. (2005a). Systems analysis of stress and positive perceptions in mothers and fathers of pre-school children with autism. *Journal of Autism and Developmental Disorders, 35*, 635–644.

Hastings, R., Kovshoff, H., Brown, T., Ward, N., degli Espinosa, F., & Remington, B. (2005b). Coping strategies in mothers and fathers of preschool and school-age children with autism. *Autism, 9,* 377–391.

Heaton, P. (2003). Pitch memory, labelling and disembedding in autism. *Journal of Child Psychology and Psychiatry, 44,* 543–551.

Heaton, P., Hermelin, B., & Pring, L. (1998). Autism and pitch processing: A precursor for savant ability? *Music Perception, 15,* 291–305.

Heaton, R.K., Chelune, G., Talley, J., Kay, G., & Curtiss, G. (1993). *Wisconsin Card Sorting Test: Revised.* Psychological Assessment Resources, Odessa, FL.

Heidgerken, A., Geffken, G., Modi, A., & Frakey, L. (2005). A survey of autism knowledge in a health care setting. *Journal of Autism and Developmental Disorders, 35,* 323–330.

Heiman, T. (2002). Parents of children with disabilities: Resilience, coping and future expectations. *Journal of Developmental and Physical Disabilities, 14,* 159–171.

Henn, J. & Henn, M. (2005). Defying the odds: You can't put a square peg in a round hole. *Journal of Vocational Rehabilitation, 22,* 129–130.

Hermelin, B. (2001). *Bright Splinters of the Mind.* London: Jessica Kingsley Publishers.

Hermelin, B. & O'Connor, N. (1967). Remembering of words by psychotic and normal children. *British Journal of Psychology, 68,* 213–218.

Hermelin, B. & O'Connor, N. (1970). *Psychological Experiments with Autistic Children.* Oxford: Pergamon Press.

Hermelin, B. & O'Connor, N. (1985). Logico-affective states and non-verbal language. In E. Schopler & G. Mesibov (Eds.), *Communication Problems in Autism* (pp. 293–309). Plenum Press: New York.

Hesmondhalgh, M. & Breakey, C. (2001). *Access and Inclusion for Children with Autistic Spectrum Disorders: 'Let Me In'.* London: Jessica Kingsley Publishers.

Hetzler, B. & Griffin, J. (1981). Infantile autism and the temporal lobe of the brain. *Journal of Autism and Developmental Disorders, 11,* 317–330.

Hewetson, A. (2002). *The Stolen Child: Aspects of Autism and Asperger Syndrome.* Westport CT: Greenwood Publishing Group.

Hill, E.L. (2004). Evaluating the theory of impairments of executive function in autism. *Developmental Review, 24,* 189–233.

Hill, E., Berthoz, S. & Frith, U. (2004). Brief report: Cognitive processing of own emotions in individuals with autistic spectrum disorder and in their relatives. *Journal of Autism and Developmental Disorders, 34,* 229–235.

Hill, E. & Russell, J. (2002). Action memory and self-monitoring in children with autism: Self versus other. *Infant and Child Development, 11,* 159–170.

Hobson, R.P. (1990). On the origins of self and the case of autism. *Development and Psychopathology, 2,* 163–181.

Hobson, R.P. (1993). *Autism and the Development of Mind.* Hove: Lawrence Erlbaum Associates.

Hobson, R.P. (2002). *The Cradle of Thought.* London: Macmillan.

Hobson, R.P., Chidambi, G., Lee, A., & Meyer, J. (2006). Foundations for self-awareness: An exploration through autism. *Monographs of the Society for Research in Child Development,* Serial No. 284, Vol. 17.

Hobson, P., Ouston, J., & Lee, A. (1988). What's in a face? The case of autism. *British Journal of Psychology, 79,* 441–453.

Hoerl, C. & McCormack, T. (2001). *Time and Memory.* Oxford: OUP.

Hoksbergen, R., ter Laak, J., Rijk, K., van Dijkum, C., & Stoutjesdik, F. (2005). Post-institution autistic syndrome in Romanian adoptees. *Journal of Autism and Developmental Disorders, 35,* 615–623.

Hollander, E., King, A., Delaney, K., Smith, C., & Silverman, J. (2003). Obsessive-compulsive behaviours in parents of multiplex autism families. *Psychiatry Research, 117,* 11–16.

Hollander, E., Phillips, A., King, B., Guthrie, D., Aman, M., Law, P., Owley, T., & Robinson, R. (2004). Impact of recent findings on study design of future autism clinical trials. *CNS Spectrums, 9,* 49–56.

Horrath, K., Cataldo, M., Wachtel, R., Spurrier, A., Papadimitriou, J., & Tildon, J. (1998). Gastrointestinal findings in autistic children: Hypersecretory response to secretin predicts behavioural improvement. *Journal of Pediatric Gastroenterology and Nutrition, 26,* 549.

Howard, M., Cowell, P., Boucher, J., Broks, P., Mayes, A., Farrant, A., & Roberts, N. (2000). Convergent neuroanatomical and behavioural evidence of an amygdala hypothesis of autism. *NeuroReport, 11,* 2931–2935.

Howlin, P. (2000). Outcome in adult life for more able individuals with autism or Asperger syndrome. *Autism, 4,* 63–83.

Howlin, P. (2003). Can early interventions alter the course of autism? In G. Bock & J. Goode (Eds.), *Autism: Neural Basis and Treatment Possibilities* (pp. 250–265). Chichester: John Wiley & Sons for the Novartis Foundation.

Howlin, P. (2005). The effectiveness of intervention for children with autism. In W. Fleischhaker & D.J. Brooks (Eds.), *Neurodevelopmental Disorders* (pp. 101–119). Vienna: Springer.

Howlin, P., Alcock, J., & Burkin, J. (2005). An 8-year follow-up of a specialist supported employment service for high-ability adults with autism or Asperger syndrome. *Autism, 9,* 533–569.

Howlin, P. & Asgharian, A. (1999) The diagnosis of autism and Asperger syndrome: Findings from a survey of 770 families. *Developmental Medicine and Child Neurology, 41,* 834–839.

Howlin, P., Goode, S., Hutton, J., & Rutter, M. (2004). Adult outcome for children with autism. *Journal of Child Psychology and Psychiatry, 45,* 212–229.

Howlin, P., Gordon, K., Pasco, G., Wade, A. & Charman, T. (2007). The effectiveness of Picture Exchange Communication System (PECS) training for teachers of children with autism: A pragmatic, group randomised controlled trial. *Journal of Child Psychology and Psychiatry, 48,* 473–481.

Hughes, C. (1996). Brief report: Planning problems in autism at the level of motor control. *Journal of Autism and Developmental Disorders, 26,* 101–109.

Hughes, C. & Russell, J. (1993). Autistic children's difficulty with mental disengagement from an object: Its implications for theories of autism. *Developmental Psychology, 29,* 498–510.

Hughes, C. Russell, J. & Robbins, T. (1994). Evidence for central impairments of executive function in autism. *Neuropsychologia, 32,* 477–492.

Hughes, P.J. (2007). *Reflections: Me and Planet Weirdo.* London: Chipmunkapublishing.

Huizink, A., Mulder, E., & Buitelaar, J. (2004). Prenatal stress and risk for psychopathology early or later in life: Specific effects of induction of general susceptibility? *Psychological Bulletin, 130,* 115–142.

Hu-Lince, D., Craig, D., Huentelman, M., & Stephan, D. (2005). The Autism Genome Project: Goals and strategies. Databases and genome projects. *American Journal of PharmocoGenomics, 5,* 233–246.

Hultman, C., Sparen, P., & Cnattingius, S. (2002). Perinatal risk factors for infantile autism. *Epidemiology, 13,* 417–423.

Hume, K. & Odom, S. (2007). Effects of an individual work system on the independent functioning of students with autism. *Journal of Autism and Developmental Disorders, 37,* 1166–1180.

Humphrey, N. & Parkinson, G. (2006). Research on interventions for children and young people on the autistic spectrum: A critical perspective. *Journal of Research in Special Educational Needs, 6,* 76–86.

Hurlburt, K. & Chalmers, L. (2004). Employment and adults with Asperger syndrome. *Focus on Autism and Other Developmental Disabilities, 19,* 215–222.

Hurth, J., Shaw, E., Izeman, S., Whaley, K., & Rogers, S. (1999). Areas of agreement about effective practices among programs serving young children with autism spectrum disorders. *Infants and Young Children, 12,* 17–26.

Hutt, S., Hutt, C., Lee, D., & Ounsted, C., (1964). Arousal and childhood autism. *Nature, 204,* 908.

Hutt, S., Hutt, C., Ounsted, C., & Lee, D. (1965). A behavioural and electroencephalographic study of autistic children. *Journal of Psychiatry Research, 3,* 181–197.

Iarocci, G. & McDonald, J. (2006). Sensory integration and the perceptual experience of persons with autism. *Journal of Autism and Developmental Disorders, 36,* 77–90.

Isager, T., Mouridsen, S., & Rich, B. (1999). Mortality and causes of death in pervasive developmental disorders. *Autism, 3,* 7–17.

Isanon, A. (2001). *Spirituality and the Autistic Spectrum: Of Falling Sparrows.* London: Jessica Kingsley Press.

Ives, M. & Munro, N. (2002). *Caring for a Child with Autism.* London: Jessica Kingsley Publishers.

Jackson, J. & Bland, B. (2005). Medial septal modulation of the ascending brainstem hippocampal synchronizing pathways in the anesthetized rat. *Hippocampus, 16,* 1–10.

Jacobsen, P. (2003). *Asperger Syndrome and Psychotherapy.* London: Jessica Kingsley Publishers.

Jäkälä, P., Hänninen, T., Ryynanen, M., Laakso, M., Partanen, K., Mannermaa, A., & Soininen, H. (1997). Fragile-X: Neuropsychological test performance, CGG triplet repeat lengths, and hippocampal volumes. *Journal of Clinical Investigation, 100,* 331–338.

Jansiewicz, E., Goldberg, M., Newschaffer, C., Denkla, M., Landa, R., & Mostofsky, S. (2006). Motor signs distinguish children with high functioning autism and Asperger's syndrome from controls. *Journal of Autism and Developmental Disorders, 36,* 613–621.

Järbrink, K., Fombonne, E., & Knapp, M. (2003). Measuring the parental, service and cost impacts of children with autistic spectrum disorders: A pilot study. *Journal of Autism and Developmental Disorders, 33,* 395–402.

Järbrink, K. & Knapp, M. (2001). The economic impact of autism in Britain. *Autism, 5,* 7–22.

Jarrold, C. (1997). Pretend play in autism: Executive explanations. In J. Russell (Ed.), *Autism as an Executive Disorder* (pp. 101–142). Oxford: Oxford University Press.

Jarrold, C., Boucher, J., & Smith, P.K. (1996). Generativity deficits in pretend play in autism. *British Journal of Developmental Psychology, 14,* 275–300.

Jemel, B., Mottron, L., & Dawson, M. (2006). Impaired face processing in autism: Fact or artifact? *Journal of Autism and Developmental Disorders, 36,* 91–106.

Jones, V. & Prior, M. (1985). Motor imitation abilities and neurological signs in autistic children. *Journal of Autism and Developmental Disorders, 15,* 37–47.

Jordan, R. (2001). Effects of culture on service provision for people with autistic spectrum disorders. *Good Autism Practice, 2,* 332–338.

Jordan, R. (2005a). Diagnosis and the identification of special educational needs for children at the 'able' end of the autism spectrum: Reflections on social and cultural influences. *Autism News: Orange County & the Rest of the World, 2,* 13–16.

Jordan, R. (2005b). Managing autism and Asperger's syndrome in current educational provision. *Developmental Neurorehabilitation, 8,* 104–108.

Jordan, R. (2008). Autism spectrum disorders: A challenge and a model for inclusion in education. *British Journal of Special Education, 35,* 11–15.

Jordan, R., Jones, G., & Murray, D. (1998). *Educational Interventions for Children with Autism: A Literature Review of Recent and Current Research*. Research Report RR77 for the Department for Education and Employment, London: HMSO.

Jordan, R. & Powell, S. (1995). *Understanding and Teaching Children with Autism*. Chichester: John Wiley & Sons.

Just, M.A., Cherkassky, V., Keller, T., & Minshew, N. (2004). Cortical activation and synchronisation during sentence comprehension in high-functioning autism: Evidence of underconnectivity. *Brain, 127*, 1811–1821.

Just, M.A., Cherkassky, V., Keller, T., Kana, R., & Minshew, N. (2007). Functional and anatomical cortical underconnectivity in autism: Evidence from an fMRI study of an executive function task using corpus callosum morphometry. *Cerebral Cortex, 17*, 951–961.

Kaminsky, L. & Dewey, D. (2002). Psychosocial adjustment in siblings of children with autism. *Journal of Child Psychology and Psychiatry, 43*, 225–232.

Kanner, L. (1943). Autistic disturbances of affective contact. *Nervous Child, 2*, 217–250.

Karmiloff-Smith, A. (1992). *Beyond Modularity*. Cambridge, MA: MIT Press.

Karmiloff-Smith, A. (1998). Development itself is the key to understanding developmental disorders. *Trends in Cognitive Sciences, 2*, 389–398.

Karmiloff-Smith, A., Scerif, G., & Thomas, M. (2002). Different approaches to relating genotype to phenotype in developmental disorders. *Developmental Psychobiology, 40*, 311–322.

Kates, W., Burnette, C., Eliez, S., Strunge, L.A., Kaplan, D., Landa, R., Reiss, A., & Pearlson, G. (2004). Neuroanatomic variation in monozygotic twin pairs discordant for the narrow phenotype for autism. *American Journal of Psychiatry, 161*, 539–546.

Keel, J.H., Mesibov, G., & Woods, A. (1997). TEACCH-supported employment program. *Journal of Autism and Developmental Disorders, 27*, 3–9.

Kemper, T. & Bauman, M. (1998). Neuropathology of infantile autism. *Journal of Neuropathology and Experimental Neurology, 57*, 645–652.

Kjelgaard, M. & Tager-Flusberg, H. (2001). An investigation of language profiles in autism: Implications for genetic subgroups. *Language and Cognitive Processes, 16*, 287–308.

Klein, K. & Diehl, E. (2004). Relationship between the MMR vaccine and autism. *Annals of Pharmacotherapy, 38*, 1297–1300.

Klein, S., Chan, R., & Loftus, J. (1999). Independence of episodic and semantic self-knowledge: The case from autism. *Social Cognition, 17*, 413–437.

Klin, A. (1991). Young autistic children's listening preferences in regard to speech: A possible characterization of the symptom of social withdrawal. *Journal of Autism and Developmental Disorders, 21*, 29–42.

Klin, A., Jones, W., Schultz, R., & Volkmar, F. (2003). The enactive mind, or from actions to cognition: Lessons from autism. In U. Frith & E. Hill (Eds.), *Mind and Brain* (pp. 127–159). Oxford: OUP.

Klin, A., Saulnier, C., Tsatsanis, K., & Volkmar, F. (2005). Clinical evaluation in autism spectrum disorders: Psychological assessment within a transdisciplinary framework. In F. Volkmar, R. Paul, A. Klin, & D. Cohen (Eds.), *Handbook of Autism and Pervasive Developmental Disorders, Vol. 2* (3rd edition) (pp. 772–798). Hoboken, NJ: John Wiley & Sons.

Klin, A. & Volkmar, F. (1995). *Asperger's Syndrome: Guidelines for Assessment and Diagnosis*. Paper published by the Learning Disabilities Association of America.

Klin, A., Volkmar, F., & Sparrow, S. (2000). *Asperger Syndrome*. New York: Guilford Press.

Klin, A., Volkmar, F., Sparrow, S., Cicchetti, D., & Rourke, B. (1995). Validity and neurological characterisation of Asperger syndrome. *Journal of Child Psychology and Psychiatry, 36*, 1127–1140.

Knowlton, B. & Squire, L. (1993). The learning of categories: Parallel brain systems for item memory and category knowledge. *Science, 262,* 1747–1749.

Kolvin, I. (1971). Studies in childhood psychoses, I: Diagnostic criteria and classification. *British Journal of Psychiatry, 118,* 381–384.

Konidaris, J. (2005). A sibling's perspective on autism. In F. Volkmar, R. Paul, A. Klin, & D. Cohen (Eds.), *Handbook of Autism and Pervasive Developmental Disorders, Vol. 2* (3rd edition) (pp. 1265–1275). Hoboken, NJ: John Wiley & Sons.

Koshino, H., Carpenter, P., Minshew, N., Cherkassky, V., Keller, T., & Just, M.A. (2005). Functional connectivity in an fMRI working memory task in high-functioning autism. *Neuroimage, 24,* 810–824.

Kraijer, D. (2000). Review of adaptive behaviour studies in mentally retarded persons with autism/pervasive developmental disorder. *Journal of Autism and Developmental Disorders, 30,* 39–48.

Krause, I., He., X., Gershwin, M., & Schoenfeld, Y. (2002). Review of autoimmune factors in autism. *Journal of Autism and Developmental Disorders, 32,* 337–345.

Krauss, M. & Seltzer, M. (2000). An unanticipated life: The impact of lifelong caregiving. In H. Bersani (Ed.), *Responding to the Challenge: International Trends and Current Issues in Developmental Disabilities* (pp. 173–188). Brookline, MA: Brookline Books.

Krauss, M., Seltzer, M., & Jacobson, H. (2005). Adults with autism living at home or in non-family settings: Positive and negative aspects of residential status. *Journal of Intellectual Disability Research, 49,* 111–124.

Krug, D. & Arick, J. (2003). *Krug Autism Disorder Index.* Austin, TX: Pro-Ed Inc.

Krug, D., Arick, J., & Almond, P. (1980). *Autism Screening Instrument for Educational Planning.* Portland, OR: ASIEP Educational.

Kyrkou, M. (2005). Health issues and quality of life in women with intellectual disability. *Journal of Intellectual Disability Research, 49,* 770–777.

Landry, L. & Bryson, S. (2004). Impaired disengagement of attention in young children with autism. *Journal of Child Psychology and Psychiatry, 45,* 1115–1123.

Lawson, J., Baron-Cohen, S., & Wheelwright, S. (2004). Empathising and systemising in adults with and without Asperger Syndrome. *Journal of Autism and Developmental Disorders, 34,* 301–310.

Lawson, W. (2001). *Understanding and Working with the Spectrum of Autism: An Insider's View.* London: Jessica Kingsley Press.

Leary, M. & Hill, D.A (1996). Moving on: Autism and movement disturbance. *Mental Retardation, 34,* 39–53.

Le Couteur, A., Bailey, A., Goode, S., Pickles, A., Robertson, S., Gottesman, I., & Rutter, M. (1996). A broader phenotype of autism: The clinical spectrum in twins. *Journal of Child Psychology and Psychiatry, 37,* 785–801.

Le Couteur, A., Baird, G., & National Initiative for Autism Screening and Assessment (NIASA) (2003). *National Autism Plan.* London: National Autistic Society.

Lee, A. & Hobson, R.P. (1998). On developing self concepts: A controlled study of children and adolescents with autism. *Journal of Child Psychology and Psychiatry, 39,* 1131–1141.

Leekam, S. (2005). Why do children with autism have a joint attention impairment? In N. Eilan, C. Hoerl, T. McCormack, & J. Roessler (Eds.), *Joint Attention: Communication and Other Minds* (pp. 205–229). Oxford: OUP.

Leekam, S., Libby, S., Wing, L., Gould, J. & Taylor, C. (2002). The Diagnostic Interview for Social and Communication Disorders: Algorithms for ICD-10 childhood autism and Wing and Gould autistic spectrum disorder. *Journal of Child Psychology and Psychiatry, 43,* 327–342.

Leekam, S., Lopez, B., & Moore, C. (2000). Attention and joint attention in preschool children with autism. *Developmental Psychology, 36,* 261–273.

Leekam, S. & Perner, J. (1991). Does the autistic child have a metarepresentational deficit? *Cognition, 40,* 203–218.

Leekam, S. & Ramsden, C. (2006). Dyadic orienting and joint attention in preschool children with autism. *Journal of Autism and Developmental Disorders, 36,* 185–197.

Leinonen, E., Letts, C., & Smith, B.R. (2000). *Children's Pragmatic Communication Difficulties.* London: Whurr.

Leslie, A. (1987). Pretense and representation in infancy: The origins of theory of mind. *Psychological Review, 94,* 412–427.

Leslie, A., Friedman, O., & German, T. (2004). Core mechanisms in 'theory of mind'. *Trends in Cognitive Sciences, 8,* 528–533.

Leslie, A. & Roth, D. (1993). What autism teaches us about metarepresentation. In S. Baron-Cohen, H. Tager-Flusberg, & D. Cohen (Eds.), *Understanding Other Minds: Perspectives from Autism* (pp. 83–111). Oxford: OUP.

Leslie, A. & Thaiss, L. (1992). Domain specificity in conceptual development: Evidence from autism. *Cognition, 43,* 225–251.

Levy, S. & Hyman, S. (2005). Novel treatments for autistic spectrum disorders. *Mental Retardation and Developmental Disabilities Research Reviews, 11,* 131–142.

Lewis, M. & Lazoritz, M. (2005). Psychopharmacology of autism spectrum disorders. *Psychiatric Times, 22,* 1–7.

Lewis, V. & Boucher, J. (1988). Spontaneous, instructed, and elicited play in relatively able autistic children. *British Journal of Developmental Psychology, 6,* 325–339.

Lewis, V. & Boucher, J. (1991). Skill, content, and generative strategies in autistic children's drawings. *British Journal of Developmental Psychology, 9,* 393–416.

Lewis, V. & Boucher, J. (1995). Generativity in the play of young people with autism. *Journal of Autism and Developmental Disorders, 25,* 105–121.

Libby, J., Sweeten, T., McMahon, W., & Fujinami, R. (2005). Autistic disorder and viral infections. *Journal of NeuroVirology, 11,* 1–10.

Lillard, A. (1994). Making sense of pretence. In C. Lewis & P. Mitchell (Eds.), *Children's Early Understanding of Mind* (pp. 211–221). Hove: Lawrence Erlbaum Associates.

Lim, M., Bielsky, I., & Young, L. (2005). Neuropeptides and the social brain: potential rodent models of autism. *International Journal of Developmental Neuroscience, 23,* 235–243.

Limoges, E., Mottron, L., Bolduc, C., Berthiaume, C. & Godbout, R. (2005). Atypical sleep architecture and the autism phenotype. *Brain, 128,* 1049–1061.

Lincoln, A.J., Allen, M., & Killman, A. (1995). The assessment and interpretation of intellectual abilities in people with autism. In E. Schopler & G. Mesibov (Eds.), *Learning and Cognition in Autism* (pp. 89–118). New York: Plenum Press.

Lincoln, A.J., Courchesne, E., Allen, M., Hanson, E., & Ene, M. (1998). Neurobiology of Asperger syndrome: Seven case studies and quantitative magnetic resonance imaging findings. In E. Schopler, G. Mesibov., & L.J. Kunce (Eds.), *Asperger Syndrome or High-functioning Autism?* (pp. 145–166). New York: Plenum Press.

Lind, S. & Bowler, D.M. (2008). Episodic memory and autonoetic consciousness in autism spectrum disorders. In J. Boucher & D.M. Bowler (Eds.), *Memory in Autism.* Cambridge: CUP.

Lopez, B.R., Lincoln, A.J., Ozonoff, S., & Lai, Z. (2005). Examining the relationship between executive functions and restricted, repetitive symptoms of autistic disorder. *Journal of Autism and Developmental Disorders, 35,* 445–460.

Lord, C., Cook, E., Blumenthal, B., & Amarel, D. (2000). Autistic spectrum disorders. *Neuron, 28,* 355–363.

Lord, C. & Costello, C. (2005). Diagnostic instruments in autistic spectrum disorders. In F. Volkmar, R. Paul, A. Klin, & D. Cohen (Eds.), *Handbook of Autism and Pervasive Developmental Disorders, Vol. 2* (3rd edition) (pp. 730–771). Hoboken, NJ: John Wiley & Sons.

Lord, C. & Paul, R. (1997). Language and communication in autism. In D. Cohen & F. Volkmar (Eds.), *Handbook of Autism and Pervasive Developmental Disorders* (2nd edition) (pp. 195–225). New York: John Wiley.

Lord, C., Risi, S., DiLavore, P., Shulman, C., Thurm, A., & Pickles, A. (2006). Autism from 2 to 9 years of age. *Archives of General Psychiatry, 63,* 694–701.

Lord, C., Rutter, M., DiLavore, P., & Risi, S. (1999). *Autism Diagnostic Observation Schedule.* Los Angeles: Western Psychological Services.

Lord, C. & Schopler, E. (1989). Stability of assessment results of autistic and non-autistic language-impaired children from preschool years to early school age. *Journal of Child Psychology and Psychiatry, 30,* 575–590.

Lord, C., Wagner, A., Rogers, S., Szatmari, P., Aman, M., Charman, T., Dawson, G., Durand, V., Grossman, L., Guthrie, D., Harris, S., Kasari, C., Marcus, L., Murphy, S., Odon, S., Pickles, A., Scahill, L., Shaw, E., Siegel, B., Sigman, M., Stone, W., Smith, T., & Yoder, P. (2005). Challenges in evaluating psychosocial interventions for autistic spectrum disorders. *Journal of Autism and Developmental Disorders, 35,* 695–708.

Loveland, K.A. (2001). Toward an ecological theory of autism. In J. Burack, T. Charman, N. Yirmiya, & P.R. Zelazo (Eds.), *The Development of Autism: Perspectives From Theory and Research* (pp. 17–38). Mahwah, NJ: Lawrence Erlbaum Associates.

Loveland, K.A., Bachevalier, J., Pearson, D., & Lane, D. (2008). Fronto-limbic functioning in children and adults with and without autism. *Neuropsychologia, 46,* 49–62.

Loveland, K.A. & Landry, S. (1986). Joint attention in autism and developmental language delay. *Journal of Autism and Developmental Disorders, 16,* 335–349.

Loynes, F. (2001). *The Rising Challenge: A Survey of Local Education Authorities on Educational Provision for Pupils with Autistic Spectrum Disorders.* London: All Party Parliamentary Group on Autism.

Luna, B., Doll, S.K., Hegedus, S., Minshew, N., & Sweeney, J.A. (2006). Maturation of executive function in autism. *Biological Psychiatry, 61,* 474–481.

Ma, D., Jaworski, J., Menold, M., Donnelly, S., Abramson, R., Wright, H., Delong, G., Gilbert, J., Pericak-Vance, M., & Cuccaro, M. (2005). Ordered-subset analysis of savant skills in autism for 15q11-q13. American Journal of Medical Genetics Part B: *Neuropsychiatric Genetics, 135B,* 38–41.

MacCulloch, M. & Williams, C. (1971). On the nature of infantile autism. *Acta Psychiatrica Scandinavica, 47,* 295–314.

Macintosh, K. & Dissanayake, C. (2004). The similarities and differences between autistic disorder and Asperger's disorder: A review of the empirical evidence. *Journal of Child Psychology and Psychiatry, 45,* 421–434.

Mackintosh, N.J. (1998). *IQ and Human Learning Abilities.* Oxford: OUP.

Magiati, I., Charman, T., & Howlin, P. (2007). A two-year prospective follow-up study of community-based early intensive behavioural intervention and specialist nursery provision for children with autism spectrum disorders. *Journal of Child Psychology and Psychiatry, 48,* 803–812.

Magiati, I. & Howlin, P. (2001). Monitoring the progress of preschoolers with autism enrolled in early intervention programmes. *Autism, 5,* 399–406.

Mahler, M. (1952). On child psychosis and schizophrenia: autistic and symbiotic psychosis. *Psychoanalytic Study of the Child, 7,* 286–305.

Mann, T. & Walker, P. (2003). Autism and a deficit in broadening the spread of visual attention. *Journal of Child Psychology and Psychiatry, 44,* 274–284.

Mansell, W. & Morris, K. (2004). A survey of parents' reactions to the diagnosis of an autistic spectrum disorder by a local service. *Autism, 8,* 387–407.

Marcus, L., Kunce, L., & Schopler, E. (2005). Working with families. In F. Volkmar, R. Paul, A. Klin, & D. Cohen (Eds.), *Handbook of Autism and Pervasive Developmental Disorders, Vol. 2* (3rd edition) (pp. 1055–1086). Hoboken, NJ: John Wiley & Sons.

Marinović, J., Terzić, C., Petković, Z., Zekan, L., Terzić, I., & Šušnjara, I. (2003). Lower cortisol and higher ACTH levels in individuals with autism. *Journal of Autism and Developmental Disorders, 33*, 443–448.

Mascha, K. & Boucher, J. (2006). Preliminary investigation of a qualitative method of examining siblings' experiences of living with a child with ASD. *The British Journal of Developmental Disabilities, 52*, 19–28.

Mawhood, L. & Howlin, P. (1999). The outcome of a supported employment scheme for high-functioning adults with autism or Asperger syndrome. *Autism, 3*, 229–254.

Mayes, A. & Boucher, J. (2008). Acquired memory disorders in adults: Implications for autism. In J. Boucher & D.M. Bowler (Eds.), *Memory in Autism*. Cambridge: CUP.

McCann, J. & Peppé, S. (2003). Prosody in autism spectrum disorders: A critical review. *International Journal of Language and Communication Disorders, 38*, 325–350.

McClelland, J. (2000). The basis of hyperspecificity in autism: A preliminary suggestion based on the properties of neural nets. *Journal of Autism and Developmental Disorders, 30*, 497–502.

McConachie, H. & Diggle, T. (2007). Parent implemented early intervention for young children with autism spectrum disorder: A systematic review. *Journal of Evaluation in Clinical Practice, 13*, 120–129.

McGill, P., Tennyson, A., & Cooper, V. (2006). Parents whose children with learning disabilities and challenging behaviour attend 52-week residential schools: Their perception of services received and expectations for the future. *British Journal of Social Work, 36*, 597–616.

McGovern, C. & Sigman, M. (2005). Continuity and change from early childhood to adolescence in autism. *Journal of Child Psychology and Psychiatry, 46*, 401–408.

McIntosh, D., Reichmann-Decker, A., Winkielman, P., & Wilbarger, J. (2006). When the social mirror breaks: Deficits in automatic, but not voluntary, mimicry of emotional facial expressions in autism. *Developmental Science, 9*, 295–302.

Medical Research Council (2001). *Review of Autism Research: Epidemiology and Causes*. London: MRC.

Meltzer, H., Gatward, R., Corbin, T., Goodman, R., & Ford, T. (2003). *The Mental Health of Young People Looked After by Local Authorities in England*. Norwich: HM Stationery Office.

Meltzoff, A. & Gopnik, A. (1993). The role of imitation in understanding persons and developing theories of mind. In S. Baron-Cohen, H. Tager-Flusberg, & D. Cohen (Eds.), *Understanding Other Minds: Perspectives from Autism* (pp. 335–366). Oxford: OUP.

Mesibov, G. & Handlan, S. (1997) Adolescents and adults with autism. In D. Cohen & F. Volkmar (Eds.), *Handbook of Autism and Pervasive Developmental Disorders* (2nd edition) (pp. 309–322). New York: John Wiley.

Mesibov, G., Schopler, E., & Shea, V. (2004). *The TEACCH Approach to Autism Spectrum Disorders*. New York: Springer.

Meyer, J. & Hobson, R.P. (2004). Orientation to self and other: The case of autism. *Interaction Studies, 5*, 221–244.

Miles, J., Takahashi, N., Haber, A., & Hadden, L. (2003). Autism families with a high incidence of alcoholism. *Journal of Autism and Developmental Disorders, 33*, 403–416.

Miller, M.T., Strömland, K., Ventura, L., Johansson, M., Bandim, J., & Gillberg, C. (2005). Autism associated with conditions characterised by developmental errors in early embryogenesis: A mini review. *International Journal of Developmental Neuroscience, 23*, 201–219.

Millward, C., Powell, S., Messer, D., & Jordan, R. (2000). Recall for self and other in autism: Children's memory for events experienced by themselves and their peers. *Journal of Autism and Developmental Disorders, 30*, 15–28.

Milne, E., Swettenham, J., & Campbell, R. (2005). Motion perception and autistic spectrum disorder: A review. *Current Psychology of Cognition, 23*, 3–36.

Minshew, N. & Goldstein, G. (1993). Is autism an amnesic disorder? Evidence from the California Verbal Learning Test. *Neuropsychology, 7*, 209–216.

Minshew, N. & Goldstein, G. (2001). The pattern of intact and impaired memory functions in autism. *Journal of Child Psychology and Psychiatry, 42*, 1095–1101.

Minshew, N., Goldstein, G., & Siegel, D. (1997). Neuropsychologic functioning in autism: Profile of a complex information processing disorder. *Journal of the International Neuropsychological Society, 3*, 303–317.

Minshew, N., Meyer, J., & Goldstein, G. (2002). Abstract reasoning in autism: A dissociation between concept formation and concept identification. *Neuropsychology, 16*, 327–334.

Minshew, N., Sweeney, J., Bauman, M., & Webb, S.J. (2005). Neurologic aspects of autism. In F. Volkmar, R. Paul, A. Klin, & D. Cohen (Eds.), *Handbook of Autism and Pervasive Developmental Disorders* (3rd edition) (pp. 473–514). Hoboken, NJ: John Wiley.

Minshew, N., Turner, C., & Goldstein, G. (2005). The application of short forms of the Wechsler Intelligence Scales in adults and children with high functioning autism. *Journal of Autism and Developmental Disorders, 35*, 45–52.

Mittler, P. (1979) *People not Patients: Problems and Policies in Mental Handicap.* London: Methuen.

Molesworth, C., Bowler, D., & Hampton, J. (2005). The prototype effect in recognition memory: Intact in autism? *Journal of Child Psychology and Psychiatry, 46*, 661–672.

Montes, G. & Halterman, J. (2007). Psychological functioning and coping among mothers of children with autism: A population-based study. *Pediatrics, 119*, 1040–1046.

Moore, C. & Lemmon, K. (2001). *The Self in Time: Developmental Perspectives.* Mahwah, NJ: Lawrence Erlbaum Associates.

Morris, J., Abbott, D., & Ward, L. (2002). At home or away? An exploration of policy and practice in the placement of disabled children at residential schools. *Children and Society, 16*, 3–16.

Morton-Cooper, A. (2004). *Healthcare and the Autism Spectrum: A Guide for Health Professionals, Parents and Carers.* London: Jessica Kingsley Publishers.

Mostert, M. (2004). Facilitated Communication since 1995: A review of published studies. *Journal of Autism and Developmental Disorders, 31*, 287–313.

Mostofsky, S., Bunoski, R., Morton, S., Goldberg, M., & Bastian, A. (2004). Children with autism adapt normally during a catching task requiring the cerebellum. *Neurocase, 10*, 60–64.

Mostofsky, S., Goldberg, M., Landa, R., & Denkla, M. (2000). Evidence for a deficit in procedural learning in children and adolescents with autism: Implications for cerebellar contribution. *Journal of the International Neuropsychological Society, 6*, 752–759.

Mottron, L. & Belleville, S. (1993). A study of perceptual analysis in a high-level autistic subject with exceptional graphic abilities. *Brain and Cognition, 23*, 279–309.

Mottron, L. & Burack, J. (2001). Enhanced perceptual functioning in the development of autism. In J. Burack, T. Charman, N. Yirmiya, & P.R. Zelazo (Eds.), *The Development of Autism: Perspectives From Theory and Research* (pp. 131–148). Hove: Lawrence Erlbaum Associates.

Mottron, L. & Burack, J. (2006). Editorial preface. *Journal of Autism and Developmental Disorders, 36*, 1–3.

Mottron, L., Dawson, M., Soulières, I., Hubert, B., & Burack, J. (2006). Enhanced perceptual functioning in autism: An update, and eight principles of autistic perception. *Journal of Autism and Developmental Disorders, 36*, 27–43.

Mottron, L., Dawson, M., & Soulières, I. (2008). A different memory: Are distinctions drawn from the study of non-autistic memory appropriate to describe memory in autism? In J. Boucher & D.M. Bowler (Eds.), *Memory in Autism.* Cambridge: CUP.

Mottron, L., Peretz, I., Belleville, S., & Rouleau, N. (1999). Absolute pitch in autism: A case study. *Neurocase, 5,* 485–502.

Moussavand, S. & Findling, R. (2007). Recent advances in the pharmacological treatment of pervasive developmental disorders. *Current Pediatric Reviews, 3,* 79–91.

Muhle, R., Trentacoste, S., & Rapin, I. (2004). The genetics of autism. *Pediatrics, 113,* 472–486.

Mundy, P. (1995). Joint attention and socio-emotional approach behaviour in children with autism. *Development and Psychopathology, 7,* 63–82.

Mundy, P. (2003). The neural basis of social impairments in autism: The role of the dorsal medial-frontal cortex and anterior cingulate system. *Journal of Child Psychology and Psychiatry, 44,* 793–809.

Mundy, P., Sigman, M., Ungerer, J., & Sherman, T. (1986). Defining the social deficit of autism: The contribution of non-verbal communication measures. *Journal of Child Psychology and Psychiatry, 27,* 657–669.

Murphy, D., DeCarli, C., Daly, E., Haxby, J., Allen, G., White, B., McIntosh, A., Powell, C., Horwitz, B., Rapoport, S., & Schapiro, M. (1993). X-chromosome effects on female brain: a magnetic resonance imaging study of Turner's syndrome. *The Lancet, 342,* 1197–1201.

Murphy, M., Bolton, P., Fombonne, E., Pickles, A., Piven, J., & Rutter, M. (2000). Personality traits of the relatives of autistic probands. *Psychological Medicine, 30,* 1411–1424.

Murray, D., Lesser, M., & Lawson, W. (2005). Attention, monotropism and the diagnostic criteria for autism. *Autism, 9,* 139–156.

Myles, B., Bock, S., & Simpson, R. (2005). *Asperger Syndrome Diagnostic Scale (ASDS).* Minneapolis, MN: AGS Publishing.

Nation, K., Clarke, P., Wright, B., Williams, C. (2006). Patterns of reading ability in children with autism spectrum disorder. *Journal of Autism and Developmental Disorders, 36,* 911–919.

National Health Service Scotland (2006). *Learning Resource on Autism Spectrum Disorders (ASDs) for GPs and Primary Care Practitioners.* www.nes.scot.nhs.uk/asd/index.htm

Nelson, K. & Nelson, P. (2005). Size of the head and brain in autism: Clue to underlying biologic mechanisms. In M. Bauman & T. Kemper (Eds.), *The Neurobiology of Autism* (2nd edition). Baltimore: The Johns Hopkins University Press.

Newson, E. (1984). The social development of the young autistic child. Paper given at the National Autistic Society Conference, Bath, UK.

Newson, E., Le Maréchal, K., & David, C. (2003). Pathological demand avoidance syndrome: A necessary distinction within the pervasive developmental disorders. *Archives of Disease in Childhood, 88,* 595–600.

Newson, J. & Newson, E. (1975). Intersubjectivity and the transmission of culture: On the social origins of symbolic functioning. *Bulletin of the British Psychological Society, 28,* 437–447.

Nicholas, B., Rudrasingham, V., Nash, S., Kirov, G., Owen, M., & Wimpory, D. (2007). Association of per1 and Npas2 with autistic disorder: Support for the clock genes/social timing hypothesis. *Molecular Psychiatry, 12,* 581–592.

Nir, I. (1995). Circadian melatonin, thyroid stimulating hormone, prolactin and cortisol levels in serum of young adults with autism. *Journal of Autism and Developmental Disorders, 25,* 641–654.

Nirje, B. (1969). The normalization principle and its human management implications. In R. Kugel & W. Wolfensberger (Eds.), *Changing Patterns in Residential Services for the Mentally Retarded* (pp. 179–195). Washington, DC: President's Commission on Mental Retardation.

Norman, D.A. & Shallice, T. (1986). Attention to action: Willed and automatic control of behaviour. In R.J. Davidson, G.E. Schwarts, & D. Shapiro (Eds.), *Consciousness and*

Self-Regulation: Advances in Research and Theory, Vol. 4 (pp. 1–18). New York: Plenum.

Nye, C. & Brice, A. (2002). Combined vitamin B12–magnesium treatment for autistic spectrum disorder. *Cochrane Database System Review, 4*, CD003497.

Oberman, L., Hubbard, E., McCleery, J.P., Altschuler, E., Ramachandran, V.S., & Pineda, J. (2005). EEG evidence for mirror neuron dysfunction in autism spectrum disorders. *Cognitive Brain Research, 24*, 190–198.

Oberman, L. & Ramachandran, V. (2007). The simulating social mind: The role of the mirror neuron system and simulation in the social and communicative deficits of autism spectrum disorders. *Psychological Bulletin, 133*, 310–327.

O'Brien, E., Shang, X., Nishimura, C., Tomblin, B., & Murray, J. (2003). The association of specific language impairment (SLI) to the region of 7q31. *The American Journal of Human Genetics, 72*, 1536–1543.

Office of Alternative Medicine Committee in Definition and Description (1997). Defining and describing complementary medicine and alternative medicine. *Alternative Therapies and Health Medicine, 3*, 49–57.

Olsson, M. & Hwang, C. (2002). Sense of coherence in parents of children with different developmental disabilities. *Journal of Intellectual Disability Research, 46*, 548–559.

Ornitz, E.M. (1974). The modulation of sensory input and motor output in children with autism. *Journal of Autism and Developmental Disorders, 4*, 197–215.

Ornitz, E.M. (1989). Autism at the interface between sensory and information processing. In G. Dawson (Ed.), *Autism: Nature, Diagnosis, and Treatment* (pp. 174–207). New York: Guilford Press.

Ornitz, E. & Ritvo, E. (1968). Neurophysiologic mechanisms underlying perceptual inconstancy in autistic and schizophrenic children. *Archives of General Psychiatry, 19*, 76–98.

Orsmond, G., Krauss, M.W., & Seltzer, M.M. (2004). Peer relationships and social and recreational activities among adolescents and adults with autism. *Journal of Autism and Developmental Disorders, 34*, 245–257.

Osterling, J. & Dawson, G. (1994). Early recognition of children with autism: A study of first birthday home videotapes. *Journal of Autism and Developmental Disorders, 24*, 247–257.

Ousley, O.Y. & Mesibov, G. (1991). Sexual attitudes and knowledge in high functioning adolescents and adults with autism. *Journal of Autism and Developmental Disorders, 21*, 471–481.

Ozonoff, S. & Griffith, E. (2000). Neuropsychological function and the external validity of Asperger syndrome. In A. Klin, F. Volkmar, & S. Sparrow (Eds.), *Asperger Syndrome* (pp. 72–96). New York: Guilford Press.

Ozonoff, S., Cook, I., Coon, H., Dawson, G., Joseph, R., Klin, A., McMahon, W., Minshew, N., Munson, J., Pennington, B., Rogers, S., Spence, M., Tager-Flusberg, H., Volkmar, F., & Wrathall, D. (2004) Performance on Cambridge Neuropsychological Test Automated Battery Subtests sensitive to frontal function in people with autistic disorder. *Journal of Autism and Developmental Disorders, 34*, 139–150.

Ozonoff, S., Pennington, B., & Rogers, S. (1991). Executive function deficits in autistics: Relationship to theory of mind. *Journal of Child Psychology and Psychiatry, 32*, 1081–1185.

Ozonoff, S., Strayer, D., McMahon, W., & Filloux, F. (1994). Executive function abilities in autism and Tourette's syndrome: An information processing approach. *Journal of Child Psychology and Psychiatry, 35*, 1015–1032.

Page, J. & Boucher, J. (1998). Motor impairments in children with autistic disorder. *Child Language, Teaching, and Therapy, 14*, 233–259.

Palmen, S., van Engeland, H., Hof, P., & Schmitz, C. (2004). Neuropathological findings in autism. *Brain, 127*, 2572–2583.

Papps, I. & Dyson, A. (2004). *The Costs and Benefits of Earlier Identification and Effective Intervention: Final Report.* Department for Education and Science.

Parish-Morris, J., Hennon, E.A., Hirsch-Pasek, K., Golinkoff, R.M., & Tager-Flusberg, H. (2007). Children with autism illuminate the role of social intention in word learning. *Child Development, 78,* 1265–1287.

Park, C.C. (2001). *Exiting Nirvana: A Daughter's Life with Autism.* Boston, MA: Little, Brown & Co.

Parsons, J. (2007). *Advocacy for Adults with Autism Spectrum Disorders.* London: National Autistic Society.

Parsons, S. & Mitchell, P. (2002). The potential of virtual reality in social skills training for people with autistic spectrum disorders. *Journal of Intellectual Disability Research, 46,* 430–443.

Paul, R., Augustyn, A., Klin, A., & Volkmar, F. (2005). Perception and production of prosody by speakers with autistic spectrum disorders. *Journal of Autism and Developmental Disorders, 35,* 205–220.

Peeters, T. & Gillberg, C. (1999). *Autism: Medical and Educational Aspects.* London: Whurr Press.

Pellicano, E., Maybery, M., & Durkin, K. (2005). Central coherence in typically developing preschoolers: Does it cohere and does it relate to mindreading and executive control? *Journal of Child Psychology and Psychiatry, 46,* 533–547.

Pellicano, E., Maybery, M., Durkin, K., & Maley, A. (2006). Multiple cognitive capabilities/deficits in children with an autism spectrum disorder: 'Weak' central coherence and its relationship to theory of mind and executive control. *Development and Psychopathology, 18,* 77–98.

Pelphrey, K., Adolphs, R., & Morris, J.P. (2004). Neuroanatomical substrates of social cognition dysfunction in autism. *Mental Retardation and Developmental Disabilities Research Reviews, 10,* 259–271.

Pennington, B., Rogers, S., Bennetto, L., Griffith, E., Reed, D., & Shyu, V. (1997). Validity tests of the impairments of executive function hypothesis of autism. In J. Russell (Ed.), *Autism as an Executive Disorder* (pp. 143–178). Oxford: OUP.

Perkins, M. (2007). *Pragmatic Impairment.* Cambridge: CUP.

Perkins, M., Dobbinson, S., Boucher, J., Bol, S., & Bloom, P. (2006). Lexical knowledge and lexical use in autism. *Journal of Autism and Developmental Disorders, 36,* 795–805.

Perner, J. (1991). *Understanding the Representational Mind.* London: MIT Press.

Perner, J., Baker, S., & Hutton, D. (1994). The conceptual origins of belief and pretence. In C. Lewis & P. Mitchell (Eds.), *Children's Early Understanding of Mind* (pp. 261–286). Hove: Lawrence Erlbaum Associates.

Perner, J. & Lang, B. (1999). Development of theory of mind and executive control. *Trends in Cognitive Sciences, 3,* 337–344.

Peterson, C.C. & Siegal, M. (1995). Deafness, conversation and theory of mind. *Journal of Child Psychology and Psychiatry, 36,* 459–474.

Peterson, D. & Bowler, D. (2000). Counterfactual reasoning and false belief understanding in children with autism. *Autism, 4,* 391–405.

Pickles, A., Starr, E., Kazak, S., Bolton, P., Papanikolaou, K., Bailey, A., Goodman, R., & Rutter, M. (2000). Variable expression of the autism broader phenotype: Findings from extended pedigrees. *Journal of Child Psychology and Psychiatry, 41,* 491–502.

Piven, J., Bailey, J., Ranson, B., & Arndt, S. (1998). No difference in hippocampus volume detected on magnetic resonance imaging in autistic individuals. *Journal of Autism and Developmental Disorders, 28,* 105–110.

Piven, J. & Palmer, P. (1997). Cognitive deficits in parents from multiple-incidence autism families. *Journal of Child Psychology and Psychiatry, 38,* 1011–1021.

Piven, J., Palmer, P., Jacobi, D., Childress, D., & Arndt, S. (1997). Broader autism phenotype: Evidence from a family history study of multiple-incidence autism families. *American Journal of Psychiatry, 154,* 185–190.

Plaisted, K., Dobler, V., Bell, S., & Davis, G. (2006). The microgenesis of global perception in autism. *Journal of Autism and Developmental Disorders, 36,* 107–116.

Plaisted, K., O'Riordan, M., & Baron-Cohen, S. (1998a). Enhanced discrimination of novel, highly similar stimuli by adults with autism during a perceptual learning task. *Journal of Child Psychology and Psychiatry, 39,* 765–775.

Plaisted, K., O'Riordan, M., & Baron-Cohen, S. (1998b). Enhanced visual search for a conjunctive target in autism: A research note. *Journal of Child Psychology and Psychiatry, 39,* 777–783.

Plaisted, K., Saksida, L., Alcantara, J., & Weisblatt, E. (2003). Towards an understanding of the mechanisms of weak central coherence effects: Experiments in visual configural learning and auditory perception. *Philosophical Transactions of the Royal Society: Biological Sciences, 358,* 375–386.

Plaisted, K., Swettenham, J., & Rees, L. (1999). Children with autism show local precedence in a divided attention task and global precedence in a selective attention task. *Journal of Child Psychology and Psychiatry, 40,* 733–742.

Pletnikov, M. & Carbone, K.M. (2005). An animal model of virus-induced autism: Borna disease. In M. Bauman and T. Kemper (Eds.), *The Neurobiology of Autism* (2nd edition) (pp. 190–203). Baltimore: The Johns Hopkins University Press.

Poirier, M. & Martin, J. (2008). Short-term and working memory: How intact are they? In J. Boucher & D.M. Bowler (Eds.), *Memory in Autism.* Cambridge: CUP.

Porges, S. (2005). The vagus: A mediator of behavioral and physiologic features. In M. Bauman & T. Kemper (Eds.), *The Neurobiology of Autism* (2nd edition) (pp. 65–78). Baltimore: The Johns Hopkins University Press.

Posserud, M.-B., Lundervold, A., & Gillberg, C. (2006). Autistic features in a total population of 7–9-year-old children assessed by the ASSQ (Autism Spectrum Screening Questionnaire). *Journal of Child Psychology and Psychiatry, 47,* 167–175.

Powell, S. & Jordan, R. (1993). Being subjective about autistic thinking and learning to learn. *Educational Psychology, 13,* 359–370.

Preece, D. & Jordan, R. (2007). Short break services for children with autistic spectrum disorders: Factors associated with service use and non-use. *Journal of Autism and Developmental Disorders, 37,* 374–385.

Preissler, M. (2008). Associative learning of words and pictures in low-functioning children with autism. *Autism.* London: Sage.

Pring, L. (2005). *Autism and Blindness: Research and Reflections.* London: Whurr Press.

Pring, L. (2008). Memory characteristics in individuals with savant skills. In J. Boucher & D.M. Bowler (Eds.), *Memory in Autism.* Cambridge: CUP.

Prior, M. (2003). *Learning and Behaviour Problems in Asperger Syndrome.* New York: Guilford Press.

Prior, M. & Hoffman, W. (1990). Neuropsychological testing of autistic children through an exploration with frontal lobe tests. *Journal of Autism and Developmental Disorders, 20,* 581–590.

Quartz, S.R. (1999). The constructivist brain. *Trends in Cognitive Sciences, 2,* 48–57.

Rajendran, G. & Mitchell, P. (2007). Cognitive theories of autism. *Developmental Review, 27,* 224–260.

Randall, P. & Parker, J. (1999). *Supporting the Families of Children with Autism.* Chichester: Wiley.

Rapin, I. (1996). Neurological issues. In I. Rapin (Ed.), *Preschool Children with Inadequate Communication* (pp. 98–112). Cambridge: Mac Keith Press.

Rapin, I. & Dunn, M. (2003). Update on the language disorders of individuals on the autistic spectrum. *Brain and Development, 25,* 166–172.

Raymaekers, R., van der Meere, J., Roeyers, H. (2004). Event-rate manipulation and its effect on arousal modulation and response inhibition in adults with high functioning autism. *Journal of Clinical and Experimental Neuropsychology, 26,* 74–82.

Redcay, E. & Courchesne, E. (2005). When is the brain enlarged in autism? A meta-analysis of all brain size reports. *Biological Psychiatry, 58,* 1–9.

Reick, M., Garcia, J., Dudley, C., & McKnight, S. (2004). NPAS2: An analog of clock operative in the mammalian forebrain. *Science, 293,* 506–509.

Renner, P., Klinger, L., & Klinger, M. (2000). Implicit and explicit memory in autism: Is autism an amnesic disorder? *Journal of Child Psychology and Psychiatry, 30,* 3–14.

Renzaglia, A., Karvonen, M., Drasgow, E., & Stoxen, C. (2003). Promoting a lifetime of inclusion. *Focus on Autism and Other Developmental Disabilities, 18*(3), 140–149.

Richdale, A. (1999). Sleep problems in autism: Prevalence, cause and intervention. *Developmental Medicine and Child Neurology, 41,* 60–67.

Richdale, A. & Prior, M.R. (1995). The sleep/wake rhythm in children with autism. *European Child and Adolescent Psychiatry, 4,* 175–187.

Richler, J., Luyster, R., Risi, S., Hsu, W-L., Dawson, G., Bernier, R., Dunn, M., Hepburn, S., Hyman, S., McMahon, W., Goudie-Nice, J., Minshew, N., Rogers, S., Sigman, M., Spence, M., Goldberg, W., Tager-Flusberg, H., Volkmar, F., & Lord, C. (2006). Is there a 'regressive phenotype' of autistic spectrum disorder associated with the measles-mumps-rubella vaccine? A CPEA study. *Journal of Autism and Developmental Disorders, 36,* 299–316.

Ricks, D.M. & Wing, L. (1975). Language, communication, and the use of symbols in normal and autistic children. *Journal of Autism and Developmental Disorders, 5,* 191–221.

Rimland, B. (1964). *Infantile Autism.* New York: Appleton-Century-Crofts.

Rincover, A. & Ducharme, J.M. (1987). Variables influencing stimulus overselectivity and 'tunnel vision' in developmentally delayed children. *American Journal of Mental Deficiency, 91,* 422–430.

Rinehart, N.J., Bellgrove, M.A., Tonge, B., Brereton, A., Howells-Rankin, D., & Bradshaw, J. (2006). An examination of movement kinematics in young people with high-functioning autism and Asperger's disorder: Further evidence for a motor planning deficit. *Journal of Autism and Developmental Disorders, 36,* 757–767.

Rinehart, N.J., Bradshaw, J., Brercton, A., and Tonge, B. (2001a). Movement preparation in high-functioning autism and Asperger disorder: A serial choice reaction time task involving motor reprogramming. *Journal of Autism and Developmental Disorders, 31,* 79–88.

Rinehart, N.J., Bradshaw, J., Moss, S., Brereton, A., & Tonge, B. (2000). Atypical interference of local detail on global processing in high-functioning autism and Asperger's syndrome. *Journal of Child Psychology and Psychiatry, 41,* 769–778.

Rinehart, N.J., Bradshaw, J., Moss, S., Brereton, A., & Tonge, B. (2001b). A deficit in shifting attention present in high-functioning autism but not Asperger's disorder. *Autism, 5,* 67–80.

Rinehart, N., Tonge, B., Iansek, R., McGinley, J., Brereton, A., Enticott, P., & Bradshaw, J. (2006). Gait function in newly diagnosed children with autism: Cerebellar and basal ganglia related motor disorder. *Developmental Medicine and Child Neurology, 48,* 819–824.

Rippon, G., Brock, J., Brown, C., & Boucher, J. (2007). Disordered connectivity in the autistic brain: Challenges for the new psychophysiology. *International Journal of Psychophysiology, 63,* 164–172.

Risi, S., Lord, C., Gotham, K., Chrysler, C., Corsello, C., Szatmari, P., Cook, E., Leventhal, B., & Pickles, A. (2006). Combining information from multiple sources in the diagnosis of autistic spectrum disorders. *Journal of the American Academy of Child and Adolescent Psychiatry, 45,* 1094–1103.

Ritvo, E. & Freeman, B. (1977). National Society for Autistic Children definition of the syndrome of autism. *Journal of Pediatric Psychology, 2,* 146–148.

Ritvo, E., Freeman, B., & Scheibel, A. (1986). Lower Purkinje cell counts in the cerebella of four autistic subjects: Initial findings of the UCLA-NSAC autopsy research report. *American Journal of Psychiatry, 143,* 862–866.

Roberts, J., Rice, M., & Tager-Flusberg, H. (2004). Tense marking in children with autism. *Applied Psycholinguistics, 25,* 429–448.

Robins, D. & Dumont-Mathieu, T. (2006). Early screening for autism spectrum disorders: Update on the Modified Checklist for Autism in Toddlers and other measures. *Journal of Developmental and Behavioural Pediatrics, 27 Supplement 2,* S111–S119.

Robins, D., Fein, D., Barton, M., & Green, J. (2001). The Modified Checklist for Autism in Toddlers. *Journal of Autism and Developmental Disorders, 31,* 131–144.

Rodier, P. & Arndt, T. (2005). The brainstem in autism. In M. Bauman & T. Kemper (Eds.), *The Neurobiology of Autism* (2nd edition) (pp. 136–149). Baltimore: The Johns Hopkins University Press.

Rogers, S., Hepburn, S., Stackhouse, T., & Wehner, E. (2003). Imitation performance in toddlers with autism and those with other developmental disorders. *Journal of Child Psychology and Psychiatry, 44,* 763–781.

Rogers, S. & Pennington, B. (1991). A theoretical approach to the deficits in infantile autism. *Development and Psychopathology, 3,* 137–162.

Rosenhall, U., Nordin, V., Sandstroem, M., Ahlsen, G., & Gillberg, C. (1999). Autism and hearing loss. *Journal of Autism and Developmental Disorders, 29,* 349–357.

Rourke, B. (1989). *Nonverbal Learning Disabilities: The Syndrome and the Model.* New York: Guilford Press.

Rourke, B. & Tsatsanis, K. (2000). Nonverbal learning disabilities and Asperger syndrome. In A. Klin, F. Volkmar, & S. Sparrow (Eds.), *Asperger Syndrome* (pp. 231–253). New York: Guilford Press.

Rubin, R. & Rubin, R. (2005). Response to 'Scientifically unsupported interventions for childhood psychopathology: A summary'. *Pediatrics, 116,* 289.

Rumsey, J. & Hamburger, S. (1988). Neuropsychological findings in high-functioning men with infantile autism, residual state. *Journal of Clinical and Experimental Psychology, 10,* 201–221.

Russell, J. (1996). *Agency: Its Role in Mental Development.* Hove: Lawrence Erlbaum Associates.

Russell, J. (1997). How executive disorders can bring about an inadequate 'theory of mind'. In J. Russell (Ed.), *Autism as an Executive Disorder* (pp. 256–299). Oxford: OUP.

Russell, J., Hala, S., & Hill, E. (2003). The automated windows task: The performance of preschool children, children with autism, and children with moderate learning difficulties. *Cognitive Development, 18,* 111–137.

Russell, J. & Hill, E. (2001). Action monitoring and intention reporting in children with autism. *Journal of Child Psychology and Psychiatry, 42,* 317–328.

Russell, J., Jarrold, C., & Henry, L. (1996). Working memory in children with autism and with moderate learning difficulties. *Journal of Child Psychology and Psychiatry, 37,* 673–687.

Russell, J., Jarrold, C., & Hood, B. (1999). Two intact executive capacities in children with autism: Implications for the core impairments of executive functions in the disorder. *Journal of Autism and Development Disorders, 29,* 103–112.

Russell, J., Mauthner, N., Sharpe, S., & Tidswell, T. (1991). The 'Windows task' as a test of strategic deception in preschoolers and autistic subjects. *British Journal of Developmental Psychology, 9,* 101–119.

Rutgers, A., Bakermans-Kranenburg, M., Ijzendoom, M., & Berckelaer-Onnes, I. (2004). Autism and attachment: A meta-analytic review. *Journal of Child Psychology and Psychiatry, 45*, 1123–1134.

Rutter, M. (1968). Concepts of autism: A review of research. *Journal of Child Psychology and Psychiatry, 9*, 1–25.

Rutter, M. (1983). Cognitive deficits in the pathogenesis of autism. *Journal of Child Psychology and Psychiatry, 24*, 513–531.

Rutter, M. (2005a). Incidence of autism spectrum disorders: Changes over time and their meaning. *Acta Paediatrica, 94*, 2–15.

Rutter, M. (2005b). Aetiology of autism: Findings and questions. *Journal of Intellectual Disability Research, 49*, 231–238.

Rutter, M., Anderson-Wood, L., Beckett, C., Bredenkamp, D., Castle, J., Groothues, C., Kreppner, J., Keaveney, L., Lord, C., & O'Connor, T. (1999). Quasi-autistic patterns following severe early global privation. *Journal of Child Psychology and Psychiatry, 40*, 537–550.

Rutter, M., Greenfield, D., & Lockyer, L. (1967). A five to fifteen year follow-up study of infantile psychosis: II. Social and behavioural outcome. *British Journal of Psychiatry, 113*, 1183–1200.

Rutter, M., Le Couteur, A., & Lord, C. (2003). *Autism Diagnostic Interview–Revised*. Los Angeles: Western Psychological Services.

Rutter, M., Silberg, J., & Simonoff, E. (1999). Genetics and child psychiatry: II Empirical research findings. *Journal of Child Psychology and Psychiatry, 40*, 19–55.

Sacks, O. (1995). *An Anthropologist on Mars*. London: Picador.

Sainsbury, C. (2000). *Martian in the Playground: Understanding the Schoolchild with Asperger's Syndrome*. Bristol: Lucky Duck Publishing Ltd.

Sakai, T., Tamura, T., Kitamoto, T., & Kidokoro, Y. (2004). A clock gene, period, plays a key role in long-term memory formation in Drosophilia. *Proceedings of the National Academy of Sciences, 101*, 16054–16063.

Sanders, J.L. & Morgan, S. (1997). Family stress and adjustment as perceived by caregivers of children with autism or Down syndrome: Implications for intervention. *Child and Family Behaviour Therapy, 19*, 15–32.

Sansosti, F. & Powell-Smith, K. (2006). Using social stories to improve the social behaviour of children with Asperger syndrome. *Journal of Positive Behavioural Interventions, 8*, 43–57.

Santangelo, S. & Tsatsanis, K. (2005). What is known about autism: Genes, brain, and behaviour. *American Journal of PharmacoGenomics, 5*, 71–92.

Scahill, L. & Martin, A. (2005). Psychopharmacology. In F. Volkmar, R. Paul, A. Klin, & D. Cohen (Eds.), *Handbook of Autism and Pervasive Developmental Disorders, Vol. 2* (3rd edition) (pp. 1102–1117). Hoboken, NJ: John Wiley & Sons.

Scambler, D., Hepburn, S., & Rogers, S. (2006). A two-year follow-up on risk status identified by the Checklist for Autism in Toddlers. *Journal of Developmental and Behavioural Pediatrics, 27 Supplement 2*, S104–S110.

Scheuffgen, K., Happé, F., Anderson, M., & Frith, U. (2000). High 'intelligence', low 'IQ'? Speed of processing and measured IQ in children with autism. *Development and Psychopathology, 12*, 83–90.

Schmahmann, J. & Caplan, D. (2006). Cognition, emotion and the cerebellum. *Brain, 129*, 290–293.

Schmitz, C., Martineau, J., Barthelemy, C., & Assaante, C. (2003). Motor control and children with autism: Deficit of anticipatory function. *Neuroscience Letters, 348*, 17–20.

Schopler, E. & Mesibov, G. (1987). *The Neurobiology of Autism*. New York: Plenum.

Schopler, E., Reichler, R., & Renner, P. (1988). *The Childhood Autism Rating Scale (CARS)*. Los Angeles: Western Psychological Services.

Schultz, R.T. (2005). Developmental deficits in social perception in autism: The role of the amygdala and fusiform face area. *International Journal of Developmental Neuroscience, 23*, 125–141.

Seal, B. & Bonvillian, J. (1997). Sign language and motor functioning in students with autistic disorder. *Journal of Autism and Developmental Disorders, 27*, 437–466.

Scott, F., Baron-Cohen, S., Bolton, P., & Brayne, C. (2002). The CAST (Childhood Asperger Syndrome Test). *Autism, 6*, 9–31.

Seltzer, M.M., Krauss, M.W., Shattuck, P., Orsmond, G., Swe, A., & Lord, C. (2003). The symptoms of autism spectrum disorders in adolescence and adulthood. *Journal of Autism and Developmental Disorders, 33*, 565–582.

Shah, A. & Frith, U. (1983). An islet of ability in autistic children: A research note. *Journal of Child Psychology and Psychiatry, 24*, 613–620.

Shao, Y., Cuccaro, M., Hauser, E., Raiford, K., Menold, M., Wolpert, C., Ravan, S., Elston, L., Decena, K., Donnelly, S., Abramson, R., Wright, H., DeLong, G., Gilbert, J., & Pericak-Vauce, M. (2003). Fine mapping of autistic disorder to chromosome 15q11-q13 by use of phenotypic subtypes. *American Journal of Human Genetics, 72*, 539–548.

Shavelle, R., Strauss, D., & Pickett, J. (2001). Causes of death in autism. *Journal of Autism and Developmental Disorders, 31*, 569–576.

Shea, V. (2004). A perspective on the research literature related to early intensive behavioural intervention (Lovaas) for young children with autism. *Autism, 8*, 349–367.

Shields, J. (2001). The NAS 'EarlyBird' programme: Partnership with parents in early intervention, *Autism, 5*, 49–56.

Siegel, B. (2004). *Early Childhood Screeners for ASDs: The Pervasive Developmental Disorders Screening Test-II:* San Antonio, TX: Harcourt Assessment.

Siegel, D., Minshew, N., & Goldstein, G. (1996). Wechsler IQ profiles in diagnosis of high functioning autism. *Journal of Autism and Developmental Disorders, 26*, 389–407.

Sigman, M. & Capps, L. (1997). *Children with Autism: A Developmental Perspective.* Cambridge, MA: Harvard University Press.

Sigman, M., Dijamco, A., Gratier, M., & Rozga, A. (2004). Early detection of core deficits in autism. *Mental Retardation and Developmental Disabilities Research Reviews, 10*, 221–233.

Sigman, M., Kasari, C., Kwon, J., & Yirmiya, N. (1992). Responses to the negative emotions of others by autistic, mentally retarded, and normal children. *Child Development, 63*, 796–807.

Singer, T. (2006). The neuronal basis and ontogeny of empathy and mind reading: Review of literature and implications for future research. *Neuroscience and Biobehavioral Reviews, 30*, 855–863.

Skuse, D. (2005). X-linked genes and mental functioning. *Human Molecular Genetics, 14*, R27–R32.

Skuse, D., James, R., Bishop, D.V., Coppin, B., Dalton, P., Aamodt-Leeper, G., Bacarese-Hamilton, M., Cresswell, C., McGurk, R., & Jacobs, P. (1997). Evidence from Turner's syndrome of an imprinted X-linked locus affecting cognitive function. *Nature, 387*, 705–708.

Slade, L. & Ruffman, T. (2005). How language does (and does not) relate to theory of mind: A longitudinal study of syntax, semantics, working memory and false belief. *British Journal of Developmental Psychology, 23*, 117–141.

Slater-Walker, G. & Slater-Walker, C. (2002). *An Asperger Marriage.* London: Jessica Kingsley Publishers.

Smart, M. (2004). Transition planning and the needs of young people and their carers. *British Journal of Special Education, 31*, 128–137.

Smith, T., Scahill, L., Dawson, G., Guthrie, D., Lord, C., Odom, S., Rogers, S., & Wagner, A. (2007). Designing research studies on psychosocial intervention in autism. *Journal of Autism and Developmental Disorders, 37*, 354–366.

Sofronoff, K., Attwood, T., & Hinton, S. (2005). A randomised controlled trial of a CBT intervention for anxiety in children with Asperger syndrome. *Journal of Child Psychology and Psychiatry, 46*, 1152–1160.

Sonuga-Barke, E. (1998). Categorical models of childhood disorder: A conceptual and empirical analysis. *Journal of Child Psychology and Psychiatry, 39*, 115–133.

South, M., Ozonoff, S., & McMahon, W. (2007). The relationship between executive functioning, central coherence, and repetitive behaviours in the high-functioning autism spectrum. *Autism, 11*, 437–451.

Sparrow, S. & Davis, S.M. (2000). Recent advances in the assessment of intelligence and cognition. *Journal of Child Psychology and Psychiatry, 41*, 117–132.

Spiker, D. & Ricks, M. (1984). Visual self-recognition in autistic children: Developmental relationships. *Child Development, 55*, 214–225.

Stachnik, J. & Nunn-Thompson, C. (2007). Use of atypical antipsychotics in the treatment of autistic disorder. *The Annals of Pharmacotherapy, 41*, 626–634.

Stehli, A. (1992). *The Miracle of Silence*. London: Doubleday.

Steingaard, R., Connor, D., and Au, T. (2005). Approaches to psychopharmacology. In M. Bauman and T. Kemper (Eds.), *The Neurobiology of Autism* (2nd edition) (pp. 79–102). Baltimore: The Johns Hopkins University Press.

Stern, D. (1985). *The Interpersonal World of the Infant: A View from Psychoanalysis and Developmental Psychology*. New York: Basic Books.

Steyn, B. & Le Couteur, A. (2003). Understanding autistic spectrum disorders. *Current Paediatrics, 13*, 274–278.

Stokes, M. & Kaur, A. (2005). High-functioning autism and sexuality: A parental perspective. *Autism, 9*, 266–281.

Stone, W.L., Coonrod, E., Turner, L., & Pozdol, S. (2004). Psychometric properties of the STAT for early autism screening. *Journal of Autism and Developmental Disorders, 24*, 691–701.

Stores, G. (1999). Children's sleep disorders: Modern approaches, developmental effects, and children at special risk. *Developmental Medicine and Child Neurology, 41*, 568–573.

Storey, A., Walsh, C., Quinton, R., & Wynne-Edwards, K. (2000). Hormonal correlates of paternal responsiveness in new and expectant fathers. *Evolution and Human Behaviour, 21*, 79–95.

Stromswold, K. (2006). Why aren't identical twins linguistically identical? Genetic, prenatal and postnatal factors. *Cognition, 101*, 333–384.

Sturm, H., Fernell, E., & Gillberg, C. (2004). Autistic spectrum disorders in children with normal intellectual levels: Associated impairments and subgroups. *Developmental Medicine and Child Neurology, 46*, 444–447.

Suddendorf, T. & Corballis, M. (1997). Mental time travel and the evolution of the human mind. *Genetic, Social, and General Psychology Monographs, 123*, 629–650.

Summers, J. & Craik, F. (1994). The effect of subject-performed tasks on the memory performance of verbal autistic children. *Journal of Autism and Developmental Disorders, 24*, 773–783.

Sweeten, T., Posey, D., & McDougle, C. (2004). Autistic disorder in three children with cytomegaloviral infection. *Journal of Autism and Developmental Disorder, 34*, 583–586.

Sutera, S., Pandey, J., Esser, E., Rosenthal, M., Wilson, L., Barton, M., Green, J., Hodgson, S., Robins, D., Dumont-Mathieu, T., & Fein, D. (2007). Predictors of optimal outcome in toddlers diagnosed with autism spectrum disorders. *Journal of Autism and Developmental Disorders, 37*, 98–107.

Szatmari, P., Bartolucci, G., Bremner, R., Bond, S., & Rich, S. (1989). A follow-up study of high-functioning autistic children. *Journal of Autism and Developmental Disorders, 19*, 213–225.

Szelag, E., Kowalska, J., Galkowski, T., & Pöppel, E. (2004). Temporal processing deficits in high-functioning children with autism. *British Journal of Psychology, 95*, 269–282.

Tager-Flusberg, H. (1991). Semantic processing in the free recall of autistic children: Further evidence of a cognitive deficit. In G. Dawson (Ed.), *Autism: Nature, Diagnosis, and Treatment.* (pp. 92–109). New York: Guilford Press.

Tager-Flusberg, H. (2000). Language and understanding minds: Connections in autism. In S. Baron-Cohen, H. Tager-Flusberg, & D. Cohen (Eds.), *Understanding Other Minds: Perspectives from Developmental Cognitive Neuroscience* (2nd edition) (pp. 124–149). Oxford: OUP.

Tager-Flusberg, H., Lord, C., & Paul, R. (2005). Language and communication in autism. In F. Volkmar, R. Paul, A. Klin, & D. Cohen (Eds.), *Handbook of Autism and Pervasive Developmental Disorders, Vol. 1* (3rd edition) (pp. 335–364). Hoboken, NJ: John Wiley & Sons.

Tager-Flusberg, H. & Sullivan, K. (2000). A componential view of theory of mind: Evidence from Williams syndrome. *Cognition, 76*, 59–89.

Tanguay, P. (1984). Towards a new classification of serious psychopathology in children. *Journal of the American Academy of Child Psychiatry, 23*, 378–384.

Tantam, D. (1988). Asperger syndrome. *Journal of Child Psychology and Psychiatry, 29*, 245–255.

Tarakeshwar, N. & Pargament, K. (2002). Religious coping in families of children with autism. *Focus on Autism and Other Developmental Disabilities, 16*, 247–260.

Teitelbaum, P., Teitelbaum, O., Nye, J., Fryman, J., & Maurer, R.G. (1998). Movement analysis in infancy may be useful for early diagnosis of autism. *Proceedings of the National Academy of Sciences, 95*, 13982–13987.

Tobing, L. & Glenwick, D. (2002). Relation of the Childhood Autism Rating Scale – Parent version to diagnosis, stress, and age. *Research in Developmental Disabilities, 23*, 211–223.

Toichi, M. & Kamio, Y. (2003). Long term memory in high functioning autism: Controversy on episodic memory reconsidered. *Journal of Autism and Developmental Disorders, 33*, 151–161.

Tomblin, J.B., Hafeman, L.L., & O'Brien, M. (2003). Autism and autism risk in siblings of children with specific language impairment. *International Journal of Language & Communication Disorders, 38*, 235–250.

Tordjmann, S., Anderson, G., Pichard, N., Charbury, H., & Touitou, Y. (2005). Nocturnal excretion of 6-sulphatoxymelatonin in children and adolescents with autistic disorder. *Biological Psychiatry, 57*, 134–138.

Toth, K., Munson, J., Meltzoff, A., & Dawson, G. (2006). Early predictors of communication development in young children with autistic spectrum disorder: Joint attention, imitation and play. *Journal of Autism and Developmental Disorders, 36*, 993–2005.

Trevarthen, C. (1980). The foundations of intersubjectivity. Development of interpersonal and co-operative understanding of infants. In D. Olson (Ed.), *The Social Foundations of Language and Thought* (pp. 316–342). New York: WW Norton.

Trevarthen, C. (1989). Development of early social interactions and the affective regulation of brain growth. In C. von Euler, H. Forssberg, and H. Lagercrantz (Eds.), *Neurobiology of Early Infant Behaviour. (Wenner-Gren Center International Symposium Series, Vol. 55)*. Basingstoke: Macmillan.

Trevarthen, C. & Aitken, K. (2001). Infant intersubjectivity: Research, theory, and clinical applications. *Journal of Child Psychology and Psychiatry, 42*, 3–48.

Trevarthen, C. & Hubley, P. (1978). Secondary intersubjectivity: Confidence, confiding, and acts of meaning in the first year. In A. Lock (Ed.), *Action, Gesture, and Symbol* (pp. 183–229). London: Academic Press.

Tuchman, R. & Rapin, I. (2002). Epilepsy in autism. *Lancet Neurology, 1*, 352–358.

Tulving, E. (1995). Organisation of memory: Quo vadis? In M. Gazzaniga (Ed.), *The Cognitive Neurosciences* (pp. 839–847). Cambridge, MA: MIT Press.

Turner, M. (1997). Towards an impairment of executive function account of repetitive behaviour in autism. In J. Russell (Ed.), *Autism as an Executive Disorder* (pp. 57–100). Oxford: OUP.

Turner, M. (1999). Generating novel ideas: fluency performance in high-functioning and learning disabled persons with autism. *Journal of Child Psychology and Psychiatry, 40*, 189–202.

Tustin, F. (1981). *Autism and Childhood Psychosis.* London: Hogarth Press. (Reprinted in 1995 and published by Karnac Books.)

Tustin, F. (1991). Revised understanding of psychogenic autism. *International Journal of Psychoanalysis, 72*, 585–591.

Uchiyama, T., Kurosawa, M., & Inaba, Y. (2007). MMR-vaccine and regression in autism spectrum disorders: Negative results presented from Japan. *Journal of Autism and Developmental Disorders, 37*, 210–217.

Ullman, M. (2001). The declarative/procedural model of lexicon and grammar. *Journal of Psycholinguistic Research, 30*, 37–69.

Ullman, M. (2004). Contributions of memory circuits to language: The declarative/procedural model. *Cognition, 92*, 231–270.

Van der Geest, J.N., Kemner, C., Camfferman, G., Verbaten, M., & van Engeland, H. (2001). Eye movements, visual attention, and autism: A saccadic reaction time study using the gap and overlap paradigm. *Biological Psychiatry, 50*, 614–619.

Varela, F., Thompson, E., & Rosch, E. (1991). *The Embodied Mind.* Cambridge, MA: MIT Press.

Vargha-Khadem, F., Gadian, D., Watkins, K., Connelly, A., van Paesschen, W., & Mishkin, M. (1997). Differential effects of early hippocampal pathology on episodic and semantic memory. *Science, 277*, 376–380.

Vidal, C., Nicolson, R., DeVito, T., Hayashi, K., Geaga, J., Drost, D., Williamson, P., Rajakumar, N., Sui, Y., Dutton, R., Toga, A., & Thompson, P. (2006). Mapping corpus callosum deficits in autism: An index of aberrant cortical connectivity. *Biological Psychiatry, 60*, 218–225.

Vincent, J.B., Melmer, G., Bolton, P., Hodgkinson, S., Holmes, D., Curtis, D., & Gurling, H. (2005). Genetic linkage analysis of the X chromosome in autism, with emphasis on the fragile X region. *Psychiatric Genetics, 15*, 83–90.

Volkmar, F. (2005). International perspectives. In F. Volkmar, R. Paul, A. Klin, & D. Cohen (Eds.), *Handbook of Autism and Pervasive Developmental Disorders, Vol. 2* (3rd edition) (pp. 1193–1252). Hoboken, NJ: John Wiley & Sons.

Volkmar, F., Klin, A., Cohen, D. (1997). Diagnosis and classification of autism and related conditions: Consensus and issues. In D. Cohen & F. Volkmar (Eds.), *Handbook of Autism and Pervasive Developmental Disorders* (2nd edition) (pp. 5–40). New York: John Wiley.

Volkmar, F., Paul, R., Klin, A., & Cohen, D. (2005). *Handbook of Autism and Pervasive Developmental Disorders, Vols. 1 and 2* (3rd edition). Hoboken, NJ: John Wiley & Sons.

Wakefield, A., Murch, S., Anthony, A., Linnell, J., Casson, D., Malik, M., Berelowitz, M., Dhillon, A., Thomson, M., Harvey, P., Valentine, A., Davies, S., & Walker-Smith, J. (1998). Ileal-lymphoid-nodular hyperplasia, non-specific colitis, and pervasive developmental disorder in children. *The Lancet, 351*, 637–641.

Wallace, G. & Happé, F. (2007). Time perception in autism spectrum disorders. *Research in Autism Spectrum Disorders, 2*, 447–455.

Waltz, M. & Shattock, P. (2004). Autistic disorder in nineteenth-century London: Three case reports. *Autism, 8*, 7–20.

Warnock, D.M. (1978). *Special Educational Needs: The Warnock Report.* London: HMSO.

Wassink, T., Brzustowicz, L., Bartlett, C., & Szatmari, P. (2004). The search for autism disease genes. *Mental Retardation and Developmental Disabilities Research Reviews, 10*, 272–283.

Wassink, T., Piven, J., Vieland, V., Pietila, Goedken, R., Folstein, S., & Sheffield, V. (2004). Examination of AVPR1a as an autism susceptibility gene. *Molecular Psychiatry, 9*, 968–972.

Waterhouse, L., Fein, D., & Modahl, C. (1996). Neurofunctional mechanisms in autism. *Psychological Review, 103*, 457–489.

Wechsler, D. (1999). *Wechsler Adult Intelligence Scale (WAIS-III-UK).* Oxford: Harcourt Assessment.

Wechsler, D. (2004). *Wechsler Intelligence Scale for Children (WISC-IV-UK).* Oxford: Harcourt Assessment.

Weiss, M. (2002). Hardiness and social support as predictors of stress in mothers of typical children, children with autism, and children with mental retardation. *Autism, 6*, 115–130.

Welch, M. (1984). Retrieval from autism through mother-child holding. In E. Tinbergen & N. Tinbergen (Eds.), *Autistic Children: New Hope for a Cure* (pp. 322–336). London: Allen & Unwin.

Welch, M. (1988). *Holding Time.* London: Century Hutchinson.

Werner, H. & Kaplan, B. (1984). *Symbol Formation.* Hillsdale, NJ: Lawrence Erlbaum Associates.

Werth, A., Perkins, M., & Boucher, J. (2001). 'Here's the weavery looming up': Verbal humour in a woman with high-functioning autism. *Autism, 5*, 111–127.

Wheeler, M., Stuss, D., & Tulving, E. (1997). Toward a theory of episodic memory: The frontal lobes and autonoetic consciousness. *Psychological Bulletin, 121*, 331–354.

Whitaker, P. (2001). *Challenging Behaviour and Autism: Making Sense – Making Progress.* London: National Autistic Society.

Whitaker, P. (2002). Supporting families of preschool children with autism: What parents want and what helps. *Autism, 6*, 411–426.

Whitaker-Azmitia, P. (2001). Serotonin and brain development: Role in human developmental diseases. *Brain Research Bulletin, 56*, 479–485.

White, B.B. & White, M.S. (1987). Autism from the inside. *Medical Hypotheses, 24*, 223–229.

Wier, M., Yoshida, C., Odouli, R., Grether, J., & Croen, J. (2006). Congenital anomalies associated with autism spectrum disorders. *Developmental Medicine and Child Neurology, 48*, 500–507.

Wilcox, J., Tsuang, M., Schurr, T., & Baida-Fragoso, N. (2003). Case-control study of lesser variant traits in autism. *Neuropsychobiology, 47*, 171–177.

Williams, D. (1994). *Somebody Somewhere.* London: Doubleday.

Williams, D., Botting, N., & Boucher, J. (in press). Language in autism and specific language disorder: Where are the links? *Psychological Bulletin.*

Williams, D.L., Goldstein, G., Carpenter, P., & Minshew, N. (2005). Verbal and spatial working memory in autism. *Journal of Autism and Developmental Disorders, 35*, 747–756.

Williams, D., Happé, F., & Jarrold, C. (2008). Intact inner speech use in autism spectrum disorder: Evidence from a short-term memory task. *Journal of Child Psychology and Psychiatry, 49*, 51–58.

Williams, J. (2005). Language is fundamentally a social affair. Commentary in *Behavioural and Brain Sciences, 28,* 146–147.

Williams, J. & Brayne, C. (2006). Screening for autism spectrum disorders: What is the evidence? *Autism, 10,* 11–35.

Williams, J., Waiter, G., Gilchrist, A., Perrett, D., Murray, A., & Whiten, A. (2006). Neural mechanisms of imitation and 'mirror neuron' functioning in autistic spectrum disorder. *Neuropsychologia, 44,* 610–621.

Williams, J., Whiten, A., & Singh, T. (2004). A systematic review of action imitation in autistic spectrum disorder. *Journal of Autism and Developmental Disorders, 34,* 285–299.

Williams, J., Whiten, A., Suddendorf, T., & Perrett, D. (2001). Imitation, mirror neurons and autism. *Neuroscience and Biobehavioural Reviews, 25,* 287–295.

Wimpory, D., Nicholas, B., & Nash, S. (2002). Social timing, clock genes and autism: A new hypothesis. *Journal of Intellectual Disability Research, 46,* 352–358.

Wing, L. (1981). Asperger's syndrome: A clinical account. *Psychological Medicine, 11,* 115–129.

Wing, L. (1988). The continuum of autistic characteristics. In E. Schopler and G. Mesibov (Eds.), *Diagnosis and Assessment in Autism* (pp. 91–110). New York: Plenum.

Wing, L. (1996). *The Autistic Spectrum.* London: Constable.

Wing, L. & Gould, J. (1979). Severe impairments of social interaction and associated abnormalities in children: Epidemiology and classification. *Journal of Autism and Childhood Schizophrenia, 9,* 11–29.

Wing, L., Leekam, S., Libby, S., Gould, J., & Larcombe, M. (2002). The Diagnostic Interview for Social and Communication Disorders. *Journal of Child Psychology and Psychiatry, 43,* 307–327.

Wing, L. & Potter, D. (2002). The epidemiology of autistic spectrum disorders: Is the prevalence rising? *Mental Retardation and Developmental Disabilities Research Reviews, 8,* 151–161.

Wolff, S. (2000). Schizoid personality in childhood. In A. Klin, F. Volkmar, & S. Sparrow (Eds.), *Asperger Syndrome* (pp. 278–308). New York: Guilford Press.

Woodbury-Smith, M., Robinson, J., Wheelwright, S., & Baron-Cohen, S. (2005). Screening adults for Asperger syndrome using the AQ: A preliminary study of its diagnostic validity. *Journal of Autism and Developmental Disorders, 35,* 331–336.

World Health Organisation (1992). *International Classification of Mental and Behavioural Disorders: Clinical Descriptions and Diagnostic Guidelines,* (10th edition) (ICD-10). Geneva: WHO.

World Health Organisation (1993). *The ICD-10 Classification of Mental and Behavioural Disorders: Diagnostic Criteria for Research.* Geneva: WHO.

Yirmiya, N., Erel, O., Shaked, M., & Solomonica-Levi, D. (1998). Meta-analyses comparing theory of mind abilities of individuals with autism, individuals with mental retardation, and normally developing individuals. *Psychological Bulletin, 124,* 283–307.

Yirmiya, N., Kasari, C., Sigman, M., & Mundy, P. (1989). Facial expressions of affect in autistic, mentally retarded and normal children. *Journal of Child Psychology and Psychiatry, 30,* 725–735.

Yirmiya, N., Sigman, M., Kasari, C., & Mundy, P. (1992). Empathy and cognition in high functioning children with autism. *Child Development, 63,* 150–160.

Yoder, P. & Stone, W. (2006). Randomised comparison of two communication interventions for preschoolers with autism spectrum disorders. *Journal of Consulting and Clinical Psychology, 74,* 426–435.

Zandt, F., Prior, M., & Kyrios, M. (2007). Repetitive behaviour in children with high-functioning autism and obsessive compulsive disorder. *Journal of Autism and Developmental Disorders, 37,* 251–259.

Zeegers, M., van der Grond, J., van Daalen, E., Buitelaar, J., & van Engeland, H. (2007). Proton magnetic resonance spectroscopy in developmentally delayed young boys with or without autism. *Journal of Neural Transmission, 114,* 289–295.

Zelazo, P.D., Burack, J., Benedetto, E., & Frye, D. (1996). Theory of mind and rule use in individuals with Down syndrome: A test of the uniqueness and specificity claims. *Journal of Child Psychology and Psychiatry, 37,* 479–484.

Zelazo, P.D., Jacques, S., Burack, J., & Frye, D. (2002). The relation between theory of mind and rule use: Evidence from persons with autism-spectrum disorders. *Infant and Child Development, 11,* 171–195.

Zelazo, P.R. & Zelazo, P.D. (1998). The emergence of consciousness. In H.H. Jasper, L. Descarries, V.F. Castellucci, & S. Rossingnol (Eds.), *Consciousness: At the Frontiers of Neuroscience. Advances in Neurology, Vol. 77* (pp. 149–165). New York: Lippincott-Raven Press.

INDEX

accidents, risk of 84, 85, 86
acquired autism 27, 76, 86, 331
action initiation 170, 176–7, 186, 199, 208
action–outcome monitoring 170, 172, 178–9, 186, 331
adaptive behaviour 14, 331
addiction 84
adolescence 79, 86
adults/adult outcomes 80–5, 86
  care needs 82, 320–3, 329
  diagnosis 268
  support for parent carers 316, 329
  see also employment
affect 44, 331
  see also emotion processing; emotions
affective agnosia 156, 331
affordances 158, 215, 331
age of onset 27, 74–7
agency 178–9, 182, 331
alcohol abuse 84, 122
amnesia 234, 235, 236, 240, 246, 338
amygdala 126, 134, 137, 138, 144, 221, 222, 230, 331
amygdala-orbitofrontal system 252, 253
animal models 119, 131, 234–5, 251, 332
anxiety 64, 68, 101, 139, 168–9, 198, 229, 268, 302
apoptosis (programmed cell death) 128, 129, 133, 332
appearance-reality test 148, 332
Applied Behavioural Analysis (ABA) 292, 299, 300
apraxia 61, 332
articulation 56, 204, 332
Asperger, Hans 5, 10, 11, 20, 21
Asperger disorder *see* Asperger syndrome
Asperger syndrome (AS) 4, 10, 11, 12, 56, 93, 327, 332
  and autistic disorder, differentiated 24, 25
  communication impairments 90
  diagnosis 26, 263, 272–3
  diagnostic criteria 13–14, 21
  educational provision 319, 324
  language ability 56, 68, 90, 203, 235
  memory abilities 235, 238
  motor abnormalities 25, 48, 93, 198–9

Asperger syndrome (AS) *cont.*
  and non-verbal learning disability (NVLD) 25–6
  prevalence 72
  screening for 277, 278
  socio-economic status and 74
  use as a term 38
Asperger Syndrome Diagnostic Interview (ASDI) 273
Asperger Syndrome Diagnostic Scale (ASDS) 273, 277
assessment 258–9, 277
  see also diagnosis; screening
association studies 119
associative learning 138, 203, 239
attachment 50, 332
attention 64–5, 101, 138, 214, 230, 288, 332
  disengagement of 170, 172, 173, 179, 182, 183, 186, 245
  monotropic 48, 189, 349
  over-selective 48, 351
  preferential 160–2, 165, 215
  selective 161, 190, 207, 357
  switching/shifting 137, 164, 170, 173–4, 179, 193, 217, 332
attentional bias 163, 214, 332
attention deficit disorder (ADD) 65, 332
attention deficit and hyperactivity disorder (ADHD) 9, 65, 285, 332
atypical autism 14, 332
auditory ability 193
  see also hearing/hearing impairment
Auditory Integration Training (AIT) 287
Autism Behaviour Checklist (ABC) 272, 278
Autism Diagnostic Interview- Revised (ADI-R) 269–70, 272, 276, 278
Autism Diagnostic Observation Schedule (ADOS) 270, 271, 272, 276, 278
Autism-Spectrum Quotient (AQ) 276
Autism Spectrum Screening Questionnaire (ASSQ) 276
autistic continuum 29, 333
autistic disorder
  and Asperger syndrome differentiated 24–5
  diagnostic criteria 12–13, 21
  use as a term 38

autistic disorder *cont.*
   see also classic autism; Kanner's
      syndrome; low-functioning autism
autistic psychopathy 10
autistic spectrum disorders (ASDs) 333
  as diagnostic description 263
  use as a term 29–30, 35, 38
autoimmune disorders 62, 123, 333
autonoetic awareness 246, 333
autonomic nervous system (ANS) 135, 333
axons 125–6, 127, 128, 129, 333

Baron-Cohen, S. 105, 122, 139, 145, 148–9,
    154, 157, 183–4, 202, 204, 207, 213,
    217, 240, 243
  'the bar game' 198
befriending schemes 314–15, 333
behavioural inertia 176–7
behavioural inflexibility 79, 89, 100, 214,
    230, 333
  brain–behaviour explanations 220
  contributory causes not specific to autism
    168–70, 186, 245
  and executive function impairments 101,
    169–83, 186, 187, 211, 218,
    220, 245
  hypersystemising and 183–4, 186, 217
  sensory-perceptual anomalies and
    184–5, 187
  uneven memory abilities and 185–6,
    187, 224, 245–7
  see also imagination, impairment of;
    restricted, repetitive behaviour
behavioural problems, challenging/anti-social
    64–6, 68, 79, 84, 282, 335
behaviourism 92, 333
behaviourist models/approaches 6, 109, 291,
    300–1, 333–4
Belmonte, M. 224–5, 227, 229–30, 231
blind children 144, 169
Block Design test 59, 192, 206
Bloom, P. 202–3, 240
body schema 48, 334
bonding 160, 222, 334
Borna virus 123, 334
Boucher, J. 33, 91, 235, 236–7, 238, 240,
    242, 243, 249–50
brain anatomy/structure(s) 98, 125–6, 132–4,
    197, 220, 222
  abnormalities of 133–4, 138, 139, 140–1,
    219, 221, 222, 223–4, 230–1
  methods of assessing 130, 132
  reversed asymmetry in 133, 356
  see also individual structures
brain bases 98, 100, 125–41, 144,
    218–27, 252–4
  links from first causes to 228–9

brain–behaviour explanations
  218–27, 230–1
brain chemistry 130, 132, 134–6,   139,
  139–40, 222, 283
brain-derived neurotrophic factor
    (BDNF) 136, 334
brain function 98, 103, 126–7, 136–8, 139,
    141, 169, 219, 220–5, 227, 283
  methods of assessing 131, 132
brain-mind development 132, 136, 139,
    197, 227
  connectionist or neural network models
    133, 214–15
  constructivist-emergence model 214, 215,
    218, 222–7, 230, 231
  dedicated-systems model 213, 214,
    218, 219–22
  dynamic systems modelling 214–15
  environmental factors and 129, 228
  genetic factors and 129, 228–9
  physical aspects of 127–9, 135
  plasticity of 129, 213, 214
brain size, abnormalities of 132–3, 138, 140,
    223, 224, 231
brain stem 126, 127, 138, 221, 252, 334
  abnormalities of 132, 133, 138, 140,
    190, 227, 253
  reticular activating system 190, 356
broader autism phenotype (BAP) 24, 334
Brock, J. 219, 223, 233
Burack, J. 185, 193, 194

care 82, 308–30
  assessments for 258, 259, 277
  crisis 314–15, 329
  families and 309–17, 328–9
  inclusive 308–9, 323, 326, 327
  respite 314–15, 329, 356
  substitute, or out-of-home 82,
    317–23, 329
catatonic states 65, 334
categorical model 6, 335
  see also subtypes model
category formation 240–1, 243
causal explanations
  importance of 98, 112
  levels of explanation 98–100, 112, 210
  hypotheses concerning links across
    228–30, 231
  'many-to-one' and 'one-to-many'
    phenomena 101–2, 113
  simplifying the search for 101–4, 113
  sources of difficulty in 98–108, 112–13
causal theories
  assessment of merits of 108–12, 113
  single common pathway 104–8, 211
  see also individual theories

cause-effect links 101–3, 112–13
cell death *see* apoptosis
central coherence 164, 214, 227, 335
  see also weak central coherence
central executive 170–1, 181, 335
cerebellar vermis 127, 335
cerebellum 126, 128, 133, 137, 138, 219,
    221, 222–5 *passim*, 227, 229, 253, 335
cerebral cortex 128, 133, 140, 335
cerebral hemispheres 128–9, 132, 335
cerebral palsy 63
Checklist for Autism in Toddlers (CHAT)
    275, 276, 278
Childhood Asperger's Screening Test
    (CAST) 277
Childhood Autism Rating Scale (CARS)
    272, 278
childhood disintegrative disorder 8, 12,
    23, 27, 335
Children's Communication Checklist
    (CCC) 54, 55
circadian rhythms 249, 250, 251, 335
classic autism 13, 38, 72, 335–6
  see also autistic disorder; Kanner's
    syndrome
clock genes 162, 250–1, 251–2, 336
clumsiness 25, 48, 197, 198–200, 208
cognition 136, 138, 336
cognitive ability 35, 52, 57
Cognitive Behavioural Therapy 302
cognitive complexity and control (CCC)
    theory 151, 336
cognitive flexibility *see* mental flexibility
cognitivist models 92, 109, 336
communication 53, 54, 336
  non-verbal 12, 33, 54, 90, 143, 350
  protodeclarative 51, 75, 78, 146, 149, 153,
    155, 157, 354
  protoimperative or 'demand'
    50–1, 354
communication impairment 10–11, 13, 21,
    31–3, 34, 54–5, 89, 100, 143
  brain-based theories 144
  emotion processing and 92
  impaired theory of mind (ToM) theory
    145–52, 164, 211, 218
  and language impairment, dissociability
    of 90–1
  manifest behaviours exemplifying 19
  mindblindness theory 152–4
  primary intersubjectivity deficit
    theories 154–64, 165
  psychodynamic theories 144
  and social interaction impairment,
    interdependence of 89–90
  time-processing and 249
communicative ability, spared 50–1

co-morbid conditions 56, 61–7, 68–9, 169,
    186, 203–4, 205, 208, 336
complementary and alternative medicines
    (CAMS) 284, 287, 288, 294, 297–8,
    304, 305, 336
comprehension 57, 68, 93, 200, 242
compulsions/obsessions 64, 65, 101, 168, 169
computational models 131, 213, 336
Computerised (Axial) Tomography (CT/CAT
    scan) 130, 336
conation/volition 176–7, 186
conjunctive search 195–6, 337
connectionism/connectionist modelling
    214, 337
  see also neural network models
connectivity 219, 337
  see also impaired connectivity theories
constructivist-emergence model 214, 215,
    218, 222–7, 230, 231
constructivists/constructivism 129, 337
corpus callosum 126, 128, 134, 140, 337
counterfactual reasoning 150, 152, 337
Courchesne, E. 223–4, 227, 231
Creak's Nine Points 7–8, 94
creativity 39, 91
  savant 52–3, 168, 185
  see also imagination
criminality 82, 84, 86, 282
critical cause, as a concept 103–4, 113, 337
cure 281, 283, 304
cyclic changes 79
cytomegaloviral (CMV) infections 122, 337

Daily Life Therapy 301
Dawson, G. 161, 164, 220–1, 227, 229,
    231, 238, 251, 253
deafness *see* hearing/hearing impairment
dedicated-systems model 213, 214, 218,
    219–22
defective agency theory 182
defective integration theories 157–8, 161
deixis/deictic terms 57, 200, 242, 338
dendrites 125–6, 127, 128, 129, 338
depression 64, 84, 268, 302
design fluency 175, 180, 338
detail, processing of 184–5, 189, 190–1, 192
  see also local processing
developmental trajectory 77–80, 86, 338
diagnosis 259–73, 277–8, 327, 338
  differential 265, 266, 273, 278, 338
  infants and young children 265, 267–8
  methods 268–73
  older children and adults 268
  overuse or misuse of 260–1, 262–4
  professionals involved in 267
  as staged process 265, 266
  stigmatising effects of 260, 261–2, 277

diagnosis *cont.*
  of subtypes 26, 271, 272–3, 278
  support for families following
    313–14, 328–9
  timing of 264–5, 277
  uses of 259–61
diagnostic criteria
  manifest behaviours in relation to
    17–18, 19–20
  see also Creak's Nine Points; DSM-III;
    DSM-IV; DSM-IV-TR; ICD-10
Diagnostic Interview for Social and
  Communication Disorders (DISCO)
  270–2, 276, 278
Diagnostic and Statistical Manual of Mental
  Disorders see DSM- III; DSM-IV;
  DSM-IV-TR
diet/dietary supplements 284, 288–9, 304, 305
disconnectivity *see* impaired connectivity
  theories
distractability 64, 65
distribution 73–4, 86
Doman Delacato method 287
dopamine 127, 135, 141, 228, 285, 339
Down syndrome 9, 27, 56, 63, 102, 105, 117,
  309, 339
drug treatments *see* medications
DSM-III 10–11, 21
DSM-IV 11–14, 17, 18, 20, 21, 90, 143, 167,
  200, 272
  and subtypes model 23, 27, 28, 29, 40–1
DSM-IV-TR 11
dyadic relating 152, 339
  see also primary intersubjectivity
dyad of impairments 91
dynamic systems modelling 214–15, 339
dyslexia 9, 66, 338
dyspraxia 61–2, 68, 247, 339

Early Intensive Behavioural Intervention
  (EIBI) 291, 292, 300
early-onset autism 74–6, 86, 339
Early Screening of Autistic Traits
  Questionnaire (EST) 276
echolalia 57, 103, 168, 239, 340
echopraxia 160, 340
ecological theory/model 215, 216, 340
education 80, 260–1, 262, 277, 310, 317,
  318–19, 323–4, 329
educational interventions *see* intervention
  methods, non- physical
efficacy studies 110, 305–6, 340
  designs and methods 295–7, 298–9
  interpretation of findings 299–300
  medications/physical interventions 130,
    134, 285–6, 288, 289, 290, 293, 294,
    295–8 *passim*

efficacy studies *cont.*
  non-physical interventions 295, 296,
    298–304, 305
electroencephalography (EEG) 8, 131,
  138, 340
embedded rules 151, 152, 340
embodied mind 214, 215
emergence model *see* constructivist-
  emergence model
emotion blindness 156, 340
emotion contagion 44, 158, 163, 340
  spared 45, 143
emotion detector 157, 340
emotion processing 43, 44–5, 92, 94, 100,
  143, 213, 214, 226
  brain-based problems in 137, 144
  impaired theory of mind (ToM) theory
    150, 151, 164
  mindblindness theory 154
  primary intersubjectivity deficit theories
    156–8, 163, 165
emotions
  basic 44, 45, 143, 158, 333
  complex 44, 45, 143, 150, 336
empathising system deficit theory
  157, 213
empathy 44, 45, 92, 143, 154, 340
employment 80–1, 324–6, 329
enactive mind theory 215, 341
enhanced discrimination-reduced
  generalisation theory 194–6, 207–8,
  211, 233, 341
enhanced perceptual function theory 52,
  185, 193–4, 196, 207, 211, 213, 225,
  230, 233, 341
environmental factors 79, 98, 116, 118, 121–
  5, 129, 140, 228, 229
epidemiology 71–4, 341
epilepsy 8, 62, 68, 79, 286
epistemic states 150, 341
etiology 98, 100, 210, 341
  single common pathway explanations
    104, 105, 106
  see also first causes
'event grammar' 245–6
evoked response potentials 138, 341
executive control 150, 151
executive function impairments 151–2, 164,
  169–70, 211, 217–18
  and behavioural inflexibility 101,
    169–70, 171–83, 186, 187, 211,
    216, 220, 245
  brain bases of 137, 139, 141, 219, 231
  causes of 181–2
executive functions 101, 164, 213,
  225, 229, 341
  and central coherence 164, 214, 227

executive functions *cont.*
   description and definitions 170–1
   as general purpose mechanisms 217
extra-dimensional shift 174, 341
extreme male brain (EMB) theory 122, 139,
   154, 184, 204, 341
eye direction detector 152, 342

face processing 33, 103, 137, 141, 160, 192,
   220, 225, 229, 238
Facilitated Communication 302
false appearances test 148, 342
false belief tasks 145, 146, 148, 149, 150,
   151, 211, 226, 342
false photographs task 148, 342
familiarity 236, 237, 238, 240, 342
families 301, 309–17, 328–9
family studies 116–17, 119, 203
feature binding 220, 229, 251, 342
Fein, D. *see* Waterhouse, L. et al
feral children 4, 309
financial help and advice 326, 329
fine cuts 49, 68, 342
first causes 98, 115–25, 140
   links to behaviour 229
   links to brain bases 228–9
   see also etiology
Flexyx therapy 287
fluency 78, 174–5, 180, 342, 362
food fads 35, 62
Fragile-X syndrome 56, 63, 69, 120,
   134, 342–3
Freeman, B. 9, 272
friendships 82–3
Frith, U. 101, 145, 146, 148–9, 184–5, 190–
   3, 202, 207, 215, 216, 219, 225
frontal lobe(s) 128, 133, 135, 137, 138, 182,
   219, 221, 222, 224, 226, 252, 253, 343
fundamental causes 107, 343
fusiform gyrus 137, 343
future thinking 34, 246

GABA (gamma-amino-butyric acid)
   120, 122, 135–6, 139, 141, 223,
   229, 343
gait and posture 48, 197, 198–200, 208
gastrointestinal disorders 62, 289, 305
gaze following 146, 147, 149, 343
gender distribution 73–4, 86, 120
general learning difficulty *see* intellectual
   disability
general purpose mechanisms 216–17, 218,
   230, 343
generativity 78, 91, 174–5, 179, 180, 181,
   183, 186, 227, 235, 245–6, 343
gene therapy 283, 304
genetic counselling 283, 304

genetic factors 98, 104, 105, 115–21, 140
   and behaviour 229
   and brain development 129, 228–9
   candidate genes 118, 119–20, 334
   susceptibility genes 119–21, 134, 203,
      283, 360
genetic screening 118–19, 343
genomes 115–16, 344
genotypes 115, 228, 344
geographical differences 74, 86
Gilliam Asperger's Disorder Scale
   (GADS) 277
glial cells 125, 128, 133, 344
global processing 189, 191, 192–3, 194,
   207, 344
glutamate 127, 344
Gould, J. 28–30, 41, 93
grammar, impairments of 57, 200, 204, 242
grey matter 126, 133, 138, 140, 344

habituation 234, 235, 239, 344
Halperidol 297
Happé, F. 192–3, 202, 207
Harris, P.L. 150, 151
Hawthorne effect 299, 344
health care 310, 323, 327, 329
hearing/hearing impairment 47, 61, 68, 101,
   149, 193, 196, 208
Hermelin, B. 157, 178, 249
herpes simplex encephalitis 76, 123, 344
high-functioning autism (HFA) 38, 139
   communication impairments 90
   diagnosis 268
   educational provision 319, 324
   employment 325–6
   IQ profiles 60, 68, 205–6
   language ability 56, 68, 90, 203, 234, 235
   memory abilities and 234, 235, 236,
      237, 238, 247, 248
   screening 277
   socio-economic status and 74
   see also Asperger syndrome
hippocampal-dorsolateral prefrontal
   system 252, 253
hippocampus 126, 129, 141, 185, 221–2, 344
   abnormalities in, and learning 132,
      134, 138, 185, 226
   and memory 132, 134, 138, 185, 226,
      234–5, 236, 237, 239, 253
historical background 4–11
Hobson, R.P. 156–7, 160–1, 201, 202, 215–
   16, 240
holding therapy 293–4, 300
Hughes, P.J. 75–6
hyperactivity 64–5, 280, 283, 285,
   286, 288
hyperacusia 47, 196, 345

hyperkinetic syndrome *see* attention deficit and hyperactivity disorder
hyperlexia 52, 345
hypersystemising 183–4, 186, 198, 205, 207, 208, 217, 240, 243, 345
hypertonia/hypotonia 61, 247, 345
hypothalamic-pituitary-adrenal axis (HPA) 135, 139, 345

ICD-10 11, 14, 20, 21, 23, 27, 28, 29, 40–1, 90, 269, 272
ideational fluency 175, 180, 345
identity *see* self, sense of
idiopathic autism 115, 140
imagination
    impairment of 30, 33–4, 39, 41, 89, 91, 100, 167–8, 187
    and executive function impairments 101, 171–83
    spared 51–3
    see also creativity
imitation 154, 155
imitation impairments 35, 49, 158–60, 163, 165, 197, 199, 204, 208, 220
immune-system disorders 62, 123, 288, 305
impaired affordances theory 158, 215
impaired connectivity theories 222–7, 231, 233, 251–2, 253
impaired interpersonal-relatedness theory 156–7
impaired theory of mind (ToM) theories 105, 111–12, 136, 145–52, 164, 191, 211, 213, 217, 218, 219, 230
incidence 71, 72, 345
inclusion 262, 308–9, 323, 326, 327, 328, 330, 345
infants
    brain development 127–8
    diagnosis 265, 267
    emotion processing 156–7
    imitative movements 154, 158–9, 163
    preferential social responsiveness 160–1, 215
    primary intersubjectivity 154–5
        impairments of 156, 157, 163–4, 227
    screening 275–6
information processing 214, 216, 217, 223, 224
information processing models 92, 109, 345
inner speech 178, 207, 243, 345
intellectual ability 24–5, 29, 43, 57–61, 93, 101
intellectual disability/impairment 9, 37, 101, 120, 149, 183, 205–7, 346
    acquired global amnesia and 234
    and language impairment 204, 206–7, 208, 243

intellectual disability/impairment *cont.*
    low-functioning autism (LFA) 93, 206–7, 213, 233
    memory and 234, 235, 243–4
    sequencing impairments 239
intelligence 57, 58–61, 217
    crystallised 58, 60, 93, 207, 243, 337
    fluid 58, 60, 206, 243–4, 342
    general ('g') 58, 60, 206, 243–4, 343
    non-verbal 58, 93, 206, 350
    see also verbal abilities/intelligence
Intelligence Quotient (IQ) 59, 68, 205–6, 346
intelligence tests 58–61, 205–6, 239, 244
intention detector 152, 346
International Classification of Diseases see ICD-10
intersubjectivity *see* primary intersubjectivity; secondary intersubjectivity
intervention
    age of individuals and 282–3
    assessments for 258, 259, 277
    family involvement in 301, 310
    goals of 280–2
    immediate aims and targets 282
intervention methods 283–90
    non-physical 287, 290, 291–2, 293–4, 305, 324
    physical 283–7, 288–9, 304–5
    see also efficacy studies
intra-dimensional shift 174, 346

Jarrold, C. 91, 181
joint/shared attention 75, 78, 146, 149, 153, 155, 165, 227, 346

Kanner, Leo 4–5, 8, 9, 10, 11, 20, 21, 28, 105, 109, 144, 156
Kanner's syndrome 13, 38, 72, 104, 346
kinaesthetic awareness 48
Krug's Asperger's Disorder Index (KADI) 277

labelling, diagnostic 260–1, 262, 277
language 53, 54, 58, 346
    acquisition 217, 239, 240–2
    brain systems 220, 225
    stereotyped/repetitive use of 13, 167
language ability 24–5, 29, 43, 53–7, 101, 226–7, 229, 234
    high-functioning autism 56, 68, 90, 203, 234, 235
language impairment 10, 11, 13, 31–3, 56–7, 68, 101, 220
    amodal 57, 68, 242
    autism-specific 201–5, 206
    brain bases of 138, 139, 220

language impairment *cont.*
  and communication impairment,
    dissociability of 90–1
  co-morbid conditions, hearing loss
    101, 208
  specific language impairment 101, 203–4,
    205, 208, 240
  high-functioning autism 56
  hypersystemising and 204, 205, 208,
    240, 243
  intellectual disability and 204, 206–7,
    208, 243
  low-functioning autism 56–7, 68,
    93, 200–5, 213, 220, 229, 233,
    235, 240–3
  memory and 234, 235, 240–3
  mindreading defects and 202–3, 205,
    208, 240
  mirror neurons and 204, 205, 208, 240
  perinatal risk factors and 122
  sequencing impairments and 201,
    208, 239, 240
  symbolising impairments and 108,
    201–2, 205, 240, 243
late-onset/regressive autism 14, 27, 76–7, 86,
    123–4, 346
learning
  associative 138, 203, 239
  hippocampal abnormalities and 132, 134,
    138, 185, 226
  maladaptive 65, 101, 169, 186,
    245, 347
learning disability
  use as a term 37, 346
  see also intellectual disability
legal advice 326, 329
Leicestershire Preschool Autism- Support
    Programme 314
leisure activities 83–4
Leslie, A. 145, 149
lesser variant autism 24, 346
lexical knowledge 241–3
life expectancy 85, 86
lifespan development 74–85
limbic system 126, 128, 132, 134, 136, 138,
    224, 227, 231, 346
  see also amygdala; hippocampus
linkage studies 118, 347
living arrangements 82
  see also care
local processing 347
  bias towards 189, 191, 192–3, 194,
    197, 206, 207
  see also detail, processing of
Lopez, B.R. 180–1
Lovaas Method 291, 300
Loveland, K.A. 158, 215, 216

low-functioning autism (LFA) 38, 104
  diagnosis 268
  hypersystemising 184, 204, 207
  intellectual disability 93, 206–7, 213,
    233, 243–4
  IQ profiles 60, 68, 205
  language impairment 56–7, 68, 93, 200–5,
    213, 220, 229, 233, 235, 240–3
  learning impairment 235
  memory abilities 234, 235, 236, 237,
    238, 243–4, 247, 248
  motor abnormalities 25, 48
  spared and savant abilities 247
  see also autistic disorder; classic autism;
    Kanner's syndrome

Magnetic Resonance Imaging (MRIs) 130,
    131, 132, 137, 228, 347, 360
Magnetic Resonance Spectroscopy Imaging
    (MRSI/MRS) 130, 134
magnetoencephalography 131, 347
maladaptive behaviour 65, 101, 169, 186,
    245, 347
manifest behaviours 14–19, 347
  as clues to diagnosis 19–20
  examples 15–17
  generalised vs. particular behaviours
    14–15, 21
  in relation to diagnostic criteria 17–18,
    19, 20
meaning, linguistic 57, 68, 93, 190,
    200, 242
medial temporal lobe (MTL) 236, 237,
    239, 347
medical conditions 43, 61–3, 68–9
medical model 6, 347
  see also subtypes model
medications 284–7, 288–9, 304, 305
  efficacy studies 130, 134, 285–6, 288, 289,
    290, 293, 294, 296, 297–8
memory 35, 52, 101, 138, 203, 217
  declarative, or explicit 226, 229, 236, 238,
    239, 240, 241–2, 243–4, 245, 246,
    251, 338, 341
  episodic 235, 236, 237, 246, 341
  hippocampal abnormalities and 132, 134,
    138, 185, 226, 234–5, 236, 237,
    239, 253
  immediate/short-term 236, 237, 239, 242,
    247, 345, 358
  intact 246–7
  language-based organisational
    strategies 178
  non-declarative, or implicit 236, 237,
    253, 345
  perceptual 236, 237, 239, 242, 247,
    253, 352

memory *cont.*
   procedural 235–6, 237, 239, 242,
      247, 253, 354
   relational 220, 253, 356
   rote 35, 52, 203, 213, 247, 356
   semantic 235, 236, 237, 243, 247, 358
   uneven abilities 234–48
   and behavioural inflexibility 185–6,
      187, 234, 245–7
   and intellectual disability 234, 235, 243–4
   and language impairment 235, 240–3
   and motor skills 247–8
   and spared and savant abilities in LFA 247
   and time-processing impairment 251
   see also working memory
mental age 59, 347
mental (cognitive) flexibility 170, 173–4,
      179, 180, 182, 183, 186, 347
mental health problems 35, 43, 63–4, 68,
      292, 302
mentalising ability 150, 347–8
mentalising deficit 148, 150, 164, 182, 186,
      191, 211
mental retardation
   use as a term 36–7
   see also intellectual disability
mental set 170, 348
mental states 152, 348
   simulation of others' 150, 159
mental time travel 246, 348
metabolic disorders 63
metacognition 151, 348
metarepresentation 112, 145, 146, 148, 149–
      50, 151, 156, 164, 348
mindblindness 152–4, 211, 242, 348
mindreading 101, 136, 141, 152–3, 157,
      164, 182, 202–3, 205, 219, 225, 240, 348
mirror neurons/mirror neuron system (MNS)
      133–4, 137, 159–60, 163, 165, 204, 205,
      208, 219, 240, 248
MMR vaccination 72–3, 77, 123–5
Modahl, C. *see* Waterhouse, L. et al.
modelling 131, 348
   animal 119, 131, 234–5, 251, 332
   computational 131
   neural network 133
Modified Checklist for Autism in Toddlers
      (M-CHAT) 276, 278
modularism/modularists 129, 348–9
monitoring 170
   self- and action–outcome 172, 178–9,
      186, 217, 331
morphemes 242, 349
mother-child relationships 7, 92, 109, 144
motor skills 43, 138, 349
   automatisation of 247–8
   fine and gross 48, 344

motor skills *cont.*
   impaired 25, 35, 48–9, 94, 197–200,
      220, 229, 250
   brain bases of 137, 139, 141, 220
   spared abilities 197
   time-processing problems and 250
   uneven 93, 101, 197–200, 208, 213,
      220, 233
   uneven memory abilities and 247–8
motor stereotypies 13, 48, 79, 167, 190,
      197, 198
Mottron, L. 185, 193–4, 207, 225
multiple difficulties 66–7, 69, 281
Music Interaction Therapy 301
mutism 55, 56, 352

National Autistic Society, UK 321–2
National Society for Autistic Children,
      USA 9
neoconstructivist model 214, 349
neologisms 57, 349
neural binding 219, 223, 233, 349
neural circuits/networks 126, 349
neural network models 133, 214–15
neurobiology 98, 100, 210, 349 single com-
      mon pathway explanations 104–5, 106
   see also brain bases
neurodevelopmental disorders 9, 64–6, 350
neuromodulators 127, 136, 350
neuromuscular problems 56, 61–2,
      198, 208
neurons 125, 126, 127, 133, 222, 350
neuropeptides 120, 139, 141, 288, 350
neuroreceptors 126, 127, 350
neurosis 7, 8, 21, 350
neurotransmitters 126, 127, 135–6, 141,
      288, 350
neurotrophins 126, 350
non-idiopathic autism 115, 134
non-verbal behaviour/communication 12, 33,
      54, 90, 143, 350
non-verbal intelligence/abilities 58, 93,
      206, 350
non-verbal learning disability (NVLD or
      NLD) 25–6, 350
norepinephrine (noradrenalin) 127, 135, 139,
      141, 351
normalisation 308, 351
normality, autism and 24, 26
novelty, response to 234, 235

obsessions/compulsions 64, 65, 101,
      168, 169
obsessive-compulsive disorder (OCD) 64, 65,
      169, 186, 351
occipital lobe 126, 128, 252, 253, 351
O'Connor, N. 157, 178, 249

opioid peptides 120, 127, 136, 351
    see also oxytocin: vasopressin
orbitofrontal cortex 137, 351
organisational strategies 170, 178, 179, 186
Ornitz, E.M. 105, 189–90, 207
oxytocin 120, 127, 136, 139, 221, 222, 229,
    286, 351

pain 47
parents *see* families
parietal lobe 126, 128, 222, 252, 253, 352
Pathological Demand Avoidance Syndrome
    (PDA) 14, 352
peptides 127, 352
    see also neuropeptides; opioid peptides
perception 45, 101, 352
    see also sensory-perceptual anomalies
performance quotients (PQs) 60,
    205, 352
perinatal risk factors 122
perirhinal cortex 236, 237, 352
perseverative behaviour 174, 352
pervasive developmental disorders (PDDs)
    12–14, 21, 23–4, 352
pervasive developmental disorders not
    otherwise specified (PDD-NOS) 12,
    14, 21, 38, 75, 225, 272–3, 352
Pervasive Developmental Disorders Screening
    Test – Stage II (PDDST-II) 276
phenotype, autism 116, 332
phenotypic traits 220, 229
phenylketonuria (PKU) 63, 102, 135,
    140, 353
phonological loop 171, 353
phonology 57, 200, 204, 242
pica 64, 353
Picture Exchange Communication System
    (PECS) 291, 302
placebo/placebo effects 299, 353
Plaisted, K. 193–6, 207–8
planning abilities 168, 170, 175–6, 179,
    183, 186, 217, 227, 245–6
Positron Emission Tomography (PET scan)
    130, 131, 353
postmortem studies 130, 132, 133
Prader-Willi syndrome 63, 69, 120, 353
pragmatic language impairment (PLI) 26, 55,
    203, 353
pragmatics 54–5, 68, 353
preferred activities 79, 84
prenatal risk factors 121–2, 229
    see also rubella, maternal
prepotent responses 150, 354
pretend play 13, 33, 34, 51, 91, 167, 169,
    175, 176, 181, 201
prevalence 71–3, 85, 86, 354
prevention 281, 283, 304

primacy, or causal precedence criterion 111–
    12, 113, 354
    executive dysfunction theories and 211
    impaired shared attention hypothesis
        and 154
    impaired theory of mind (ToM) and
        152, 211
    primary intersubjectivity deficit theories
        and 165
primary intersubjectivity 101, 154–5, 164,
    213, 222, 227, 250, 354
primary intersubjectivity deficit theories
    154–64, 219, 230, 231, 233
prognosis 27, 354
proprioceptive awareness 48, 354
prosody 33, 129, 354
protodeclaratives 51, 75, 78, 146, 149, 153,
    155, 354
protoimperatives 50–1, 354
pseudo-autism 76, 355
psychic akinesia 177, 355
psychoanalysis 7, 92, 355
psychoanalytic models/theories 6, 92, 109,
    144, 355
psychodynamic theories 144
psychogenic autism 144, 355
psychological explanations/ theories 99,
    100, 210
    and brain bases *see* brain–behaviour
        explanations
    single (deficit) common pathway 105, 106,
        107, 211
    'three theories' explanation 211–13,
        217–18, 230
    see also individual theories
psychosis 7–9, 21, 355
psychosocial interventions *see* intervention
    methods, non- physical
psychotherapy 302
Purkinje cells 127, 133, 136, 223, 224, 229,
    253, 355

quantitative trait loci (QTL) studies 119,
    229, 231, 355
quasi-autism *see* pseudo-autism

racial differences 74, 86
reading
    mechanical 52, 347
    see also dyslexia
Real-Life Rating Scale (RLRS) 272
recall, tests of 238
recollection 236, 237, 238, 240, 355
reelin 122, 136, 355
referral 267, 278
regressive autism 14, 27, 76–7, 86,
    123–4, 355–6

relationships 82–3
representation(s) 146, 148, 151, 356
  of self 137
  see also metarepresentation
research studies 109–11
  diagnosis and comparability of
    participants in 261, 277
response inhibition 137, 152, 170, 171–3,
  179, 180, 181, 186, 198, 217, 356
restricted, repetitive behaviour 13, 21,
  34, 79, 89, 100, 101, 103,
  167–8, 234–5
  causes not specific to autism 168–70,
    186 245
  chromosome 15 abnormalities and 120
  Co-morbid conditions associated with
    169, 186
  executive function impairments and 101,
    171–83, 186, 187
  hypersystemising and 183–4, 186
  interventions 285, 286, 292
  manifest behaviours exemplifying 20
  memory abilities and 185–6, 187,
    234, 246–7
  sensory-perceptual anomalies and
    184–5, 187, 196
Rett syndrome 8, 12, 23, 27, 356
Ricks, D.M. 105, 201, 207, 240, 243
rights 308, 323–6, 328
Rimland, B. 104, 190, 235
Risperidone 285, 297, 305
Ritvo, E. 9, 272
rote memory/learning 35, 52, 203, 213,
  247, 356
routines/rituals, inflexible adherence to 13,
  167, 239, 247
rubella, maternal 8, 347
Russell, J. 150, 171, 172, 178–9, 182
Rutter, M. 9, 201, 240

'Sally and the marble' task 145, 146,
  150, 151
sameness, insistence on 168, 229, 235
savant abilities 52–3, 68, 168, 185,
  193–4, 233, 247, 356
savants 39, 357
schizophrenia/schizoid personality 7, 8, 21,
  26, 27, 64, 357
screening 72, 73, 273–7, 278, 357
  genetic 118–19, 343
Screening Tool for Autism in Two-year-olds
  (STAT) 276
sculpting, brain 128, 129, 357
secondary intersubjectivity 154, 155, 158,
  162, 164, 165, 201, 357
second-order beliefs 148, 357
secretin 284, 293, 294, 357

selective serotonin reuptake inhibitors
  (SSRIs) 285
self
  representation of 137
  sense of 94, 182, 186, 215–16, 246
self-activation 177, 357
self-injurious behaviours (SIBS) 47, 65, 168,
  283, 285, 286, 357
self-monitoring 170, 172, 178–9, 186,
  217, 357
self-other equivalence 199, 357
self-regulation 216, 217, 357
semantics 57, 68, 200, 242, 358
sensory deprivation 144, 169, 186, 198
sensory inputs, exposure to 284, 304
Sensory Integration Therapy 287, 305
sensory modulation 189–90, 358
sensory-perceptual anomalies 43,
  45–8, 93–4, 101, 189–97, 207–8,
  214, 220
  and behavioural inflexibility 184–5, 187
  brain–behaviour explanations 220
sensory-perceptual 'overload' 47, 64, 189,
  190, 197
sequencing, impairment of 201, 208, 239,
  240, 249
serotonin 127, 135, 139, 141, 228, 358
services
  provision and financing of 72, 260,
    277, 327
  see also care; education; health care;
    support services
sexual relationships 82
shared attention *see* joint/shared attention
shared attention mechanism (SAM) 152–3,
  153, 154, 164, 358
shifting attention *see* attention
  switching/shifting
shutdown 48, 358
siblings 312, 315
simulation 150, 152, 159, 164, 358
single (deficit) common pathway theories
  104–8, 211
Single Photon Emission Computed
  Tomography (SPECT) 131, 359
slave system 171, 359
sleep disturbance 35, 66, 68, 249, 280,
  283, 288
'smarties task' 148
smell 47
smoking during pregnancy 122
social behaviours, progress in 78–9
social brain 136–7, 138, 139, 141, 157, 163,
  216, 219, 226, 230, 359
social class differences 74, 86
social cognition system 136, 219, 225
  see also social brain

social interaction impairment 12–13, 14, 21,
    30–1, 54, 89, 100, 143, 214
    brain-based theories 144
    and communication impairment,
        interdependence of 89–90
    emotion processing and 92
    impaired theory of mind (ToM) theory
        145–52, 164, 211, 218
    manifest behaviours exemplifying 18
    minblindness theory 152–4
    primary intersubjectivity deficit theories
        154–64, 165
    psychodynmic theories 144
    time-processing and 162, 165, 249
social orienting 161–2, 163, 165, 359
social reward 119, 137, 220, 229
social stimuli, responsiveness to 155, 160–2,
    165, 215
Social Stories materials 301–2
Son-Rise (Option) programme 291, 300, 301
spared abilities 49–53, 68, 94, 101, 143,
    234, 247
    overuse of, and behavioural
        inflexibility 184–7
special educational needs, as a term 37, 359
specificity criterion 111, 113, 359
    executive dysfunction theories and 211
    impaired theory of mind (ToM) and
        49, 211
specific language impairments (SLI) 9, 66,
    101, 119, 203–4, 205, 208, 240, 359
specific learning difficulty/ disability 37,
    66, 359
spectrum concept 28–36, 41, 43, 72, 359
speech 33, 54, 56, 129, 359
    inner 178, 207, 243, 345
speech and language therapy 302
speech processing, brain bases of impaired
    138, 141
SPELL approach 301
starting 170, 174–7
stereotyped behaviour/interests 13, 14,
    48, 167
stigmatisation 260, 261–2, 277, 310
'Stockings and Cambridge' test 175–6
stopping 170, 171–3
stress 168, 186
    families 310–12
    over-reactivity to 135
    in pregnancy 122, 229
stuck-in-set behaviour 174, 180, 360
subtypes model 29, 35, 36, 360
    defense of 27–8
    definitions based on 9–14
    origins of 5–6
    theoretical and practical problems
        23–8, 40–1

suicide 84
superior temporal sulcus 137, 360
supervisory attentional system (SAS) 171,
    181, 360
support needs, families 313–17
support services 313–17
    access to 277, 323–6, 329–30
    cost of 327
symbolising, defective 34, 201–2, 205, 207,
    208, 240, 243
sympathy 44, 360
synaesthesia 47, 189, 197, 360
synaptic pruning 128, 129, 133, 361
synaptogenesis 128, 129, 133, 361
systemising 184, 204, 217, 361
    see also hypersystemising

Tager-Flusberg, H. 162, 203–4
Tanguay, P. 105, 201, 240
taste 47
TEACCH 292, 300–1, 313, 324
temporal lobes 126, 128, 129, 133, 134, 138,
    222, 224, 252, 253, 361
    see also medial temporal lobe
teratogens 121, 229, 361
terminology 36–40
    cultural differences 36–7
    and social attitudes, changes in
        37, 41
testosterone levels 122
thalidomide 121, 140, 361
theory of mind 158–9, 213, 361
    impaired 155, 156, 164
    see also impaired theory of mind
        (ToM) theories
theory of mind tests 148, 211, 226
    see also false belief tasks
thimerosal 123, 361
thirst, excessive (polydipsia) 35, 62, 353
time-processing 155, 162, 165,
    234, 248–52
touch 47
Tourette's syndrome 73, 169, 186, 361
Tower tests 175–6, 180
triadic relating 152–3, 154, 201, 219
    see also secondary intersubjectivity
triad of impairments 30–4, 41, 89, 90, 361
trichotillomania 64, 361
tuberous sclerosis 61, 63, 134, 226, 361
Turner, M. 175, 180, 181
Turner's syndrome 63, 120, 134, 362
twins
    dizygotic (DZ) 115, 116, 117,
        118, 339
    monozygotic (MZ) (identical) 115,
        116, 117, 118, 122, 140, 349
twin studies 116, 118, 119

universality criterion 111, 113, 362

valproic acid 121, 362
vasopressin 120, 127, 136, 139,
    229, 362
ventromedial prefontal cortex 137, 362
verbal abilities/intelligence 58, 93, 205,
    206–7, 362
    see also language
verbal fluency 175, 180, 362
verbal mediation *see* inner speech
verbal quotients (VQs) 60, 205, 362
viral infections 123
vision 47, 61, 196
visual recognition 238
visual search tests 47, 363
visual-spatial sketchpad 171, 363
visual stimuli, enhanced processing of 193–4
volitional states 150
volition/conation 176–7, 186, 363

Warnock Report (1978) 37
Waterhouse, L. et al. 221–2, 227, 231, 253

weak central coherence (WCC) 148, 149,
    164, 184–5, 190–3, 211, 216–17, 218,
    230, 233, 363
    brain abnormalities and 219–20, 223
    and executive functions 164, 214, 227
Wechsler scales 58–60, 205–6, 239
White Lodge Centre 315
white matter 126, 128, 133, 138, 140,
    222, 363
Williams syndrome 63, 66, 117, 363
windows task 171, 172
Wing, L. 10, 28–35, 41, 73, 90, 91, 93, 105,
    167, 201, 207, 240, 243
Wisconsin Card Sorting Test (WCST) 173–4,
    180
word recognition 238, 240, 242, 243
working memory 137, 179, 186, 236, 237,
    239, 363
    central executive in 170–1, 181, 335
    spatial 137, 239, 359
    verbal 172

X-chromosome 120, 134

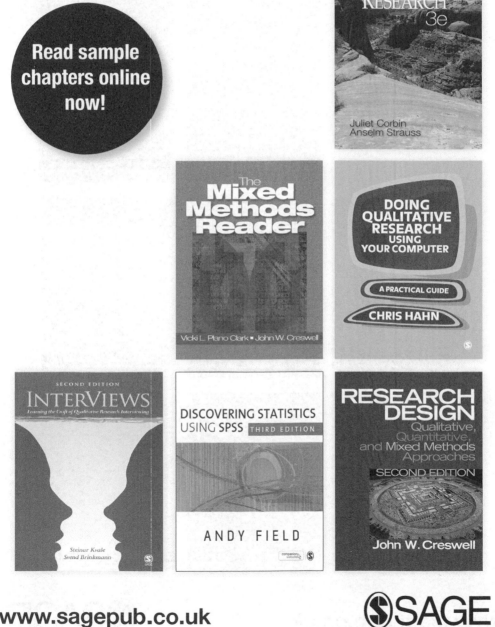

The Qualitative Research Kit

Edited by Uwe Flick

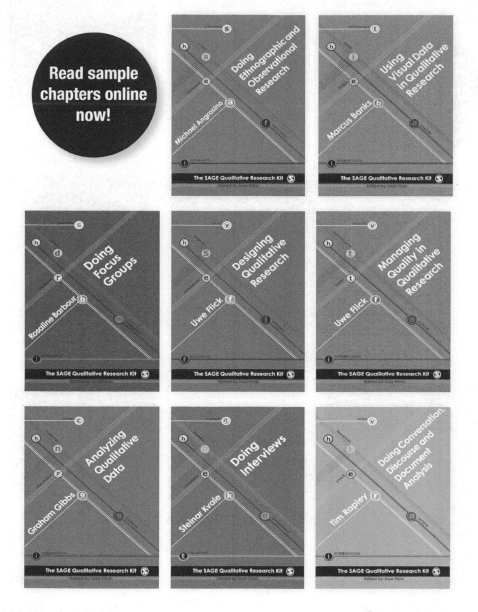

Read sample chapters online now!

Doing Ethnographic and Observational Research — Michael Angrosino

Using Visual Data in Qualitative Research — Marcus Banks

Doing Focus Groups — Rosaline Barbour

Designing Qualitative Research — Uwe Flick

Managing Quality in Qualitative Research — Uwe Flick

Analyzing Qualitative Data — Graham Gibbs

Doing Interviews — Steinar Kvale

Doing Conversation, Discourse and Document Analysis — Tim Rapley

The SAGE Qualitative Research Kit
Edited by Uwe Flick

www.sagepub.co.uk

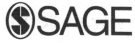